The Role of Membranes
in Metabolic Regulation

Symposia on Metabolic Regulation

Editors

Myron A. Mehlman   Richard W. Hanson

ACADEMIC PRESS RAPID MANUSCRIPT REPRODUCTION

The Role of Membranes in Metabolic Regulation

Edited by

Myron A. Mehlman

Department of Biochemistry
University of Nebraska College of Medicine
Omaha, Nebraska

Richard W. Hanson

Fels Research Institute and Department
of Biochemistry
Temple University Medical School
Philadelphia, Pennsylvania

Proceedings of a Symposium held at the
University of Nebraska Medical School
Omaha, Nebraska, May 8-9, 1972

Academic Press   New York and London   1972

ACADEMIC PRESS, INC.
111 Fifth Avenue, New York, New York 10003

United Kingdom Edition published by
ACADEMIC PRESS, INC. (LONDON) LTD.
24/28 Oval Road. London NW1

LIBRARY OF CONGRESS CATALOG CARD NUMBER: 72-88344

PRINTED IN THE UNITED STATES OF AMERICA

CONTENTS

CONTENTS

CONTENTS

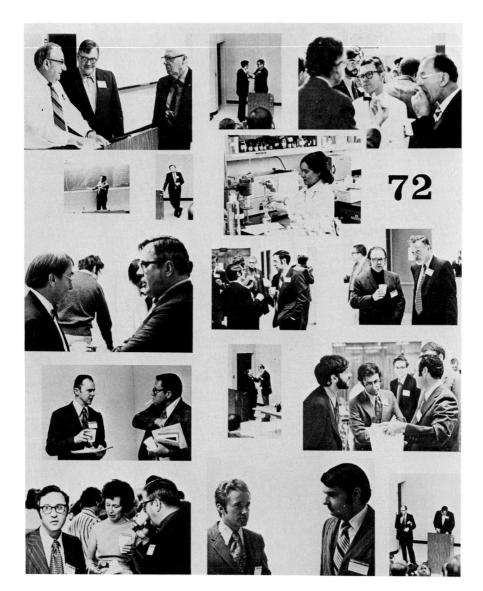

CONTRIBUTORS

Eugene Barrett, Department of Radiation Biology and Biophysics, University of Rochester School of Medicine & Dentistry, Rochester, New York 14642

Carolyn D. Berdanier, Nutrition Institute, Agricultural Research Service, United States Department of Agriculture, Beltsville, Maryland 20705

Ivan Bihler, Department of Pharmacology & Therapeutics, University of Manitoba, Winnipeg, Canada R3E OW3

Melvin Blecher, Department of Biochemistry, Georgetown University School of Medicine, School of Dentistry, Washington, D. C. 20007

Charles R. Burghardt, Biochemical Pharmacology Section, Hoffmann-LaRoche Inc., Nutley, New Jersey 07110

K.-J. Chang, Department of Biochemical Pharmacology, School of Pharmacy, State University of New York, Buffalo, New York 14214

Morton Civen, Department of Physiology, University of California, Irvine and Veterans Administration Hospital, Long Beach, California 90801

Oscar B. Crofford, Department of Physiology, Vanderbilt University School of Medicine, Nashville, Tennessee 37232

James F. Danielli, Center for Theoretical Biology, State University of New York, Amherst, New York 14226

David W. Deamer, Department of Zoology, University of California, Davis, California 95616

Charles Elson, Departments of Medicine & Nutritional Science, University of Wisconsin and the Veterans Administration Hospital, Madison, Wisconsin 53706

Nicholas A. Giorgio, Jr., Department of Biochemistry, Georgetown University School of Medicine, School of Dentistry, Washington, D. C. 20007

Carl B. Johnson, Department of Biochemistry, Georgetown University School of Medicine, School of Dentistry, Washington, D. C. 20007

Howard M. Katzen, Merck Institute for Therapeutic Research, Department of Biochemistry, Rahway, New Jersey 07065

Lalita Kaul, Department of Nutrition, University of Maryland, College Park, Maryland 20705

George Kimmich, Department of Radiation Biology and Biophysics, University of Rochester School of Medicine & Dentistry, Rochester, New York 14642

Tetsuro Kono, Department of Physiology, Vanderbilt University School of Medicine, Nashville, Tennessee 37232

Henry A. Lardy, Institute for Enzyme Research, University of Wisconsin, Madison, Wisconsin 53706

Robert J. Lefkowitz, Department of Medicine (Cardiac Unit), Massachusetts General Hospital, Department of Medicine, Harvard Medical School, Cambridge, Massachusetts 01451

Robert Leonard, Department of Zoology, University of California, Davis, California 95616

Edith Lerner, Departments of Medicine & Nutritional Science, University of Wisconsin and the Veterans Administration Hospital, Madison, Wisconsin 53706

Gerald S. Levey, Division of Endocrinology and Metabolism and the Department of Medicine, University of Miami School of Medicine, Miami, Florida 33152

Howard E. Morgan, Department of Physiology, Pennsylvania State University, Hershey, Pennsylvania 17033

James R. Neely, Department of Physiology, Pennsylvania State University, Hershey, Pennsylvania 17033

Takami Oka, Section on Intermediary Metabolism, NIAMDD, National Institutes of Health, Bethesda, Maryland 20014

Stephen L. Pohl, Department of Internal Medicine, Metabolism Division, Barnes & Wohl Hospitals, St. Louis, Missouri 63110

Berton C. Pressman, Department of Pharmacology, University of Miami, Miami, Florida 33152

Joan Randles, Department of Radiation Biology & Biophysics, University of Rochester School of Medicine & Dentistry, Rochester, New York 14642

Peter W. Reed, Institute for Enzyme Research, University of Wisconsin, Madison, Wisconsin 53706

Herbert Sheppard, Biochemical Pharmacology Section, Hoffmann-LaRoche Inc., Nutley, New Jersey 07110

Earl Shrago, Departments of Medicine & Nutritional Science, University of Wisconsin and the Veterans Administration Hospital, Madison, Wisconsin 53706

Austin Shug, Departments of Medicine & Nutritional Science, University of Wisconsin and the Veterans Administration Hospital, Madison, Wisconsin 53706

Denis D. Soderman, Merck Institute for Therapeutic Research, Department of Biochemistry, Rahway, New Jersey 07065

Richard B. Tobin, Departments of Biochemistry and Medicine, University of Nebraska College of Medicine and the Veterans Administration Hospital, Omaha, Nebraska 68105

Yale J. Topper, Section on Intermediary Metabolism, NIAMDD, National Institutes of Health, Bethesda, Maryland 20014

D. J. Triggle, Department of Biochemical Pharmacology, School of Pharmacy, State University of New York, Buffalo, New York 14214

Anne Marie Tucker, Department of Radiation Biology and Biophysics, University of Rochester School of Medicine & Dentistry, Rochester, New York 14642

Carol F. Whitfield, Department of Physiology, Pennsylvania State University, Hershey, Pennsylvania 17033

PREFACE

Metabolic regulation is a highly diversified field in which research ranges from the control of mRNA synthesis in bacteria to the regulation of specific metabolic pathways in man. This book is the second in a series of in-depth reviews of specific areas of metabolic regulation. Based on a symposium held at the University of Nebraska Medical School, it brings together important information and concepts previously scattered throughout the literature. This volume emphasizes membrane structure and function as well as utilization of affinity chromatography for purification of biologically important cellular components, in this case membrane receptors. The future symposia will deal with other aspects of metabolic regulation. Contributors include investigators with many years of research experience as well as younger scientists, who often bring new ideas and approaches to the field. Articles range from strict journal-style presentations to broader and more speculative personal statements on a given topic. Workers in research institutes and industrial laboratories as well as biochemists, physiologists, pharmacologists, physicians, and all others interested in current concepts in metabolic regulation will find this series of great value.

The chapters in this book are drawn together from people engaged in some aspect of research on membrane regulation. Their contributions vary in style, scope, and method of presentation. In contrast to the previous symposium, we have not attempted to dictate the content of these chapters. The responsibility for the scientific content of each chapter lies with the individual author.

We wish to express special appreciation to Beverly Friend for editorial assistance in preparing these manuscripts for publication, and to Larry Garthoff for his photographic work. At the University of Nebraska Medical Center, we also had the kind encouragement and assistance of Professor W. R. Ruegamer, Chairman, Department of Biochemistry, Professor R. B. Tobin, and the Department of Continuing Education. These meetings at Omaha are part of an overall goal to bring excellence to the graduate education in biochemistry. We have been greatly assisted by Dr. Howard Katzen as well as the other Chairmen for help in the selection of participants for this meeting.

We would like to acknowledge the fine financial support of the following: Hoffmann-LaRoche, Inc.; The Upjohn Company; G. D. Searle and Company; The Kroc Foundation; CIBA-GEIGY Pharmaceuticals; Charles Pfizer and Company, Inc.; Merck Sharp and Dohme; The Eli Lilly Research Laboratories; Schering Corporation; Smith Kline and French Laboratories; Celanese Corporation; Boehringer Mannheim Corporation; Mead Johnson Research Center; and The Bly Foundation.

Myron A. Mehlman
Richard W. Hanson

The Role of Membranes
in Metabolic Regulation

EXPERIMENT, HYPOTHESIS AND THEORY IN THE DEVELOPMENT OF CONCEPTS OF CELL MEMBRANE STRUCTURE

J. F. Danielli

Introduction

Many of the basic hypotheses concerning membrane structure were developed in the period 1900 to 1945. Over the period since 1945, there has been intensive experimental study of these hypotheses. This study has left our concepts of the role of lipids in the membrane largely unchanged since 1945. It has also greatly extended the evidence for a variety of roles for proteins in the membrane, but information about the way in which proteins enter into membrane structure, and how they carry out these roles, is still rudimentary. In this review, we shall analyze this development in terms of the interplay between hypothesis, experiment and theory.

The functions of hypothesis, experiment and theory are quite different. *Hypothesis* is an expression of intuition, which serves as a guide for development of experiment and of theory. Experiment and theory are alternative, and complementary, methods of testing the validity of a hypothesis. Without such testing, although a hypothesis may be aesthetically satisfying, it is largely useless and by providing a degree of satisfaction may actually retard the development of true understanding.

Experiment provides a test for hypothesis by establishing quantities which can be seen to be compatible, or incompatible, with the hypothesis. For example, from experiment we may be able to say, *e.g.*, 60% of the lipid in a particular membrane is in the bilayer configuration; or, receptors are present for norepinephrine; *etc.*

Theory provides a definition of process and relationship, preferably in quantifiable terms which permit prediction, such as: if the lipid bilayer hypothesis is correct, permeation of the membrane must be by activated diffusion and will be given by (*e.g.*)

$$p = \frac{ae}{nb + 2e}$$

or *e.g.* a particular model is impossible because its free energy is so much higher than that of other configurations of the same molecules.

Early work

Over the period 1900 to 1930 substantial amounts of qualitative evidence was developed indicating that the surface layers of the cell must be predominantly lipid. This arose partly from the work of such investigators as Overton (1) and Osterhaut (1), who made permeability studies and partly from studies of the conductance of the membrane made *e.g.* by Höber, Fricke and Cole (2). The impedance studies also showed clearly that the membrane could not be more than a few molecules. For reviews of this work see *e.g.* Hober (1) and Harvey and Danielli (2). Although there was a considerable measure of agreement that the membrane must contain lipid components there was much doubt as to whether the membrane was a homogeneous lipid layer, or a mosaic of different structures or could perhaps contain substantial pores. It was not possible to resolve this problem at the time, because although quantitative data were available, methods for analyzing the data were in the main qualitative. In 1934, drawing upon work by Harvey (2), I was able to show that protein absorbed strongly to lipid surfaces, even when these lipid surfaces are of low initial surface free energy (3). The concept that proteins might be an essential part of cell membranes was novel, and the question thus arose as to how both the proteins and the lipid molecules were arranged to constitute membranes. To solve this problem, I turned to the theory of amphipathic molecules. Thanks to the work of investigators such as Langmuir, Adam and Rideal the general behavior of amphipathic molecules was quite well understood at that time, and led readily to appropriate hypotheses.

Discussion

The Development of the Paucimolecular Layer Theory.

The first hypothesis concerning the arrangements of
the molecule was put forward in 1934 and is shown in Fig. 1.
In this hypothesis the interactions between the lipid and
protein was postulated to be polar (4). It must be remember-
ed that at this time extraordinarily little was known of the
structure of proteins. The α-helix structure for example
had not been suggested at that time. In Fig. 2 are shown
a number of the other possible arrangements of molecules
which were considered. Calculation of surface free energies
indicated structures such as (b) and (h) were the most probable since they would have the lowest surface free energies
(5). Structures such as (h) were based on the supposition
that part of the membrane could be made of protein molecules
which were held together by nonpolar forces forming a bilayer structure in which the bilayer component was protein.
Little attention was paid to this suggestion, but it has
now become of renewed interest for reasons which will appear
later.

The question immediately arose: Was the configuration
of proteins, as shown *e.g.* in Fig. 1, correct or was there
some other configuration of proteins which would be more
appropriate? Studies of the surface properties of proteins
made between 1934 and 1937 showed that the suggested interaction between protein and lipid was not likely to be correct.
It was found that when proteins such as ovalbumin were adsorbed at surfaces a surface free energy was available from
nonpolar forces which was of the order of 100,000 calories
per molecule. The nonpolar groups responsible for this non-
polar energy were normally concentrated in the interior of
the protein, with the polar groups on the surface of the
protein molecule thus providing a stabilizing force for the
globular protein. However, when absorption took place on
the surface, which promoted unrolling of the protein structure, these forces became available for stabilizing the
adsorbed protein at the interface (2,6). Thus the hypothesis
proposed in 1934 was replaced by 1937 by a second hypothesis,
in which the organization of the lipid components remained as
in the 1934 hypothesis but protein was postulated to be
arranged in a primary layer which involved nonpolar interactions between lipid and protein and a secondary layer in

3

which the protein molecules of the second layer were mainly
involved through nonpolar forces. Figure 3 shows the general arrangement postulated for molecules at the membrane surface, and Fig. 4 shows the arrangement of individual molecule in the lipid and first protein layer (7). Thus, the
first hypothesis put forward for membrane structure was almost immediately disproved by a set of experimental observations combined with a set of calculations.

The question now arose: Was it possible to show that
such structures are indeed stable by making artificial membranes having analogous structure? Artificial membranes
having these structures were made as spherical shell membranes, in which the lipid phase was a mixture of triolein,
oleic acid and lecithin and the protein component was egg
albumin (5). These membranes were stable for several days
and were demonstrated at Princeton at a meeting of the
Society for General Physiology in 1935.

Could These Structures Account for Cell Membrane Permeabilities?

The fact that model membranes having the postulated
structure were in fact stable was gratifying, but the extent
to which this model really corresponded to the structure of
cell membranes needed much further examination. For this I
turned to a quantitative study of the permeability properties
of natural membranes. To do this I utilized the theory of
activated diffusion, which was itself developed in the 1930's
in the fields of physics and physical chemistry. To obtain
a quantitative treatment of permeability data, it was necessary to obtain a model of the energy barriers to diffusion
which would correspond to the postulated structure of the
membrane. The model which was used is shown in Fig. 6. It
led to the following general equation for the permeability
of such membranes:

$$p = \frac{ae}{nb + 2e}$$

In this equation p is the permeability; a , b and e are
the free energies of activation for diffusion through the
corresponding energy barrier; and n is a measure of the

4

thickness of the membrane. It was shown using especially
data of Jacobs and Collander that this equation correctly
described the rate of permeation of most molecules. This
was true for a range of 10^2 in molecular weight, 10^4 in
permeability and 10^5 in oil-water partition coefficients.
In the model, it is assumed that the only significant barrier to diffusion was caused by the hydrocarbon layer of
the bilayer, and that the free energies which restrict the
rate of diffusion arise from the existence of this hydrocarbon layer. The fact that the great majority of molecules behave in a way which fits the equation which was
developed indicates that these molecules see only CH_2 groups
when they are passing through the membrane. The evidence
for this was published in 1943 (7). However, although most
molecules behaved as though they saw only a hydrocarbon
layer, certain other types of molecules, *e.g.* sugars,
phosphate and amino acids, behave differently. They diffused
faster than would be predicted by the above equation; they
behaved as though they were involved in an enzyme-like process, interacting with a polar component of the membrane.
And it was found that, whereas with molecules which obey
the above equation structural detail is of secondary importance, in the case of molecules which permeate faster than
is predicted by this equation, structural detail was of
outstanding importance so that even methylation of a single
hydroxyl group at times made a profound difference to the
permeability constant.

Thus by 1943 the evidence was quite clear that the
membrane must contain at least two types of structure which
are fundamentally different. One of these structures is
essentially hydrocarbon in nature. The other structure is
essentially polar in nature. It was suggested that the
closest analogy known at the time to the polar structures
was enzymes, and that these structures should in fact be
regarded as enzyme-like in nature. Since extremely little
was known of protein structure at that time, particularly
lipophilic proteins, all that could be said of the protein
membrane structure was that it must extend through the
thickness of the membrane (8), as was indicated in diagramatic
form by Fig. 7.

The theoretical study of permeability constants showed
quite clearly that the second hypothesis which had been developed for the structure of the membrane was wrong and
the membrane must in fact contain at least two strikingly

different structures, *i.e.* by that time the interaction between hypothesis, theory and experiment had led to the discarding of two hypotheses, and the generation of a third hypothesis. It is this third hypothesis which is largely substantiated at this time.

We may summarize the situation by saying that up to about 1940 experiment had been well ahead of theory, that over the period 1930 to 1940 theoretical examination of data and hypotheses moved ahead of experiment. Over the period approximately 1940 to 1970 the theoretical studies remained more effective than experimental studies, and that only over the last few years have the experimentalists substantially broken new ground.

Developments 1940-1970

Over this period there was a tremendous development of experimental studies of cell membranes and a corresponding remarkable development of new techniques. Particularly outstanding was the demonstration by electron microscopy that the type of membrane which had hitherto been supposed to exist only at the surfaces of cells was also an integral part of many organelle structures. Taking the period as a whole, it was characterized by certain qualities:

(1) a remarkable development of new techniques, including electron microscopy, spin resonance, nuclear magnetic resonance, calorimetry, freeze-fracture and X-ray diffraction studies;

(2) a great elaboration of hypotheses which were not very satisfactorily related to either theory or to experiment;

(3) a general failure to realize that the membrane has more than one structure;

(4) an undue concentration on the bilayer aspect of membranes, which led to a considerable struggle to demonstrate that the model which I put forward in 1934 was or was not right when in fact it had been shown to be incorrect already by 1940.

(5)   a rather desperate struggle over the nature and role of membrane protein, which has still had no very effective outcome;

(6)   an intensive development of the theory of bilayers and of experimental study of lipid bilayers;

(7)   a clarification of the differences between simple diffusion, facilitated diffusion, active transport and exchange diffusion;

(8)   a rapid development of understanding of the wide range of receptor molecules which are present in membrane structure, culminating in the understanding of the role of cyclic AMP.

So far as membrane structure is concerned, the outcome of these studies has been to produce a satisfactory volume of evidence that the uniform component of all or most cell membranes is a lipid bilayer. Thus the theory of amphipathic molecules, as it was used in the 1930's, did in fact give the right answer for the main lipid component of membrane. The question of the structures into which proteins enter in membranes still remains open, though from the X-ray data it seems reasonably clear that in many membranes there is a substantial protein component on either side of the bilayer, and from the diffusion studies and from freeze-fracture studies it seemed evident that protein molecules in some cases extend through the thickness of the membrane.

The Use of Free Energy Calculations.

When a new structure is suggested as a component of cell membranes, it is often difficult to find an experimental approach to discover whether the suggestion has any validity. Under these circumstances it is very often of value to consider the free energy of the proposed arrangement of molecules in comparison with the free energies of other possible structures. Indeed, this is a valuable procedure, even when experimental techniques are also available for testing a hypothesis. For example, consider the hypothesis that the lipid layer of cell membrane is micellar as was proposed by some electron microscopists. If one considers neutral phospholipids, three alternative structures are available: the bilayer structure; cylindrical micelles; and

7

spherical micelles. Calculations of the differences in free
energy for these structures shows that the cylindrical micelle has a free energy in aqueous phases about 6 kcal greater than that of the bilayer structure and the spherical micelle has a free energy of about 12 kcal greater than the
bilayer structure. Thus the conclusion emerges very clearly
that, in aqueous media, bilayers have the least free energy
and consequently bilayer structures will predominate. On
the other hand, it also follows that since the free energy
differences between these structures are not huge all three
structures will coexist. If no other molecular components
affecting the free energy of the three types of structure
are present, the bilayer will predominate. It is also clear
from free energy calculations that dehydration of a bilayer
system will cause tremendous changes in the free energies
of the different structures and that consequently it is
extremely difficult from studies of anhydrous systems to
make determinations about the detail of the same systems
in the aqueous state.

In this particular case the conclusion which was reached
was that the "either/or" approach to the structure of a lipid
component of cell membranes is wrong. The question is not
whether the membrane consists of bilayer or of micelle, but
of how much of each type of component is present at a particular time. Furthermore, since the free energy differences
are not huge we can ask what sorts of molecules can provide
a free energy term which will stabilize an alternative structure at particular locations in the membrane.

It is probable that the cyclic antibiotics and other
"small" molecules which greatly increase the permeability
of membranes to ions do so by stabilizing alternative arrangements of the lipid molecules, the necessary free energy being
derived from interaction between the "small" molecules and
the lipid.

Considerations Based Upon Evolution by Natural Selection.

Insight about cell membranes, and what we may expect to
find in them, can also arise from consideration of the process
of evolution. Let us first ask the question: Why is it
that over a period of about 3 billion years of evolution the
bilayer element has come to be selected as a universal membrane component? The first important consideration is probably that it provides a remarkably efficient barrier to free

diffusion, *i.e.* it provides a very economical restraint from free mixing of the interior of a cell with the external medium. I calculated in 1940 that a membrane 100 times thicker would not be significantly more efficient than is a bilayer structure. A second and perhaps more important consideration is that a lipid bilayer, being liquid crystalline in nature at physiological temperatures, provides an undemanding two-dimensional matrix in which a great variety of functional molecules may be embedded and associate with one another without significant need for isomorphous properties, except insofar as they are required by necessary physiological interactions between macromolecules. If the membranes were made of proteins only, or of some other type of macromolecule, in order to derive a satisfactory diffusion barrier it would be necessary for the molecules to be substantially isomorphous. Most membranes probably contain over 100 macromolecular species, and it is rare for more than 10% of the macromolecules composing a membrane to be of any one species. Thus if the membrane were to be isomorphous it would be a great constraint on evolution, since whenever a mutation occurred which modified one of the macromolecular species it would be necessary for others to be modified simultaneously. Thus in order to get a significant change in membrane function it would be necessary to have simultaneous mutations involving a number of macromolecular species. Now the rate of favorable mutation for any one gene is probably not greater than 10^{-10}: probably lower. Favorable mutations are in themselves uncommon events. If it were necessary for say five molecules to change simultaneously, we could expect a favorable change in macromolecular structure to occur at the rate of say 10^{-50}. Thus we very soon reach the point at which no change is possible in geological time. It is evident that the fact that macromolecules may embed in the lipid bilayer, and thereby avoid the necessity for being isomorphous, confers an extraordinary evolutionary advantage upon the cell since independent molecular evolution is possible for each membrane function.

We may illustrate this point by saying that because the bilayer structure is an undemanding matrix it can readily incorporate structures which selectively modify the barrier to diffusion which is initially imposed by the presence of the bilayer. This permits selective transport, including active transport, and the development of excitability, without the necessity for profound modification of membrane structure, except locally in terms of specific macromolecules which are embedded in the membrane.

We can now turn to the question which has sometimes been asked as to which family of molecules is primarily responsible for establishing the structure outside of the membranes, *i.e.* is the prime mover a protein or is the prime mover a lipid? When we think of this question from the point of evolution we see it is not really a sensible question. Over the 2-3 billion years of evolution natural selection must have acted continuously to produce complementarity between protein and lipid. Thus by this time the protein and lipid found in membranes must be closely adapted to one another and one can no more assign the function of prime mover to protein or to lipid than one can assign the function of prime mover to chicken or egg.

These same considerations, which limit the likelihood of membranes in general being composed of isomorphous molecules, also limit the likelihood of cooperative phenomena occurring in membrane. A cooperative process, involving dozens of types of macromolecule, is quite improbable. Thus if we are to see cooperative changes in membranes they are likely to occur only in regions of membranes which are composed of a very small variety of macromolecules.

Cell Assembly Techniques

Artificial cell assembly techniques are now moving to the point at which it will be possible to use these techniques to study some of the dynamic properties of cell membranes. One of the most interesting of such properties is the rate of replacement of molecules in cell membranes and the control of membrane composition. The techniques essentially involve taking the components of cells and reorganizing them so as to obtain a new cell. The simplest technique of this type is cell fusion, which *e.g.* permits the study of the rate of mingling of the antigens of the separate cells after fusion has taken place. The second set of techniques involves the addition of nuclei, viruses, or single chromosomes to cells or cytoplasms. The addition is made in such a way as to change the genetic control of cell behavior and composition. A third type of technique involves taking a membrane, natural or artificial, and filling it with those components whose function it is desired to test in relation to *e.g.* a membrane composition.

During the next ten years we can expect to see great advances based upon the combination of techniques such as these, with immunochemical analytic techniques.

Conclusion

To sum up, I would say that at the present time the general existence of the bilayer component of cell membranes is well established. The *presence* of protein (and glycoprotein) components is equally well established. But the details of the way in which proteins form part of the membrane can be described only in the most general terms *e.g.* by saying that some proteins extend through the thickness of the membrane, some are embedded in one surface, some are adsorbed on a surface, and that their behavior indicates that the continuous phase of the membrane is the liquid crystalline bilayer and the proteins are the disperse phase. The interactions between proteins and lipids involve polar bonding and non-polar bonding to an extent which varies from protein to protein.

Little theoretical work can be done on the membrane proteins until the three-dimensional structure of some of these proteins are known.

Optimal progress, and optimal use of resources, will require careful study of the relation between hypothesis, theory and experiment, and if this is done much of the confusion which characterised the field over the period 1950-1970 can be avoided.

Presented by J. F. Danielli. This paper was prepared with the aid of NASA grant NGR 33-015-002. My thanks are due to innumerable friends and colleagues with whom I have discussed concepts of membrane structure over forty years.

References

1. This work is well reviewed by R. Hober, Physical chemistry of cells and tissues, Churchill, London (1945).
2. Harvey, E. N. and J. F. Danielli. Properties of the cell surface. Biol. Rev. Cambridge Phil. Soc. 13: 319-341 (1938).

3. Danielli, J. F. and E. N. Harvey. The tension at the surface of Mackeral Egg Oil, with remarks on the nature of the cell surface. J. Cell. Comp. Physiol. 5: No. 4, 483–494 (1935).

4. Danielli, J. F. and H. Davson. A contribution to the theory of permeability of thin films. J. Cell. Comp. Physiol. 5: 495–508 (1935).

5. Danielli, J. F. Some properties of lipoid films in relation to the structure of the plasma membrane. J. Cell. Comp. Physiol. 7: 393–408 (1936).

6. Danielli, J. F. The nature of the forces maintaining the specific structure of globular proteins. Proc. Roy. Soc. B 127: 34–35 (1939).

7. Davson, H. and J. F. Danielli (Editors), In: The Permeability of Natural Membranes, Cambridge University Press (1943).

8. Danielli, J. F. Cell permeability and diffusion across the oil–water interface. Trans. Faraday Soc. 37: Pt.3, 121–124 (1941).

EXTERIOR

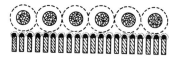

LIPOID

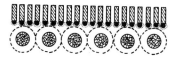

INTERIOR

Fig. 1. *The first paucimolecular layer model suggested for plasma membranes (1934).*

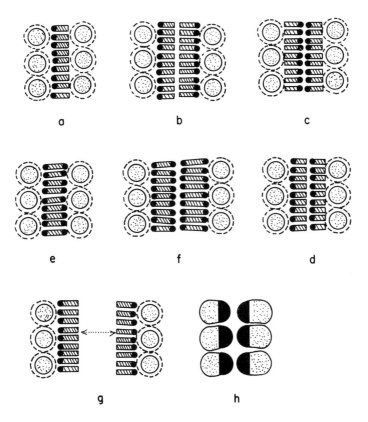

Fig. 2. *Some alternative arrangements of lipids and proteins (1936).*

13

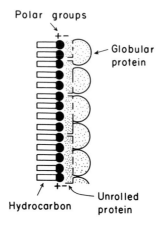

Fig. 3. *The second paucimolecular model: general organiza-*
tion (1938).

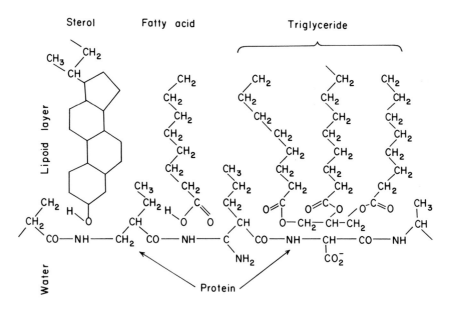

Fig. 4. *The second paucimolecular model: to show non-*
polar interactions between lipid and protein molecules
(1938).

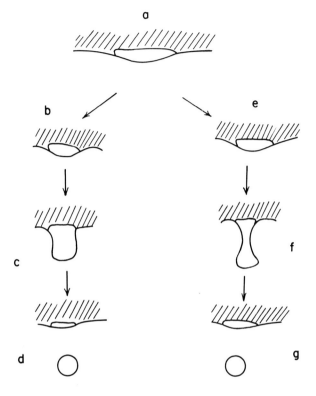

Fig. 5. *Experimental formation of lipoprotein spherical shell membranes (1936).*

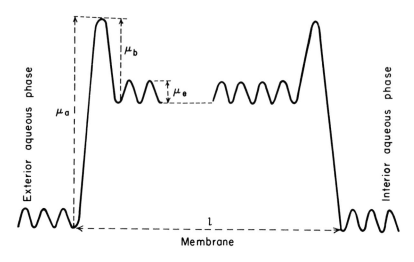

Fig. 6. *Model of the energy barriers to diffusion across the second paucimolecular model (1941).*

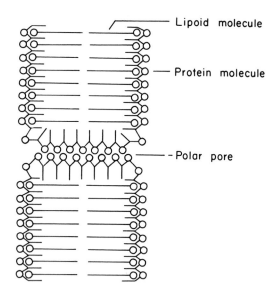

Diagram of pore of membrane

Fig. 7. *Third paucimolecular model: to show protein extending through the membrane (1943).*

16

FREEZE-ETCH IMAGES OF AN ION TRANSPORTING MEMBRANE

David W. Deamer and Robert Leonard

Introduction

New approaches to the problem of membrane structure have increased our confidence in discussing the molecular organization of lipid and protein in membranes. Several strong lines of evidence, including X-ray diffraction (1), calorimetry (2) and optical methods (3) have reached mutual agreement that most lipid hydrocarbon chains in a time-averaged membrane associate principally with one another, rather than with protein. The simplest explanation of this result is that much of the lipid in membranes is in the form of a lipid bilayer, as originally envisaged by Danielli and Davson (4).

The problem that now emerges is to determine more precisely the nature of the association between lipid and protein in membranes. There are a number of possible modes by which lipid-protein interaction may occur. Although in the past some of these have been proposed as general models for membrane structure, most membranes probably have several kinds of association between lipid and protein.

Possible structural relations between lipid and protein in membranes.

We will briefly discuss several proposed models for lipid-protein interaction in membranes. In each of these it is assumed that most of the membrane lipid forms a bilayer to which protein must somehow be attached. The two most general models of interaction fall into the categories of polar and non-polar ("hydrophobic") interactions. Polar lipid-protein interactions are probably the best understood, and several proteins apparently bind to membranes in this manner, including cytochrome c and some of the mitochondrial and chloroplast coupling factors. In this model it is assumed that charged groups on the protein interact electrostatically with charged lipid head groups (or any other charged group firmly attached to the membrane) either directly or through divalent ion bridges. It is typical of this type of interaction that the bound protein may be solubilized by varying the ionic strength, pH or divalent ion concentration. The isolated proteins contain no firmly bound lipid and are soluble in aqueous solutions.

Non-polar interactions between lipid and protein have been defined as yet only by the properties of a second distinct class of membrane proteins. Some fraction of the protein of most membranes may be solubilized by the techniques mentioned above, but there is usually a residual amount of protein, often well over half the original protein, which is still tightly bound to the membrane. For lack of a better term this association is called non-polar, or hydrophobic interaction, and it is generally considered that the stabilizing forces result from interactions of lipid chains with non-polar portions of protein molecules.

Protein bound to membranes by non-polar forces can be solubilized only by rather drastic procedures such as treatment with detergents, high or low pH ranges or organic solvents. This class of isolated protein is water insoluble, sometimes forming membranous aggregates, and often has a full complement of lipid firmly attached.

There are three possible manners in which non-polar interactions between lipid and protein may occur in membranes:

1. Protein penetration into lipid. It has long been known that protein can penetrate lipid monolayers (5, 6) and recent studies have provided evidence that protein may also penetrate lipid bilayers (7). When this knowledge is extended to membranes as a model for lipid-protein interaction, it is assumed that the major portion of a bound protein molecule remains at or near the surface of the membrane, with only a small segment actually penetrating the lipid phase and being stabilized there by non-polar forces.

2. Lipid penetration into surface protein. A second model for lipid-protein interaction suggests that some of the membrane phospholipid exists in an extended chain configuration, with chains directed into binding sites on the protein (8). The chains are

presumed to fit into binding sites on the protein, analogous to the sites on serum albumin, and non-polar forces again stabilize the association between the chains and the protein. There is no direct evidence for this type of interaction, although Hybl and Dorset (9) have found that some lipids exist in an extended chain conformation in crystals.

3. Protein embedded in lipid bilayers. Sjostrand (10), Green and Perdue (11) and Benson (12) originally proposed that some membrane protein may be embedded entirely within the lipid matrix of various membranes. In recent reviews, Branton (13) and Branton and Deamer (14) concluded that freeze-etch electron microscopy may reveal structures of this nature. Singer and Nicolson (15) proposed the term "fluid mosaic" to describe such a model, suggesting that embedded protein may form a mosaic of embedded particles floating freely within the fluid structure of lipid bilayers. Embedded proteins are of particular interest from the viewpoint of freeze-etch electron microscopy, since only embedded protein would necessarily be resolved in membrane fracture surfaces visualized by the freeze-etch technique. In the discussion to follow, we will examine the evidence that freeze-etch microscopy can reveal such structures, and in particular focus on the calcium transport ATPase of sarcoplasmic reticulum as a possible example of an embedded protein.

Freeze-etch electron microscopy

A diagrammatic sequence of the freeze-etch method is shown in Fig. 1. A small piece of biological material is frozen as rapidly as possible by immersion in liquid Freon. Usually the specimen is equilibrated with 20-50% glycerol prior to freezing to prevent damage by extensive ice crystal formation. The specimen is then fixed to the stage of a freeze-etch apparatus and fractured by repeated strokes with a cooled cutting edge. The fractured surface is shadowed and replicated with platinum-carbon and the replica is cleaned in a solvent such as commercial bleach solution. The replica may then be studied by standard electron micoscopic methods. In some instances, the fracture surface is "etched" by permitting ice to sublime from the surface for a minute or longer before shadowing. This may provide additional information, but is not a requirement of the technique.

Numerous studies (16, 17, 18) of the freeze-etch method have determined that the fracture passes along hydrophobic planes within cell membranes as originally suggested by Branton (16). Thus, the freeze-etch technique has the potential to reveal structures within the hydrophobic region of a membrane. Freeze-etch images from a variety of membranes are shown in Figs. 2-9. We will not discuss these micrographs individually, but have provided the collection in order for the reader readily to compare freeze-etch images from a wide range of structures. When making this type of comparison, it becomes apparent that one of the most striking and constant features of freeze-etch images are particulate structures on the fracture faces which occupy a considerable area of the membrane surface. Only myelin and some nuclear membranes are largely devoid of such structures. A rough generalization from such comparative studies is that membranes with metabolic and transport functions produce freeze-etch images with obvious particulate structures, whereas membranes which lack such functions, for instance myelin, also lack particles. The question naturally arises as to the significance of the particles. Could these represent a visualization of enzymatic lipoprotein structures such as cytochromes, transport proteins, or light-trapping centers in photosynthetic membranes?

Tests of the freeze-etch method

Lipid crystals

In order to place this question on a firmer foundation, it was necessary to test the freeze-etch method itself. There was no guarantee that particles were not some artifact of the freeze-etch process that occurred during freezing of cell structures. Secondly, even if the possibility of artifacts could be ruled out, one could not be certain that the technique was capable of resolving lipoprotein particles which might be present in membranes. In the discussion to follow, we will discuss two tests of the freeze-etch technique, one involving lipid crystals, and the second a study of a crystalline lipoprotein system.

20

Since hydrocarbon planes in membrane lipid layers guide fracture planes during fracturing of frozen biological material, it seemed reasonable to view pure lipid systems in order to determine whether particulate structures could be produced as artifacts of the freezing process in lipids. This study was carried out by Deamer *et al.* (18) on a series of lipid systems which were also characterized by X-ray diffraction analysis. In this manner it was possible to compare physical dimensions of the lipid crystals derived from freeze-etch and X-ray analysis. We attempted to answer the following questions:

1. Can lipid phases be preserved intact by the freeze-etch method?
2. Are any particulate structures found in lipid systems that could account for the particles found on biological membranes?

Some typical results from this study are shown in Figs. 10 and 11 which compare images obtained from lamellar and hexagonal phase lipid crystals. All lamellar phase lipids which were studied showed smooth planar regions mixed with regions where the fracture plane passed at an angle through the lamellar lipid layers (Fig. 10). Occasionally, fracture was nearly normal to the plane of the lamellae and it was possible to determine repeat distances between lipid lamellae. When hexagonal phase lipids were examined, fracture faces were not smooth, but instead contained repeating linear structures of indefinite length (Fig. 11). The simplest interpretation of this image is that the linear structures represent the lipid rods characterized by X-ray analysis of hexagonal lipid phases (19). Figure 12 shows how lamellar and hexagonal lipid phases might give rise to the observed freeze-etch images during fracture. In this analysis, it is assumed that the fracture plane always follows non-polar planes in the region of lipid hydrocarbon tails.

Table I gives some of the freeze-etch parameters for various lipids compared with X-ray data for the same lipids. The results from the two different methods are in good agreement.

We were able to draw two conclusions from this study. First, the freeze-etch method is capable of preserving lipid phases and resolving their dimensions. Second, lamellar lipid fracture faces were invariably smooth when effectively protected from contamination after fracture. We could

21

conclude that particulate structures do not arise as an un-controllable artifact of the freeze-etch method itself, and that some other explanation must be found for the particles seen on biological membranes.

Lipoprotein crystals

A second question which arises in regard to freeze-etching is whether the technique has the capacity to reveal lipoprotein particles which may be present in membranes. We were fortunate to find a system to test this point. Yolk platelets are crystalline structures found within eggs of many species of amphibia. Two proteins, phosvitin and lipo-vitellin, are organized in a crystal which is readily visu-lized in sections through the egg. Phospholipids account for approximately 15% of the dry weight of the platelet.

The function of yolk platelets is unknown, although dur-ing development of newt embryos the platelet has been found to undergo a process of dissolution with the formation of literally hundreds of lamellar membranes surrounding the platelet in concentric layers (20). This suggests that yolk platelets may be a storage depot for basic membrane compon-ents which are utilized during embryo development.

Since the yolk platelet has also been studied by X-ray diffraction analysis for one species of amphibian (21), it is again possible to compare freeze-etch and X-ray param-eters, but this time in a lipoprotein system. The results of this study were reported by Leonard, Deamer and Armstrong (22) and several of the relevant results are shown in Figs. 13 and 14 and Table II. A sectioned platelet is shown in Fig. 13. The crystallinity is readily apparent, but the sectioning technique reveals only heavy metal deposits, rather than membrane components, and the results are there-fore at best indirect and not readily interpretable. A freeze-etch image of the interior of a yolk platelet is shown in Fig. 14. We found that freeze-etching does in fact reveal the subunit structure of yolk platelets, and that the dimensions of the crystal as determined by freeze-etching are comparable to those determined by X-ray analysis (Table II). This result established that the freeze-etch method is capable of visualizing lipoprotein particles, and that if such particles are present in membranes we could ex-pect to see them in a freeze-etch replica.

Sarcoplasmic reticulum

A major difficulty in characterizing the particulate
structures revealed by freeze-etching is that most membranes
have several known functions. For instance, mitochondria
contain electron transport proteins, coupling factors and
other transport enzymes. Chloroplasts have light trapping
systems, as well as electron transport proteins. It would
obviously be a difficult task to sort out which of the many
possible enzymes might account for a freeze-etch particle
in such membranes. In reviewing several systems which might
permit simpler analysis, one membrane which appeared to be
monofunctional was sarcoplasmic reticulum isolated from
muscle as microsomes. The only known major metabolic activity of this membrane *in vitro* is an ATP-dependent uptake of
calcium ions. Typical calcium uptake and related ATPase
activity in lobster muscle microsomes is shown in Fig. 15.
Note that as calcium uptake proceeds, there is a simultaneous hydrolysis of ATP, and that approximately two calciums
are transported inward per ATP hydrolysed. This stoichiometry has been well established by previous studies (23).
The dashed line shows a similar experiment with a mammalian
preparation at the same protein concentration. It is readily
apparent that the lobster preparation has an uptake rate
approximately six times that of the mammalian system.
    Deamer and Baskin (24) first viewed sarcoplasmic retic-
ulum by freeze-etch techniques. The early experiments with
mammalian muscle preparations demonstrated that the microsomal preparations, like many other membranes, produced
highly particulate fracture faces containing randomly array-
ed particles 80-90 Å in diameter (Fig. 16a). On the basis
of the molecular weight determined by other investigators
for sarcoplasmic reticulum ATPase (25), and the fact that
the surface density of the particles was in the range of
that required to account for calcium binding (26), Deamer
and Baskin suggested that the particles may represent the
ATPase site of sarcoplasmic reticulum.

Isolation and properties of the ATPase

It soon became apparent that mammalian muscle microsomes
were highly heterogeneous, with only 20-30% of the membranes
capable of calcium transport (27, 28). Mammalian preparations had the additional drawback of losing activity within
a few hours of isolation. These problems were at least

23

partially overcome when Van der Kloot (29) demonstrated that lobster tail preparations were capable of much more rapid calcium uptake rates, as illustrated in Fig. 15. Furthermore, the preparations were stable up to 10 days in the presence of dithiothreitol. We have since confirmed these findings, and Baskin (30) has demonstrated that crustacean sarcoplasmic reticulum preparations are more homogeneous, since the majority of vesicles can be shown to transport calcium. Lobster microsomes also contain particles (30) similar to those in mammalian preparations (Fig. 16b). Therefore, we turned to lobster preparations for the work to be described here.

One approach to the problem of attaching a functional significance to freeze-etch particles would be to isolate a major enzymatic protein from a membrane and then view the isolated material by the freeze-etch method. The isolated enzyme should have a particulate structure very similar to the particles on the original membranes. On the basis of the work described above, the ATPase activity of sarcoplasmic reticulum seemed to be a good candidate for such a study, and we began to search for a suitable isolation method. Martonosi (31) used sodium deoxycholate to solubilize the ATPase of mammalian microsomal membranes, and Maclennen (32) recently succeeded in a 3.5 fold purification of ATPase activity over that of isolated washed microsomes, also with deoxycholate. However, Martonosi (31) noted that deoxycholate strongly inhibited ATPase activity at concentrations only slightly higher than those required to solubilize the membranes. In an attempt to provide a more "natural" lipid environment in working out an isolation procedure, we decided to use lysolecithin to solubilize the membranes.

Lysolecithin is derived from lecithin by enzymatic hydrolysis of fatty acids at the 2 position. Lysolipids in general are minor components of most membranes and are precursors for double-chained lipids. Lysolecithin is relatively water soluble, and is known to solubilize membranes such as myelin (33). We reasoned that sarcoplasmic reticulum treated with lysolecithin may break down into smaller lipoprotein complexes which could perhaps be separated by various techniques of protein chemistry. In preliminary experiments it was found that lysolecithin did not inhibit ATPase activity at concentrations which apparently solubilized the membranes. Furthermore, the preparations treated with lysolecithin could still form centrifugal pellets at high g forces, and the pellets had enhanced ATPase activity. Since it was possible that this relatively simple procedure might provide a purification of the ATPase , we extended these experiments by titrating the preparations with lysolecithin and measuring the pellet protein and lipid composition and ATPase activity. These results are shown in Fig. 17.

It is apparent in Fig. 17 that at 1 to 2 mg of lyso-lecithin per mg protein, approximately half the protein of the sarcoplasmic reticulum is solubilized, and the other half can be found in the pellet. Most of the ATPase activity can also be found in the pellet and the specific activity therefore was increased 2 fold. At lysolecithin concentrations higher than 2 mg per mg protein, all the protein was solubilized. Figure 18 shows the distribution of lipids in the pellet with increasing lysolecithin concentrations. As more lysolecithin was added to the microsomes, choline lipids in the pellet decreased from 0.75 to 0.2 μmoles lipid per mg protein, while ethanolamine lipids remained constant at 0.3 μmoles per mg protein. This suggests the interesting possibility that perhaps ethanolamine lipids are specifically associated with the ATPase activity of sarcoplasmic reticulum. Lysolecithin in the pellet increased to a maximum level of 1.4 μmoles per mg protein. This figure is approximately twice the original lipid content, and represents a large portion of the lysolecithin that was added to the microsomes. For instance, at the ratio of 1 mg lysolecithin per mg protein, a total of 16 μmoles lysolecithin was added and 7 μmoles appeared in the pellet. Since lysolecithin by itself does not form centrifugal pellets under the conditions employed here, we may conclude that the lysolecithin was firm-ly bound to the pellet protein.

In a second series of experiments, acrylamide gels containing sodium dodecyl sulfate were used to follow the distribution of proteins during lysolecithin treatment of the microsomes. A comparison of the protein composition of the pellet and supernatant proteins is shown in Fig. 19. The pellet was greatly enhanced in the amount of protein in a slowly migrating major band, and the supernatant contained larger amounts of protein in approximately 16 faster moving bands. We concluded that the pellet protein, while not a completely pure preparation, contained a single major protein or class of proteins of uniform molecular weight. Since the ATPase activity of the pellet and the amount of protein in this band were both increased, it seems reasonable to assign to it the ATPase activity of the pellet.

25

Freeze-etch studies were carried out on pellets derived
from several concentrations of lysolecithin (Fig. 20 a,b,c).
The most striking alteration with increasing lysolecithin
concentration was a decrease in the size of the vesicles.
Control vesicles averaged approximately 0.17 μ in diameter,
while those treated with 2 mg lysolecithin per mg protein
decreased to 0.06 μ. The concave faces of all the vesicles
were particulate, with the particles ranging from 70-90 Å
in diameter. The particles could not be distinguished from
the particles found on the original microsomal membranes.
In one instance, the vesicles apparently merged into lamellar
structures containing highly particulate fracture faces
(Fig. 21). The physical mechanism of vesicle and lamella
formation is not yet understood.

Comparison with previous studies

Martonosi (31) first attempted to isolate and study the
properties of ATPase from a mammalian (rabbit) source. It
was found that sodium deoxycholate would solubilize the
membranes, but also inhibited ATPase at concentrations only
slightly greater than those required for solubilization.
The original calcium dependent ATPase activity varied from
3-5 μmoles/mg/min. Martonosi was unable to demonstrate an
increased specific activity of the enzyme following several
purification procedures, but did observe that the solubilized
membrane components would reform vesicles upon removal of
the deoxycholate. The reformed vesicles had ATPase activity
of 0.6-0.9 μmoles/mg/min. It was reported that the vesicles,
if provided with any of several lipids, including lysolecithin, could accumulate up to 0.9 μmoles calcium per mg protein in the presence of oxalate.

Maclennan (32) repeated and extended these experiments,
and had considerable success in attaining a protein fraction
with increased specific activity of ATPase. Starting with
a specific activity of 8.3 μmoles ATP/mg/min for a washed
preparation, the final activity reached 31 μmoles ATP/mg/
min, which represents a 3.5 fold purification. Maclennan
also found that vesicles formed upon removal of deoxycholate,
but was unable to demonstrate significant calcium binding
in the reconstituted vesicles, in spite of the fact that the
lipid composition of the purified vasicular ATPase was almost
identical to that of the starting material. The control
value for calcium uptake was 0.75 μmoles/mg/min, and the

reconstituted vesicles could apparently accumulate 0.06 μmoles/mg/min. Maclennan *et al.* (34) characterized the vesicles by several electron micrographic techniques, including freeze-etching, and found that the freeze-etched vesicles were highly particulate.

Since the present results are from a different animal source, we will not be able to comment in detail on the apparent inconsistencies between the two previous studies and our own. There is general agreement that solubilized ATPase is able to participate in membrane formation under certain conditions. We also agree with the observation of Maclennan *et al.* (34) that the vesicles so formed are particulate in character when viewed by the freeze-etch method. The two major inconsistencies have to do with calcium uptake and ATPase rates in the reconstituted vesicles. We will first discuss calcium uptake.

Martonosi (31) reported that lysolecithin and other lipids are effective in reconstituting calcium uptake in deoxycholate solubilized membranes. However, when we add even small amounts (0.2 mM) of lysolecithin to lobster muscle microsomes, calcium transport is completely inhibited, and the purified ATPase by itself has no calcium binding capacity. Maclennan (32) also found that the purified ATPase had little calcium transport. It is possible that lipids other than lysolecithin will reconstitute calcium transport, and we are presently undertaking such experiments.

The second area of disagreement concerns the ATPase rates reported. Our results are in accord with those of Martonosi (31) for ATPase activity in the original microsomes. For instance, the ATPase activity in lobster preparations during calcium transport is 1.6 μmoles/mg/min, and the calcium uptake measured under the same conditions is 3.3 μmoles/mg/min. This results in a calcium/ATP ratio of approximately 2:1, in agreement with previous studies. Maclennan (32) reports a much more rapid calcium-activated ATPase activity of from 3 to 8 μmoles ATP/mg/min (depending on whether the membranes had undergone an extra washing procedure) and reported a calcium uptake rate of 0.75 μmoles/mg/min. This results in a calcium/ATP ratio of nearly 1:5, which does not agree with previous studies. One factor which may partially account for some of the difference between activities of mammalian and lobster ATPase preparations is that the mammalian values were obtained at 37°, whereas the lobster preparations were measured at 25°. This does not explain the variations in Ca/ATP ratios.

27

Summary

Muscle microsomes contain particles 70–90 Å in diameter which may be visualized by freeze-etching. The estimated molecular weight and distribution of the particles corresponds to independent estimates of the molecular weight and distribution of an ATPase enzyme in the microsomes associated with calcium transport. An ATPase preparation could be obtained from the microsomes by treatment with lysolecithin, followed by centrifugation. The ATPase had approximately twice the specific activity of the original membrane ATPase, and produced a single major band on acrylamide gels. Freeze-etch images of the purified ATPase showed it to consist of particles similar to those found on the original membranes.

Figure 22 shows a diagrammatic representation of our understanding of the isolation procedure and resulting freeze-etch images. Lysolecithin apparently causes displacement of considerable lipid from the membrane and is in turn tightly bound. Within a narrow range of lysolecithin concentration, some of the membrane protein containing ATPase activity forms vesicles of smaller diameter than the original microsomes. Freeze-etching of the vesicles reveals the particles. The data supports the suggestion that the particulate structures on muscle microsomes represent sites of ATPase activity (24), and is in accord with the result of Maclennan *et al.* (34) that purified ATPase from muscle microsomes is particulate when viewed by freeze-etching.

Presented by David W. Deamer. The authors wish to thank Mr. Larry Long for his excellent technical assistance. This investigation was supported by NSF Grant GB-32353.

References

1. Wilkins, M.H.F., A.E. Blaurock and D.M. Engelman. X-ray diffraction from membrane dispersion: bilayer structure in membranes. Nature New Biology 230:72–76 (1971).
2. Steim, J.M., M.E. Tourtellotte, J.C. Reinert, R.N. McElhaney and R.L. Rader. Calorimetric evidence for the liquid-crystalline state of lipids in a biomembrane. Proc. Nat. Acad. Sci. (U.S.) 63:104–109 (1969).

28

3. Glaser, M., H. Simpkins, S.J. Singer, M. Sheetz and S. I. Chan. On the interaction of lipids and proteins in the red blood cell membrane. Proc. Nat. Acad. Sci. (U.S.) 65:721-728 (1970).

4. Danielli, J.F. and H. Davson. A contribution to the theory of permeability of thin films. J. Cell Comp. Physiol. 5:495-508 (1935).

5. Matalon, R. and J.H. Schulman. Formation of lipo-protein monolayers: mechanism of adsorption, solution and penetration. Disc. Faraday Soc. 6:27-39 (1949).

6. Quinn, P. and R.M.C. Dawson. The penetration of serum albumin into phospholipid monolayers of different fatty acid chain length and interfacial charge. Biochem. J. 119:21-25 (1970).

7. Kimelberg, H. K. and D. Papahadjopoulos. Phospholipid-protein interactions: membrane permeability correlated with monolayer penetration. Biochim. Biophys. Acta 233:805-809 (1971).

8. Deamer, D.W. An alternative model for molecular organization in biological membranes. J.Bioenergetics 1:237-246 (1970).

9. Hybl, A. and D. Dorset. The crystal structure of the 1,3-diglyceride of 11-bromoundecanoic acid. Acta Crystallogr. B27:977-986 (1971).

10. Sjostrand, F.S. A new ultrastructural element of the membranes in mitochondria and of some cytoplasmic membranes. J. Ultrastruct. Res. 9:340-361 (1963).

11. Green, D.E. and J.F. Perdue. Membranes as expressions of repeating units. Proc. Nat. Acad. Sci. (U.S.) 55: 1295-1302 (1966).

12. Benson, A.A. On the orientation of lipids in chloroplast and cell membranes. J. Amer. Oil Chem. Soc. 43:265-270 (1966).

13. Branton, D. Membrane structure. Ann. Rev. Plant Physiol. 20:209-238 (1969).

14. Branton, D. and D.W. Deamer. Membrane structure. Protoplasmatologia II E 1, Springer-Verlag, Wien-New York. 70 pp. (1972).

15. Singer, S.J. and G. Nicolson. The fluid mosaic model of the structure of cell membranes. Science 175:720-731 (1972).

16. Branton, D. Fracture faces of frozen membranes. Proc. Nat. Acade. Sci. (U.S.) 55:1048-1056 (1966).

17. Deamer, D.W. and D. Branton. Fracture planes in an ice-bilayer model membrane system. Science 158:655-657 (1967).

18. Deamer, D.W., R. Leonard, A. Tardieu and D. Branton. Lamellar and hexagonal lipid phases visualized by freeze-etching. Biochim. Biophys. Acta 219:47-60 (1970).

19. Luzatti, V. X-ray diffraction studies of lipid-water systems. In "Biological membranes, physical fact and function." D. Chapman, ed. Academic Press, New York (1968).

20. Honjin, R., T. Nakamura and S. Shimasaki. X-ray diffraction and electron microscopic studies on the crystalline lattice structure of amphibian yolk platelets. J. Ultrastruct. Res. 12:404-419 (1965).

21. Jurand, A. and G. G. Selman. Yolk utilization in the notochord of newt as studied by electron microscopy. J. Embryol. Exp. Morph. 12:43-50 (1964).

22. Leonard, R., D.W. Deamer and P.B. Armstrong. Amphibian yolk platelet ultrastructure visualized by freeze-etching. J. Ultrastruct. Res. (in press, 1972).

23. Weber, A., R. Herz and I. Reiss. Study of the kinetics of calcium transport by isolated fragmented sarcoplasmic reticulum. Biochem. Zeit. 345:329-369 (1966).

24. Deamer, D.W. and R.J. Baskin. Ultrastructure of sarcoplasmic reticulum preparations. J. Cell Biol. 42:296-307 (1969).

25. Vegh, K., P. Spiegler, C. Chamberlain and W.F.H.M. Mommaerts. The molecular size of the calcium-transport ATPase of sarcotubular vesicles estimated from radiation inactivation. Biochim. Biophys. Acta 163:266-268 (1968).

26. Martonosi, A. Role of phospholipids in ATPase activity and Ca transport of fragmented sarcoplasmic reticulum. Fed. Proc. 23:913-921 (1964).

27. Baskin, R.J. and D.W. Deamer. Comparative ultrastructure and calcium transport in heart and skeletal muscle microsomes. J. Cell Biol. 43:610-617 (1969).

28. Greaser, M.L., R.G. Cassens, W.G. Hoekstra and E.J. Briskey. Purification and ultrastructural properties of the calcium accumulating membranes in isolated sarcoplasmic reticulum preparations from skeletal muscle. J. Cell Physiol. 74:37-50 (1969).

29. Van der Kloot, W. Calcium uptake by isolated sarcoplasmic reticulum treated with dithiothreitol. Science 164:1294-1295 (1969).

30. Baskin, R.J. Ultrastructure and calcium transport in crustacean muscle microsomes. J. Cell Biol. 48:49-60 (1971).
31. Martonosi, A. Solubilization of microsomal adenosine triphosphatase. J. Biol. Chem. 243:71-81 (1968).
32. Maclennan, D.H. Purification and properties of an adenosine triphosphatase from sarcoplasmic reticulum. J. Biol. Chem. 245:4508-4518 (1970).
33. Gent, W.L.G., N.A. Gregson, D.B. Gammack and J.H. Raper. The lipid-protein unit in myelin. Nature 204:553-555 (1964).
34. Maclennan, D.H., P. Seeman, G.H. Iles and C.C. Yip. Membrane formation by the adenosine triphosphatase of sarcoplasmic reticulum. J. Biol. Chem. 246:2702-2710 (1971).
35. Davis, B.J. Disc electrophoresis. Ann. N.Y. Acad. Sci. 121:404-427 (1964).
36. Fairhurst, A.S. and D.J. Jenden. Spectrophotometric monitoring of calcium uptake by skeletal muscle particles. Analyt. Biochem. 16:294-301 (1966).

TABLE I

COMPARISON OF FREEZE-ETCH AND X-RAY DIFFRACTION
PARAMETERS OF LIPID SYSTEMS

Phase	Repeat distance ($\overset{o}{A}$)	
	Freeze-etch	X-ray
Lamellar		
Strontium laurate	44	43
Dipalmitoyl phosphatidyl		
choline	54	55
Egg lecithin (anhydrous)	57	50–60
Hexagonal		
Calcium cardiolipin	52	52
Lecithin-cholesterol		
(anhydrous)	48	48.5
Lysolecithin	60	66

TABLE II

COMPARISON OF FREEZE ETCH AND X-RAY DIFFRACTION
PARAMETERS OF AMPHIBIAN YOLK PLATELETS

*Freeze-etch parameters were measured from freeze-etch micrographs of hexagonal (not shown)
and square (Figure 14) pattern fracture surfaces within yolk platelets. X-ray data are
taken from Ref. 20 for the equivalent X-ray spacings. X-ray data are not available for
Xenopus, and some of the difference in spacing may result from comparing two different
amphibian genera.*

Structural surface pattern	Repeat distance ($\overset{\circ}{A}$)	
	Freeze-etch (Xenopus)	X-ray (Rhacophorus)
Hexagonal	80–108	110
Square	85	110

33

Table III

COMPARISON OF THE PROPERTIES OF ATPase ENZYMES
DERIVED FROM MAMMALIAN AND CRUSTACEAN MUSCLE

Properties	Martonosi (31)	Maclennan et al. (32,34)	Present Study
A. Microsomal ATPase rate ($\mu moles$ ATP/ mg protein/min)	1.25 (37°)	8.3 (37°)	1.6 (25°)
ATPase rate in reconstituted vesicles ($\mu moles$ ATP/mg protein/ min)	0.71 (37°)	31 (37°)	3.0 (25°)
Calcium uptake in microsomes ($\mu moles$/ mg/min)	---	0.75	3.3
Calcium uptake in reconstituted vesicles ($\mu moles$/ mg/min)	0.9	0.06	N.D.

Table III

COMPARISON OF THE PROPERTIES OF ATPase ENZYMES
DERIVED FROM MAMMALIAN AND CRUSTACEAN MUSCLE

Properties	Martonosi (31)		Maclennan *et al.* (32,34)		Present Study	
	Microsomes	ATPase	Microsomes	ATPase	Microsomes	ATPase
B. Phospholipid composition ($\mu moles$ *lipid P/mg protein*)						
Phosphatidyl choline	0.182	0.203	0.37	0.39	0.72	0.25
Phosphatidyl ethanolamine	--	--	0.10	0.10	0.28	0.28
Phosphatidyl serine	--	--	0.065	0.065	0.10	--
Other lipid phosphate	0.086	0.112	--	--	--	--
Cholesterol (mgs/mg protein)	--	--	0.057	0.059	0.09	--
Percent lipid in membranes	--	--	33*	33*	40*	--

*Calculated assuming phospholipid M. W. = 800.

35

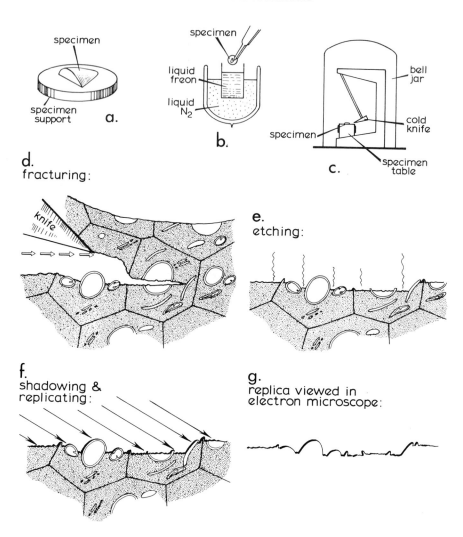

Fig. 1. *Diagram of steps involved in the freeze-etch method.* See text for details. Reprinted courtesy of Springer-Verlag, New York.

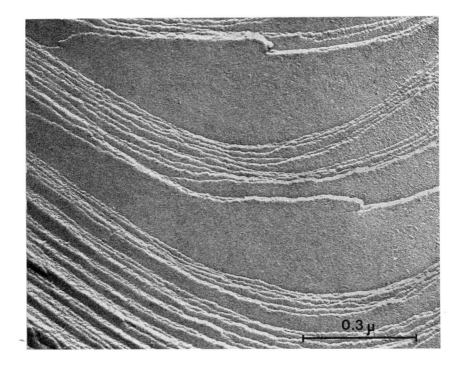

Fig. 2. *Five-day old rat sciatic nerve myelin.* Exposed fracture faces are smooth. Courtesy Daniel Branton.

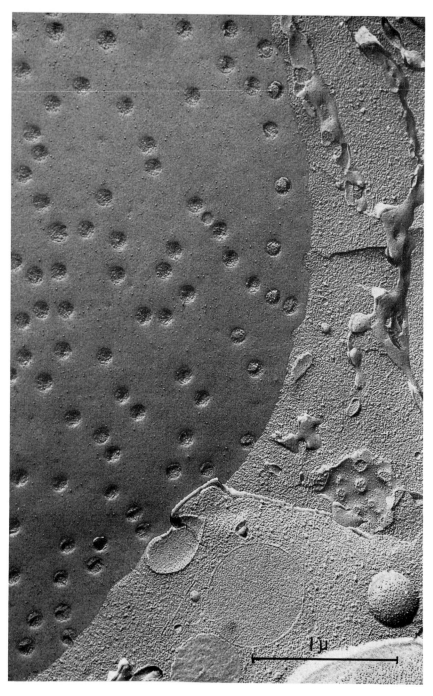

Fig. 3. *Nuclear membrane of onion root tip*. Particles are relatively sparse on membrane fracture faces between the large nuclear pores. Courtesy Daniel Branton.

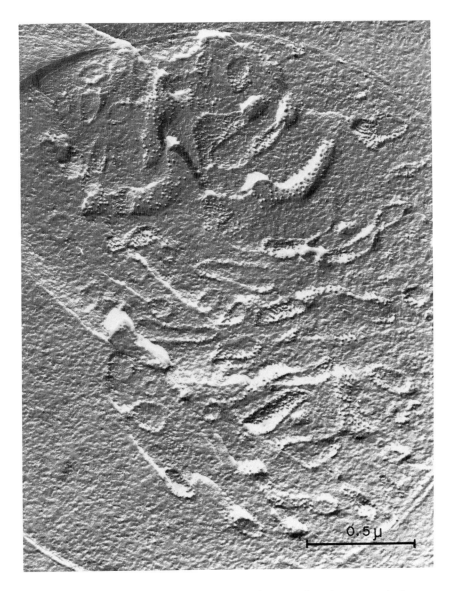

0.5 μ

Fig. 4. *Mitochondrion from beef heart showing particles on faces of cristae.*

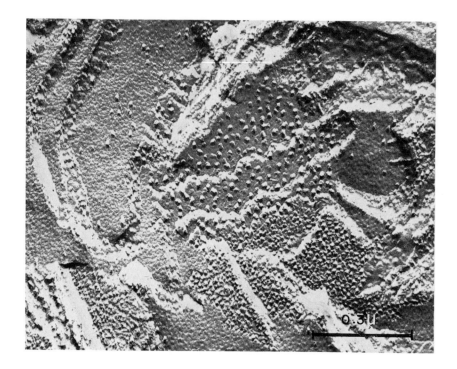

Fig. 5. *Inner membrane fracture faces of a chloroplast from wheat.* Three different fracture faces can be distinguished on the basis of particulate structures.

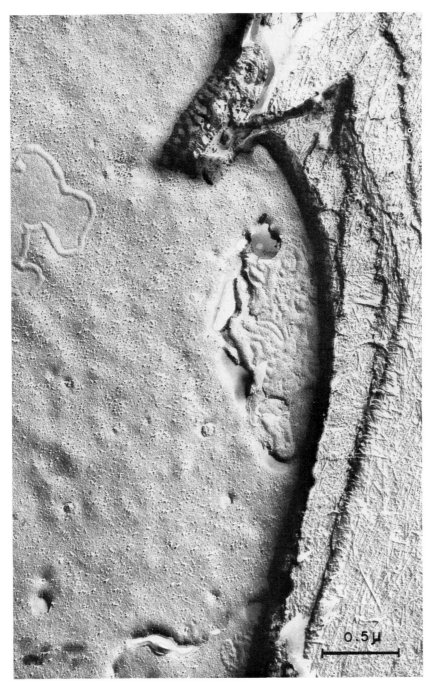

Fig. 6. *Particle-covered plasmalemma and adjacent cell wall from wheat mesophyll.*

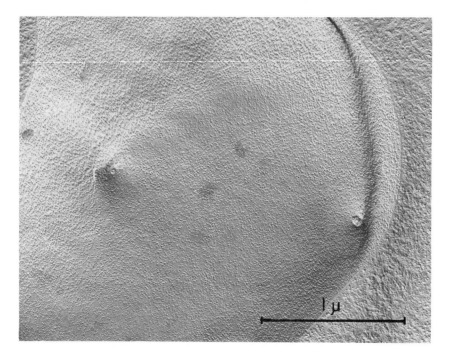

Fig. 7. *Particle-covered beef erythrocyte ghost membrane.*

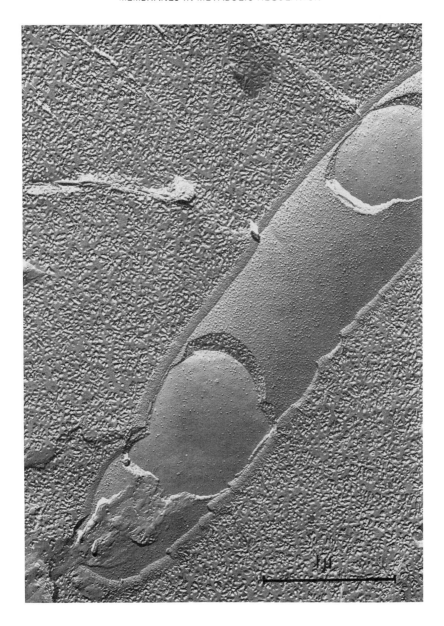

Fig. 8. *Membrane faces in an unidentified filamentous lacustrine bacterium.*

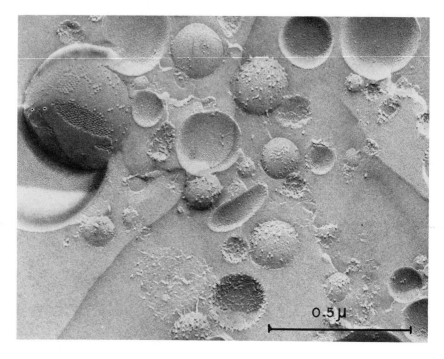

Fig. 9. *Microsomes prepared from beef heart muscle.*
Occasionally the particles are organized into a semicrystal-
line array on the microsome membranes. These are probably
the remains of a cell junction.

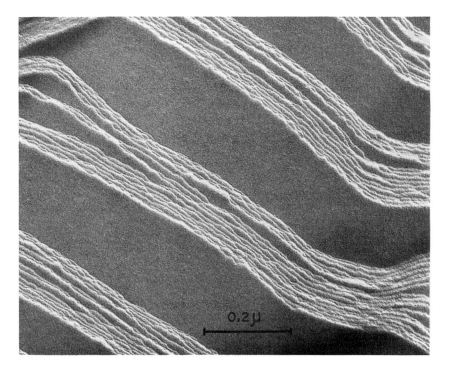

Fig. 10. *Smooth fracture faces of lamellar phase lipid (L-α-dipalmitoyl phosphatidyl choline).*

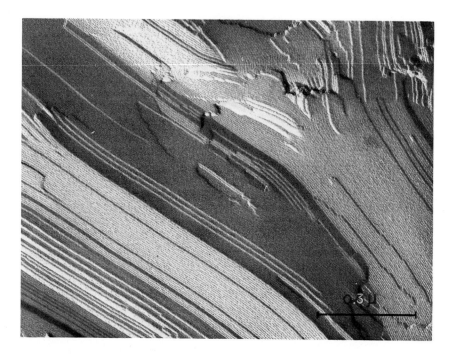

Fig. 11. *Ribbed fracture faces of hexagonal II phase lipid (calcium cardiolipin).*

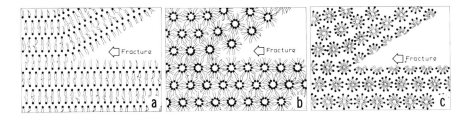

Fig. 12. *Possible fracture modes in the various lipid phases:* a. *Lamellar.* b. *Hexagonal II.* c. *Hexagonal I.* From Deamer *et al.* (15).

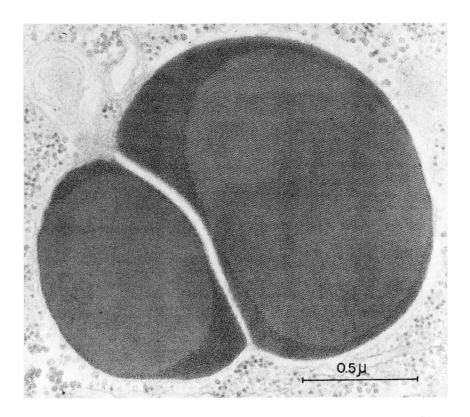

Fig. 13. *Sectioned yolk platelet from fertile egg of the African frog,* Xenopus laevis, *showing a hexagonal pattern of stained elements.* Courtesy Peter Armstrong

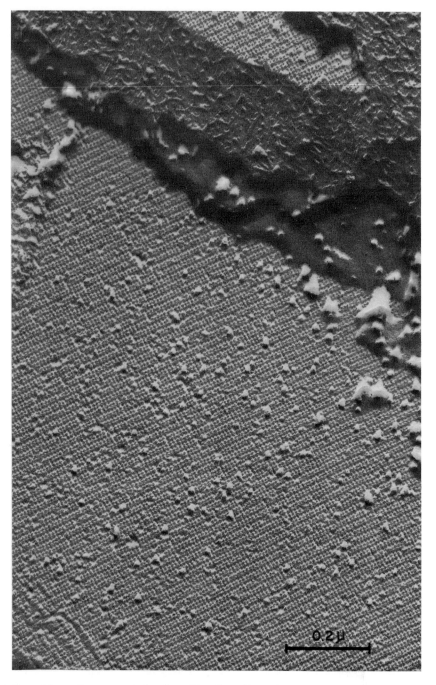

Fig. 14. *Freeze-etched yolk platelet from egg of Xenopus laevis showing a rectangular array of lipoprotein particles.* From Leonard *et al.* (22).

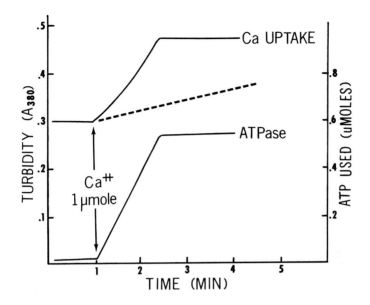

Fig. 15. *Calcium uptake and ATP hydrolysis in muscle microsomes.* The measurements were made in 2 ml of 4 mM potassium oxalate, 5 mM $MgCl_2$, 2.5 mM ATP and 0.25 mg microsomal protein per ml (pH 7.2). One micromole of $CaCl_2$ was added at 1 min. Calcium uptake was followed by the method of Fairhurst and Jenden (36) using turbidity increase at 380 nm. ATP hydrolysis was measured by calibrating the pH change during hydrolysis (about 0.1 pH unit) with a known quantity of NaOH. When all the calcium which was added was taken up by the microsomes (after 1.4 min in this experiment) no further increase in turbidity occurred and ATP hydrolysis stopped simultaneously.

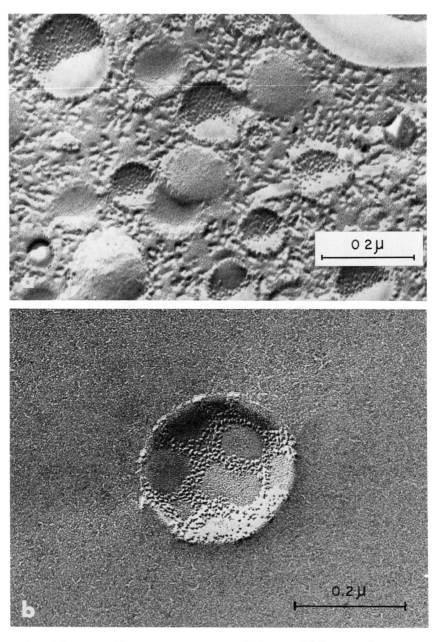

Fig. 16. *a. Microsomes prepared from rabbit muscle.* Most vesicles are covered with a random array of particles (24).

Fig. 16. *b. Microsome from lobster tail muscle.* Particles were in a more ordered array in these microsomes which were frozen during calcium uptake. In resting microsomes particles are generally in random orientations.

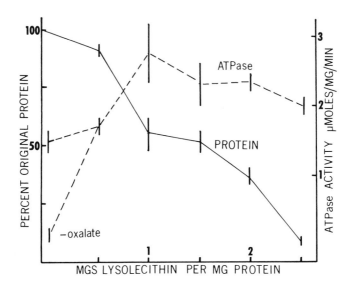

Fig. 17. *Purification of ATPase by lysolecithin treatment.*
Lobster muscle microsomes (5 ml of 5 mg protein/ml) were
titrated with increasing amounts of lysolecithin (Sigma) up
to 2.5 mg lysolecithin/ mg protein. The buffer was 10 mM
TES (pH 7.0). After a 10 sec sonication (Biosonik 1 cm
probe, maximum intensity) the suspensions were centrifuged
30 min at 108,000 x g. Protein (Lowry) and ATPase activity
were measured in the resulting pellet. Bars represent range
of values from three experiments. Note that in the absence
of oxalate, the calcium activated ATPase rate was very low.
However, upon addition of lysolecithin, the rate increased
to the level found in the presence of oxalate. This represents approximately a six fold activation of the ATPase
activity. Previous studies (32) have also noted activation
by deoxycholate at low concentrations.

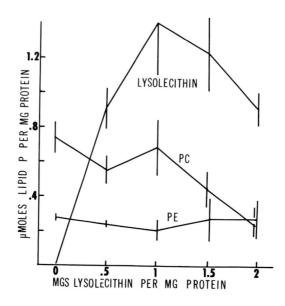

Fig. 18. *Lipid composition of pellets obtained from lysolecithin treated microsomes.* Pellets were prepared as
described in Fig. 17. Lipid classes in chloroform–methanol
extracts of the pellets were measured by quantitative thin
layer chromatography and analysis for lipid phosphate. Bars
represent range of values for two experiments. In a second
series of experiments it was found that the total amount of
phosphatidyl choline (PC) and phosphatidyl ethanolamine (PE)
appearing in the pellet treated with 2 mg lysolecithin/mg
protein decreased to 20% and 30% of their original values
in the absence of lysolecithin. Apparently a major portion
of the microsomal lipid is dissolved in the supernatant.

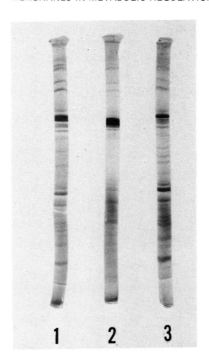

1   2   3

Fig. 19. *Acrylamide gels of microsomal protein during lysolecithin treatment.* Gels containing 0.5% sodium dodecyl sulfate were run according to the method of Davis (35). 1. Stock microsomes, showing approximately 20 detectable bands and one slowly migrating major band. 2. Pellet from 1 mg lysolecithin/mg protein and containing enhanced ATPase activity. The major band is enhanced and other bands are reduced. 3. Supernatant from 2. The major band is reduced and other bands are enhanced. All gels contained 50 µg protein dissolved in 1% SDS prior to application. The apparent molecular weight of the major band was 190,000, when compared with known protein standards.

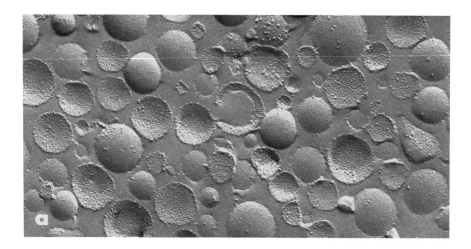

Fig. 20. *a.* *Microsomes prepared from lobster tail muscle.*
Concave faces contain a moderate concentration of particles,
and convex faces are smooth.

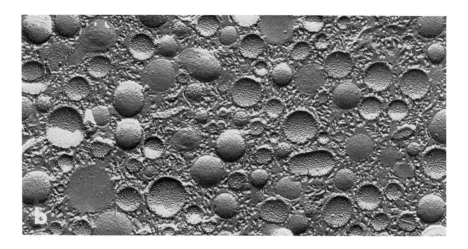

Fig. 20. *b.* *Vesicles from a pellet which had been treated*
with 1.5 mg lysolecithin/mg protein.

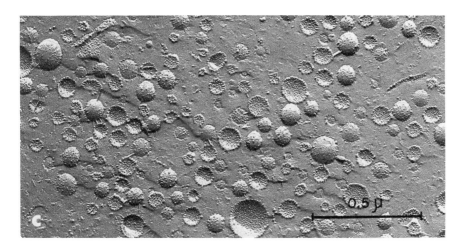

Fig. 20. *c*. *Vesicles from a pellet treated with 2.0 mg lysolecithin/mg protein.*

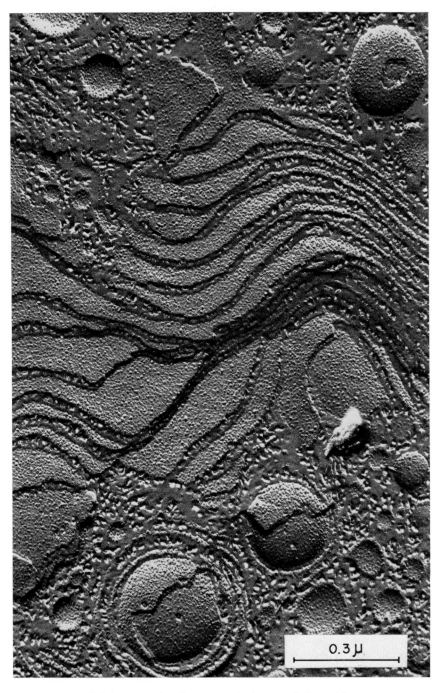

Fig. 21. *Highly particulate vesicles and lamellae.* In this instance some of the vesicles apparently merged to form extensive lamellae covered with particles. The concentration of lysolecithin was approximately 2 mg/mg protein.

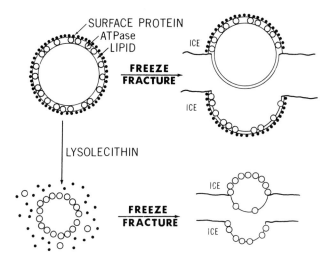

Fig. 22. *Interpretation of the effect of lysolecithin on microsomal proteins and resulting freeze-etch images.* See text for details.

MEMBRANAL Ca^{++} TRANSLOCATION AND CHOLINERGIC RECEPTOR ACTIVATION

K. -J. Chang and D. J. Triggle

Introduction

A problem of fundamental concern to an understanding of
membrane regulatory function is that of chemical excitability
whereby a variety of chemical messengers, neurotransmitters,
hormones, pheromones and other agents, physiological and
nonphysiological in origin, initiate characteristic and
specific cellular responses. An important component to the
solution of this problem will be the determination of the
transduction mechanisms by which the initial messenger-
receptor interaction becomes translated into the physiological
response. An increasing weight of experimental evidence
suggests for neurotransmitters and polypeptide hormones that
receptors forming discrete components of the cell membrane
are the sites of initial interaction (1-9).

If, for the purpose of this discussion we confine our
attention to the actions of neurotransmitters and vasoactive
polypeptides (agonists) in inducing tension responses in
muscle cells, then, because of the well established role of
Ca^{++} in excitation-contraction coupling (10-12), we may
formulate the basic transduction equations as follows:

1) $\quad A + Rec \rightleftharpoons A\text{---}Rec \xrightarrow[\text{steps}]{\text{intermediate}} Ca^{++}_{INT} \uparrow\downarrow$

2) $\quad Ca^{++}_{INT} + M \rightleftharpoons Ca^{++}\text{---}M \longrightarrow$ Contraction (C)

Increases or decreases in the level of free intracellular Ca^{++} (Ca_{INT}^{++}) serve to control the activity of the contractile machinery (M) though the Ca^{++}-sensitive component (troponin). From equations 1 and 2 several important questions can be raised: what is the source of the mobilized Ca^{++}; what are the intermediate steps through which the initial agonist-receptor interaction produces alterations in the level of Ca_{INT}^{++}; and what is the linkage between the observed concentration-response relationship and the initial agonist-receptor interaction.

In the work to be described we have sought the answers to these questions for a particular system, namely the acetylcholine-sensitive receptor system of guinea-pig ileal longitudinal muscle. From the data so obtained we have advanced a mechanism for the transduction sequence that we believe may have quite general implications and which assigns a fundamental regulatory and functional role to membrane-bound Ca^{++} (Ca_{MEM}^{++}).

Regulatory and functional roles of membrane-bound Ca^{++} (Ca_{MEM}^{++}).

As far as Ca^{++} requirements are concerned, smooth muscle contrasts with fast skeletal muscle since the small size of the smooth muscle cell and its often slower mechanical responses removes the obligatory requirement for utilization of bound Ca_{INT}^{++} that exists for fast skeletal muscle (11-14). Similarly, there is a relative paucity of sarcoplasmic reticulum particularly in visceral smooth muscle, (15, 15a, 15b) further suggesting the possibility of utilization of Ca_{EXT}^{++}, at least in part, for the excitation-contraction coupling in smooth muscle. However, in view of

the diversity of properties exhibited by smooth muscle, it
is quite likely that there will exist a broad range of
dependence upon Ca^{++}_{EXT} / Ca^{++}_{INT} for satisfaction of the E-C
coupling requirements. Additionally, there is steadily
increasing evidence that the spike generation mechanism
in mammalian visceral smooth muscle utilizes Ca^{++} as the
inward current carrying species. This follows from the
insensitivity of the spike to $[Na^{+}_{EXT}]$ (16,21), the sensitivity and overshoot dependence on $[Ca^{++}_{EXT}]$ (16-19), the
sensitivity of the spike to inhibition by Mn^{++} (18, 22, 23)
and its insensitivity to inhibition by tetrodotoxin (19, 22,
24, 25). In these properties visceral smooth muscle shows
many similarities to crayfish (26), barnacle (27-29), locust
(30), earthworm (31), amphioxus (32, 33) and frog heart (34,
35) in all of which Ca^{++}_{EXT} plays an important role as a current
carrier. We may note here, too, the importance of Ca^{++}_{EXT}
in "stimulus-secretion" coupling (36) and will make more
detailed reference subsequently to Ca^{++}-induced neurotransmitter release.

While the above studies all indicate the importance of
Ca^{++}_{EXT} they have not, in general, distinguished between free
extracellular Ca^{++} and membrane-bound (or membrane-associated)
Ca^{++} (Ca^{++}_{MEM}). This distinction appears to be of fundamental
importance in the light of many observations demonstrating
the regulatory function of Ca^{++}_{EXT} in the control of ion
permeation and excitation phenomena. Voltage clamp studies
on squid axon (37), lobster axon (38), frog medullated nerve
fibers (39) and ganglion cells (40) reveal that elevated
Ca^{++}_{EXT} displaces the curves relating activation of the Na^{+}
conductance to the membrane potential along the voltage axis

so that a greater input depolarization is required to produce a given increase in Na^+ conductance.

Elevated Ca^{++} serves to increase the fraction of the Na^+ conductance in the activated state (37) and appears to act similarly for Ca^{++} conductance (18,19,29,31). Quite generally, in nerve and muscle systems elevated concentrations of Ca_{EXT}^{++} serve to maintain or increase the resting membrane potential, raise the threshold for excitation and increase membrane resistance while reduced Ca_{EXT}^{++} decreases membrane potentials [inter alia, (18-21,40-50)]. Many other divalent and trivalent cations appear to behave in these regards similarly to elevated Ca_{EXT}^{++}. In general, the stabilizing and destabilizing effects of increased and reduced Ca_{EXT}^{++} respectively may be considered essentially similar to the effects produced by increased and decreased membrane potential (37). In Frankenhaeuser and Hodgkin's original discussion (37) of the Ca^{++}- dependent voltage shift was a suggestion advanced by A. F. Huxley that the mechanism of action of Ca^{++} might involve binding to the neural membrane outer surface thus modifying the electric field and so altering the potential dependent ion channels. There is substantial evidence for the existence of significant negative charge density at the membrane surface (39,50-57) and, although recent calculations of McLaughlin et al. (58) suggest that some of the voltage shift may occur by a screening rather than a binding process, where experimental evidence is available it appears that all membranes do bind substantial quantities of Ca^{++} (56,57,59-63).

The obvious analogy between low Ca_{EXT}^{++} (reduced Ca_{MEM}^{++}) and excitability and high Ca_{EXT}^{++} (increased Ca_{MEM}^{++}) and stability makes attractive the concept, expressed by a number of authors (18,23,40,47,62,64-67), that excitation may involve membrane changes initiated by removal of Ca_{MEM}^{++}. Quantitative formulations of axonal conduction involving M^+/M^{++} exchange on a cooperative ion exchange lattice are well known (40,67), but it is perhaps unlikely that chemical and electrical stimulation necessarily share the same source of Ca_{MEM}^{++}. Thus, in guinea-pig taenia coli replacement of Ca^{++} by Sr^{++} or Ba^{++} results in maintained or increased spike activity with an ultimate decrease in tension; however, chemical excitation by norepinephrine, acetylcholine, histamine or angiotensin was completely ineffective in modifying either electrical or mechanical responses when Ca^{++} was replaced by Sr^{++} or Ba^{++} (68).

For those systems that appear to utilize Ca^{++} or Ca^{++} and Na^+ as the inward current sources, the distinct possibility exists that the Ca^{++} translocated is derived, at least in part, from the Ca_{MEM}^{++} store. For such systems Ca_{MEM}^{++} would serve the dual function of a regulator of membrane excitability (through control of inward current pathways) and, upon displacement by the stimulating agent, could also serve, either wholly or partially, as the inward current source. This possibility appears likely for several systems. Hagiwara and Takahashi (29) found that the behavior of the Ca^{++} spike threshold and overshoot in barnacle muscle fiber did not conform to a simple Ca^{++} electrode but rather fitted a model in which the Ca_{MEM}^{++} density determined these parameters. This may also be true for crustacean (26) and amphioxus muscle (32).

Evidence for the participation of Ca_{MEM}^{++} rather than Ca_{EXT}^{++} in smooth muscle spikes is largely indirect but,

63

nonetheless, highly suggestive. Thus, from determinations of Ca^{++} bound in mammalian intestinal smooth muscle and knowledge of the surface area to volume ratio, it may be calculated that the Ca^{++} required for spike activity and for activating the contractile machinery could be supplied by "stripping" a very small fraction of the total Ca_{MEM}^{++} (56,57, 69). Several other lines of evidence are also consistent with this conclusion (20). The loss of spike activity upon removal or reduction of Ca_{EXT}^{++} appears to be very much slower than would be anticipated from the simple loss of Ca^{++} from the extracellular space (70) and, furthermore, the effects of Ca_{EXT}^{++} removal are highly temperature dependent being much slower in onset at low temperatures [Jones, unpublished observations, cited by Bülbring and Tomita (29)]. The effects of Na_{EXT}^{+} reduction are very similar to increases in Ca_{EXT}^{++} levels, namely suppression of spontaneous activity, membrane hyperpolarization and increased rate of rise and amplitude of the spike (17-19). This observation together with the direct measurements by Goodford (56,57) of the effects of cations on Ca^{++} binding in guinea-pig taenia coli and observations that the effects of Ca^{++} removal are much less dramatic in Krebs solution than in Locke solution (18,20) are all consistent with the idea of interactions among Ca^{++}, Na^{+}, K^{+} and Mg^{++} and are difficult to rationalize save on the basis of competitive interactions for membrane binding sites (56,57).[1]

[1]*There would thus seem to be an obvious analogy to the well documented Na:Ca interaction on frog heart contractility (71,72) and K:Ca^{++} interaction on Paramecium locomotor control (73,74).*

The recent studies by Goodford and Wolowyk (75) demonstrate directly the existence of cation binding sites on the smooth muscle plasma membrane. Uranyl ions are bound in pH-dependent fashion and this binding can be reduced by K^+, Na^+, Ca^{++} and Mg^{++}.

Considering the interrelationships between Ca^{++} and chemical excitation of mammalian intestinal smooth muscle, Bülbring and her colleagues have shown quite clearly that Ca^{++}_{EXT} is essential for the stabilizing actions of catecholamines exerted at both the α- and β-adrenergic receptors (23,76) and for the destabilizing effects of acetylcholine (76). Acetylcholine fails to depolarize and accelerate spike discharge in the absence of Ca^{++}_{EXT} and increased Ca^{++}_{EXT} potentiates these effects of ACh. Similarly, a reduction in Ca^{++}_{EXT} increases membrane resistance and greatly reduces the ability of epinephrine to hyperpolarize and reduce the electrotonic potential while an increase in Ca^{++}_{EXT} potentiates these effects of epinephrine. These findings would appear to be quite consistent with the general hypothesis that chemical labilization and stabilization of membranes involves decreased and increased Ca^{++}_{MEM} binding respectively [for further discussion *see* (62)].

There is an obvious analogy between the role of Ca^{++} in excitation-contraction coupling and its role in stimulus-secretion coupling (36). In the present context we may note the intriguing similarities between the muscle systems just discussed and Ca^{++}-induced neurotransmitter release at the skeletal neuromuscular junction and the squid giant synapse (77). Neurotransmitter release in the above systems is independent of $[Na^+_{EXT}]$, is unaffected by tetrodotoxin (77-80), is inhibited by Mn^{++} (77, 81) and, as with vertebrate visceral smooth muscle (21), is converted from graded responses to all-or-none processes by tetraethylammonium (TEA)(79,80). Furthermore, Mg^{++} serves as an inhibitor of Ca^{++} action in both systems although the action of Mg^{++} is much weaker in smooth muscle (21,82,83). Valuable experiments by Katz and Miledi (84) on the timing of Ca^{++} action in neurotransmitter release at the vertebrate junction reveals that Ca^{++} is only effective if it precedes the depolarizing pulse by as little as 50-100 μsec. This is highly suggestive of a role of Ca_{MEM}^{++} and is further supported by studies on neuromuscular facilitation (85,86). Of particular significance to an understanding of the mechanism of the Ca^{++}-dependent excitation-contraction coupling in visceral smooth muscle (69) and frog heart (87,88) and of Ca^{++}-induced neurotransmitter release (77,79,89-91) is the highly non-linear relationship between response and $[Ca_{EXT}^{++}]$ found in all of these systems suggesting that a similar cooperative Ca^{++} translocation process may be operative.

The function of this paper is to analyze the inter-relationships between Ca^{++}, membranal activation and the responses induced by a series of cholinergic agonists in smooth muscle in terms of the roles of Ca^{++} thus far outlined. We shall show a highly cooperative dependence of the tension response upon $[Ca_{EXT}^{++}]$ and indicate, albeit indirectly, a fundamental role of Ca_{MEM}^{++} in this response and in determining the fundamental features of the agonist-induced response.

Results

Parameters of agonist and Ca^{++} interaction in guinea-pig *ileal longitudinal muscle.*

The four agonists selected for use in this study were cis-2-methyl-(CD); 2,2-dimethyl-(DMD); 2,2-diethyl-(DED) and 2,2-di-isopropyl-4-dimethylaminomethyl-1,3-dioxolane methiodide (DPD). These agonists were selected because they present a wide spread of activities, have selective muscarinic effects and CD is at least as potent as acetylcholine (92,93). The close structural analogy between CD, muscarine and acetyl-β-methylcholine is very apparent. Values of their apparent affinities ($-\log ED_{50}$) and intrinsic activities (relative ability to produce maximum contraction) are summarized in Table I. Inspection of the concentration-response curves of these agonists showed that they are steeper than predicted from a simple mass action theory of binding and, since there is no evidence of significant threshold behavior, some element of cooperativity in the total transduction sequence is indicated (69). This is more clearly realized in the double-logarithmic plots of the concentration-response curves (Table II) which also reveal the high dependence of the cooperativity upon $[Ca_{EXT}^{++}]$.

Several experiments revealed the complex character of the dependence of contractile response upon $[Ca_{EXT}^{++}]$. Figure 1 shows what are essentially concentration-response curves for Ca^{++} obtained in the presence of fixed concentrations of agonists. What is most noteworthy is that the maximum responses obtained with Ca^{++} in the presence of the partial agonists DED and DPD are less than in the presence of the full agonists CD and DMD and that a reduced response to Ca^{++} is revealed in the presence of a submaximum concentration of the full agonist CD. Hence, both the apparent cooperativity of the response system *and* the extent to which it can be activated (intrinsic activity) are dependent upon Ca_{EXT}^{++}. Interesting features are revealed in the time course of contractile development at various Ca_{EXT}^{++} levels (Fig. 2a) and, again, significant differences between full and partial agonists are revealed. At high levels of agonist and Ca_{EXT}^{++} ($3.6 \times 10^{-3}M$), all agonists show the same pattern of response, namely, an initial and rapid phasic component followed by a sustained tonic component. The phasic component appears to be more rapid with the full agonists. As the Ca_{EXT}^{++} concentration is lowered, differences between the full and partial agonists become very apparent and the full agonists (CD and DMD) show a triphasic response in which an initial phasic component is followed by relaxation and then by a delayed contraction approximating in magnitude the initial phasic component. In contrast, DPD does not show any intermediate relaxant phase and behaves very similarly to a submaximal concentration of CD. Similar differences have been revealed between full and partial agonists in experiments in which the agonist was added to Ca^{++}-depleted tissue strips and Ca^{++} was added either simultaneously with or subsequent to the agonist. In the absence of Ca_{EXT}^{++} no responses are observed. The effects of Ca^{++} addition at 0, 1, 2, 4 and 6 min after agonist addition were then compared with control experiments in which the same concentrations of agonists were added to tissues previously equilibrated with Ca^{++}. The results showed that delayed Ca^{++} addition virtually eliminates the responses induced by full agonists but has very little effort on the responses induced by partial agonists (69). Figure 2b shows the effects of varied agonist concentrations at a fixed Ca_{EXT}^{++} concentration. It is interesting to note the transitions from a slow to a fast response as the agonist concentration is increased, the development of a triphasic pattern of response with the full agonists and the fact that with increasing agonist concentrations the response reaches a maximum level and then decreases again. Partial agonists do not show these last two characteristics.

Ca^{++} and Receptor Desensitization.

The latter results suggested that fundamental differences may exist between the full and partial agonists additional to their different intrinsic activities and affinities. Figure 3 reveals one such difference in that the full agonists desensitize the tissue (reduce the response to subsequently added agonist) whereas the partial agonists lack this property.

Differences between agonists and partial agonists continue to be revealed by the use of the spasmolytic agent papaverine which has been reported previously to preferentially eliminate in smooth muscle the tonic component of response induced by several stimulants (95,96). The data (Table III) confirm this finding for the full agonists CD and DMD but reveal that the selectivity is markedly reduced, and even inverted, with the partial agonists DED and DPD. Furthermore, with CD, the extent and selectivity of inhibition by papaverine of the tonic component of response becomes more marked with increasing agonist concentration (Fig. 4). Additional experiments (94) revealed that the rate of onset of papaverine action increases with increasing agonist concentration and that papaverine increases the desensitization produced by a maximal concentration of CD.

Sources of Ca^{++} Involved in Contractile Responses.

The experiments with papaverine indicate that the Ca^{++} mobilized for generation of the phasic and tonic components of the contractile response is likely to arise from at least two sources (95-98). However, it is also clear that the actions of papaverine are complex and, as will be discussed later, may not be confined to a single mechanism or locus of action. To obtain further evidence on the origins of the Ca^{++} mobilized some simple experiments were carried out in which the Ca^{++} concentration of the bathing media serving to maintain an equilibrium level of Ca^{++} within the tissue was abruptly changed at the same time as the agonist was introduced to the tissue. Figure 5a shows an experiment in which the equilibrating concentration of Ca^{++}, $[Ca_{EXT}^{++}]_E$, was 1.8 mM. At the time of introduction of the agonist CD this concentration of Ca^{++}, $[Ca_{EXT}^{++}]_S$, was abruptly altered and maintained at levels between 0 and 1.8 mM. This treatment had very little effect on the phasic component but drastically modified the tonic component which decreased with decreasing concentrations of the stimulus level of Ca^{++}, $[Ca_{EXT}^{++}]_S$. Figure 5b shows an experiment in which $[Ca_{EXT}^{++}]_E$ was varied between 0.0 to 1.8 mM while the $[Ca_{EXT}^{++}]_S$ was held constant at 0.2 mM. The tonic component is substantially reduced while the phasic component steadily increases with increasing $[Ca_{EXT}^{++}]_E$. Figure 5c shows a similar experiment in which the equilibrating level of Ca^{++} was held constant at 0.1 mM while the stimulus level was varied from 0 to 1.8 mM. In this instance, both the phasic and tonic components of response steadily increase with increasing $[Ca_{EXT}^{++}]_S$. These experiments demonstrate quite clearly the differentiating effects exhibited by changes in Ca_{EXT}^{++} concentrations particularly on the tonic component of the response.

Finally, La^{+++}, an agent that has achieved recent prominence because of its presumed ability to interfere with Ca^{++} binding and Ca^{++} transport across cell membranes (99-102), shows at low concentration some preferential elimination of the phasic component of response induced by CD (Fig. 6).

The effects of La^{+++} are not as obviously selective as those of papaverine and higher concentrations of La^{+++} inhibit both phasic and tonic components of response. Figure 7 shows that the combined effects of papaverine and La^{+++} are nicely additive.

Discussion

There are three principal aspects to the problem of the linkage between acetylcholine receptors and Ca^{++} that we have endeavored to analyze, namely, the relationship between Ca^{++}, co-operativity and the intrinsic activity of the agonists; the role of agonists and Ca^{++} in the desensitization process; and the interrelationships between Ca^{++}, La^{+++}, papaverine and the agonist-induced responses. We believe, as the introduction to this paper suggests, that these three aspects relate to an integral role for Ca_{MEM}^{++}.

To interpret the apparent co-operativity of response and its obvious dependence upon Ca_{EXT}^{++}, we have constructed a model which, in terms of the sequence of events, is essentially similar to that advanced recently by Hurwitz and Suria (103). We include, however, the possibility that co-operative concentration-response relationships could arise at

any or all stages of the sequence. The basic transduction
sequence may be represented as:

3) $A + R \rightleftharpoons AR \longrightarrow T_{TOT}$

4) $Ca^{++}_{EXT} + T \rightleftharpoons Ca^{++} -T \longrightarrow Ca^{++}_{INT}$

5) $Ca^{++}_{INT} + M \rightleftharpoons Ca^{++}_{INT} -M \longrightarrow Response$ (C)

where,

A is the agonist concentration,

R is the receptor concentration,

AR is the concentration of agonist-receptor complex,

T_{TOT} is the total concentration of Ca^{++} translocation
sites,

Ca^{++} -T is the concentration of the Ca^{++}-translocation
complex,

M is the concentration of calcium reactive sites in the
contractile protein and,

Ca^{++}_{INT} -M is the concentration of calcium-contractile
protein complex.

No molecular specifications are laid down by this model as
to the nature of the Ca^{++} translocation process. In its
simplest form, the model predicts a hyperbolic relationship between agonist or Ca^{++}_{EXT} concentrations and response
(103), but this is clearly not the case for the results
that we have described. However, by applying mass-action
treatment to equations 3-5 and assuming that reaction
orders >1 may occur at any step, then,

6) $\quad T_{TOT} = \gamma \, [AR]^o = \gamma \left[\dfrac{[R_{TOT}]}{1 + \dfrac{K_R}{[A]}} \right]^o$

7) $\quad Ca_{INT}^{++} = \beta \, [Ca^{++}T]^n = \cdot \beta \left[\dfrac{[T_{TOT}]}{1 + \dfrac{K_T}{[Ca_{EXT}^{++}]}} \right]^n$

8) $\quad C = \alpha \, [Ca^{++}M]^m = \alpha \left[\dfrac{[M_{TOT}]}{1 + \dfrac{K_M}{[Ca_{INT}^{++}]}} \right]^m$

From equations 6-8 an expression can be obtained for the relative response

9)

$$a = \dfrac{C}{C_{MAX}} = \dfrac{1}{\left[1 + \dfrac{K_M}{\beta^n \gamma^n [R_{TOT}]^{no}} \left(1 + \dfrac{K_T}{[Ca_{EXT}^{++}]} \right)^n \left(1 + \dfrac{K_R}{[A]} \right)^{n.o} \right]^m}$$

which upon simplification and collection of terms[2] into

[2]At maximum (saturating) concentrations of A or Ca_{EXT}^{++} eqn. 9 may be written as,

$$a = \dfrac{1}{\left[1 + E \left(1 + \dfrac{K_T}{[Ca_{EXT}^{++}]} \right)^n \right]^m} = \dfrac{1}{\left[1 + F \left(1 + \dfrac{K_R}{[A]} \right)^{n.o} \right]^m}$$

where $\quad E = \dfrac{K_M}{\beta [R_{TOT}]^{n.o} \gamma^n} \left(1 + \dfrac{K_R}{[A_{MAX}]} \right)^{n.o}$

$$and\ F = \frac{K_M}{\beta\ [R_{TOT}]^{n.o}}\gamma^n\left(1 + \frac{K_T}{[Ca^{++}_{MAX}]}\right)^n$$

When $[A]$ or $[Ca^{++}_{EXT}] \longrightarrow \infty$ then $1 + \dfrac{K_R}{[A_{MAX}]}$ and $1 + \dfrac{K_T}{[Ca^{++}_{MAX}]} \to 1$

and the only factor that can affect a is γ, the proportionality constant relating the ability of the preformed AR complex to activate the Ca^{++} translocation system.

the constants E and F (94) yields

10) $\sqrt[n]{\dfrac{1}{\sqrt[m]{a}} - 1} = \sqrt[n]{E\left[1 + \dfrac{K_T}{[Ca^{++}_{EXT}]}\right]}$ and

11) $\sqrt[n.o]{\dfrac{1}{\sqrt[m]{a}} - 1} = \sqrt[n.o]{F\left[1 + \dfrac{K_R}{[A]}\right]}$

for the Ca^{++}-induced responses in the presence of constant agonist concentration and agonist-induced responses in the presence of constant Ca^{++}_{EXT} concentration respectively.

We have elected to set m = 2 on the basis that much evidence indicates that this best describes the stoichiometry of Ca^{++} interaction with the contractile proteins (11, 104-106). Hence, from equations 10 and 11, it is possible to determine n and n.o by plotting the expressions on the left.

against $K_T/[Ca_{EXT}^{++}]$ or $K_R/[A]$ and varying n or n.o until
linearity is obtained (Fig. 8). The data thus obtained are
collected in Table IV. Since n.o $\neq$ n, it is apparent that
o = 1 and hence that the cooperativity of the agonist-res-
ponse relationship is dependent primarily upon the Ca^{++}
translocation step (eqn. 7).

There are striking similarities between these results
and the power dependence of frog heart contractility (87,88)
and synaptic transmitter release (77,89-91) upon $[Ca_{EXT}^{++}]$.
It would be interesting to know how similar the mechanisms
of calcium translocation are in these varied systems. The
basic finding common to all of the systems is that, with a
given input, the output (measured as tension, contractile
response or transmitter release) varies with Ca_{EXT}^{++} in a
highly non-linear fashion. Thus, for each of the systems,

12) response $\propto [CaX]^n$, n > 1

where X (= T in this discussion) represents the binding site
for Ca^{++}. For the guinea-pig ileal longitudinal muscle under
discussion n = 6. Of the several mechanisms that might be
advanced to accomodate this finding two seem to deserve
attention. The translocation sites (T) may be arranged in
interacting clusters of 6 so that the probability of translocation is greatly enhanced when all six sites are occupied
by Ca^{++} (83,90,107)[3]. Alternatively, the binding of Ca^{++} to

---

[3]*Since agonists and partial agonists do not differ in
their parameters of cooperativity (Table IV) they must differ
in ability of the preformed AR complex to activate the
Ca^{++} translocation system: the latter must, therefore, be
activated in discrete units.*

75

the T sites might be a cooperative function of Ca_{EXT}^{++} so that,

13) $[Ca^{++}T] \propto [Ca_{EXT}^{++}]^6$

which, if either of these mechanisms is correct and whether
the same mechanism holds for guinea-pig ileal muscle, frog
heart and synaptic transmitter release remains to be determined. However, both of these mechanisms predict a key role
to Ca_{MEM}^{++} in determining the form of the relationship between
response and Ca_{EXT}^{++} and this is certainly consistent with
available data for all of these systems.

A fundamental role for Ca_{MEM}^{++} in the excitation-contraction coupling in the guinea-pig ileal muscle is also strongly
indicated by much of the remaining data that we have described. The experiments shown in Figs. 5a-c appear particularly
instructive in this regard. Figure 5a shows that when
tissues are equilibrated in 1.8 mM Ca^{++} and then abruptly
switched for agonist-induced stimulation to Ca^{++} levels varying between 0.0 to 1.8 mM Ca^{++}, it is primarily the tonic
component of response that is affected. This suggests that
the Ca^{++} utilized for the generation of the phasic component
is derived from a compartment the concentration of which is
determined by the Ca^{++} concentration of the equilibrating
media, $[Ca_{EXT}^{++}]$, rather than by the Ca^{++} concentration of the
stimulating media, $[Ca_{EXT}^{++}]_S$. In contrast, the tonic component of response utilizes a Ca^{++} compartment affected very
directly by $[Ca_{EXT}^{++}]_S$ and which may therefore be the extracellular Ca^{++} proper. The results shown in Fig. 5b lead to
essentially the same conclusion; namely, that the phasic
component is regulated by $[Ca_{EXT}^{++}]_E$ and the tonic component
by $[Ca_{EXT}^{++}]_S$. However, Fig. 5c, which shows an experiment

where $[Ca_{EXT}^{++}]_E$ was held very low while $[Ca_{EXT}^{++}]_S$ was almost always higher, indicates that both the phasic and tonic components are equally affected by the Ca^{++} concentration of the stimulating medium. This suggests rather clearly, eventhough the experiments of Figs. 5a and 5b indicate different Ca^{++} compartments for the phasic and tonic components, that the compartment utilized by the phasic component is nonetheless very rapidly equilibrated with Ca_{EXT}^{++}. It is, therefore, most unlikely to be an intracellular source since such exchange of Ca^{++} is significantly slower than these results would indicate (108). It appears very probable, therefore, that the phasic component of response utilizes membrane-bound Ca^{++} while the tonic component utilizes free extracellular Ca^{++}.

The effects of La^{+++} in producing a partially selective inhibition at lower concentrations and a nonselective inhibition at higher concentrations of the phasic component of the CD-induced response are quite consistent with this interpretation in light of the many observations that La^{+++} binds to cell and artificial membranes to prevent Ca^{++} influx (99-102). Papaverine, however, shows selectivity for the tonic component of response (Fig. 4, Table III) and this strengthens the thesis that the phasic and tonic components of response do utilize different Ca^{++} compartments.

These considerations lead us to propose the model for excitation-contraction coupling shown in Fig. 9. According to this model, the acetylcholine receptor exists in a Ca^{++}-associated state and activation produces a transition to the dissociated permeable state. We suggest that during this agonist-induced transition the associated Ca_{MEM}^{++} is translocated to the cell interior to generate the phasic component and that while in the Ca^{++}-dissociated permeable state, free Ca_{EXT}^{++} can enter to generate the tonic component. This proposal would accomodate the association between Ca^{++} spike activity and tension development and the following calculations show that mobilization of only a small fraction of the total Ca_{MEM}^{++} could suffice to generate the Ca^{++} spikes and tension development. Assuming that 1g (wet weight) of longitudinal muscle contains 6×10^8 cells (109) and that the amount of Ca^{++} bound is 1.7 μ mole/g (56,110), then there are 1.7×10^9 Ca^{++}/cell; one cell has a surface area of at least 0.83×10^{-5} cm^2 (56) so that about 2×10^{14} Ca^{++}/cm^2 or approximately one Ca^{++} /50 $Å^2$ is bound. This does not appear too unreasonable since the membrane surface area has probably been under-estimated. Lullmann and Mohns (110) have shown for electrical stimulation that 6×10^{11} Ca^{++}/cm^2 are taken up per stimulus and this will generate an intracellular Ca^{++} concentration of $10^{-5}M$, which is adequate to generate tension development. Goodford's calculations (57) show that a flow of 5×10^{-6} g moles / Ca^{++}/kg (wet weight) will produce a 60 mV depolarization of a membrane of $3\mu Fcm^{-2}$ capacity.

The model of receptor activation shown in Fig. 9 possesses an additional component of conversion to a desensitized state. Although well known, the phenomenon of pharmacological desensitization cannot be said to be well understood (111,112). It is however, generally assumed to involve an agonist-induced conformational change of the receptor to a new "inactive conformation" (111,112). We may presume that this conformational transition is initiated from the activated receptor state (Fig. 9) since it is normally most obvious with high concentrations of agonists. Our data show rather clearly that in the series of muscarinic agonists under discussion the production of desensitization is confined to the full agonists (CD and DMD) only. Desensitization may also be presumed to accomodate the experimental results shown in Fig. 2. A characteristic of the time course of contractions induced by the full agonists is that of the intermediate relaxant phase which is enhanced by high agonist and low Ca_{EXT}^{++} concentrations; partial agonists show either none, or at most, a very small intermediate relaxant phase (Figs.2a,b). This phenomenon may well be due to desensitization enhanced by the combination of high agonist and low Ca_{EXT}^{++} concentrations and is not observed with the partial agonists. Figure 2b also shows that the full agonists behave anomalously in that with increasing concentration at fixed $[Ca_{EXT}^{++}]$ the magnitude of response first increases and then decreases. This is also likely to be related to desensitization becoming important at high A and low Ca_{EXT}^{++} levels. The partial agonists do not exhibit this behavior. Desensitization may also account for the effects of delayed Ca^{++} addition upon agonist-induced responses described in Results. In these experiments the addition of Ca^{++} either simultaneously with or subsequently to maximum concentrations of the full agonists CD and DMD resulted in greatly reduced responses whereas similar treatment with the partial agonists DED and DPD does not result in any significant reduction in response (69). Presumably, desensitization produced by the full agonists in the absence of Ca_{EXT}^{++} produces an inactive desensitized receptor incapable of utilizing subsequently added Ca^{++}.

We believe that this process of desensitization is

intimately concerned with the effects of papaverine that we have described. Papaverine is a typical spasmolytic agent affecting responses induced by several stimuli and hence is unlikely to act at the receptor but rather must act at some subsequent step in the transduction pathway that may be common to a variety of stimulating agents. It is improbable that papaverine acts directly on the contractile machinery since phasic and tonic components of responses have long been known to be differentially eliminated (95-98). Two proposals of papaverine action currently dominate the literature. One mechanism proposes that papaverine inhibits the translocation of Ca_{EXT}^{++} (95-98) and the other proposes that, since papaverine is an inhibitor of phosphodiesterase, its relaxant actions are mediated through accumulation of adenosine-3',5'-monophosphate (113,114).

Figure 4 shows that papaverine selectively inhibits the tonic phase of the CD-induced contractions but that when submaximum concentrations of CD are employed this selectivity is lost. We have also shown that the time of onset of papaverine-induced relaxation is markedly decreased with increasing concentration of CD (94). These data are not easy to reconcile with either of the proposals of papaverine action noted. Furthermore, the results of Table III show that when agonists and partial agonists are compared then the selective inhibition by papaverine of the phasic component is reduced and even inverted with the partial agonists.

These findings show intriguing parallels with the phenomenon of receptor desensitization and lead us to suggest that the selective inhibitory action of papaverine is produced by the same factors that initiate receptor desensitization. One possibility is that papaverine binds selectively to the desensitized conformation of the acetylcholine receptor. We reject this explanation, however, since papaverine shows essentially similar selective inhibition of the tonic components of response induced by K^+ (97) and histamine [K. J. Chang and D. J. Triggle, unpublished data] and since Tashiro and Tomita (115) have shown that tension reduction by papaverine in the electrically stimulated guinea-pig taenia coli develops more rapidly and to a greater extent with high than with low strength stimuli. It is difficult to see why papaverine should have similar effects on a variety of receptor systems unless interaction at some common site or component of action is involved. The possibility thus exists that the selective actions of papaverine are associated with some component of membrane excitation common to all of these excitatory events. A likely common component may well be Ca_{MEM}^{++}-depletion which we have proposed to be responsible for the initial phasic response to muscarinic agonists and to be the determinant of intrinsic activity. We propose that papaverine selectively inhibits the tonic component of response by binding to and stabilizing Ca^{++}-depleted membrane areas. The extent of Ca_{MEM}^{++} depletion will be a function of stimulus strenth (activator concentration or intrinsic activity, current strength) and will become greater at high stimulus strength. The data of Fig. 4 indicate that papaverine binding may be a cooperative function of Ca_{MEM}^{++} depletion. We do not, of course, propose this to be the total explanation of the spasmolytic activity of papaverine and other explanations, possibily those noted already, must be invoked to explain the remaining less selective components of action.

These comments on the action of papaverine suggest also a basis for our finding that only full agonists produce desensitization and that partial agonists or low concentrations of full agonists do not desensitize. Since we have related the property of intrinsic activity to the ability to activate the Ca_{MEM}^{++} translocation system and hence "strip" Ca^{++} from its receptor-associated membrane bound locus, the phenomenon of agonist-induced receptor desensitization may be similar to papaverine action in that it involves selective binding of agonist to Ca^{++}-depleted membrane areas. Since partial agonists and low concentrations of full agonists do not, according to our proposals, produce the complete Ca_{MEM}^{++}-depletion characteristic of full agonists binding desensitization will be reduced.

The studies that we have discussed attempting to link the agonist-receptor interaction, Ca^{++} mobilization and the contractile response in the longitudinal smooth muscle of the guinea-pig ileum have led us to formulate a quantitative treatment of agonist-receptor interactions. According to this model two compartments of Ca^{++} are utilized in the E-C coupling process: membrane-bound Ca^{++} (Ca_{MEM}^{++}) and extra-cellular Ca^{++} (Ca_{EXT}^{++}). Ca_{MEM}^{++} is cooperatively translocated to the cell interior following activation of the transloca-tion system by the agonist-receptor interaction and the extent of this activation determines intrinsic activities of the agonists.

The basic feature of the model is a transition between Ca^{++}-associated and Ca^{++}-dissociated states. Additionally, a further transition can be induced by full agonists to the desensitized state. The desensitized state is believed to be associated with Ca_{MEM}^{++} depletion and it is this process that is, at least in part, responsible for the selective inhibitory action of papaverine (and possibly other spasmolytics) towards the tonic component of contraction. This model emphasizes the critical role of Ca_{MEM}^{++} as a regulatory ligand and as a current carrier in guinea-pig intestinal smooth muscle. The latter role may not be as important for other smooth muscles where mobilization of Ca_{INT}^{++} may be more important.[4] However, in view of the apparently widespread regulatory function of Ca_{MEM}^{++}, it is tempting to speculate that the fundamental control of chemically and electrically excitable membranes may be achieved through control of Ca_{MEM}^{++}.

[4]*An interesting example from an entirely different system indicating the linkage between Ca^{++} and intrinsic activity is to be found in the work of Krejci, Polacek and Rudinger (116) who found in rat and rabbit uterus that the oxytocin-like, but relatively weak, activity of 2-0-methyltyrosineoxytocin was converted from partial agonistic to antagonistic character with decreasing concentrations of Ca_{EXT}^{++}. At the same Ca_{EXT}^{++} concentrations oxytocin still behaved as an agonist. Since it is highly probable that uterine contractions utilize Ca_{INT}^{++} one explanation of these findings would be that reduction of Ca_{MEM}^{++} progressively reduces the ability of the agonist-receptor complex to mobilize Ca_{INT}^{++}. The partial agonist, 2-0-methyltyrosine-oxytocin, which presumably mobilizes less Ca_{MEM}^{++} than full agonists should then lose agonistic activity before a full agonist.*

Although the discussion in this paper has been essentially confined to the role of Ca^{++}_{MEM} in regulating electrical and neurotransmitter-induced events, there is increasing evidence to suggest that polypeptides and other hormones may also possess as an integral feature of their ability to initiate physiological responses the capacity to modulate Ca^{++}_{MEM} binding. In studies with model membranes Kafka and Pak (117,118) have demonstrated that insulin, oxytocin, vasopressin and thyrocalcitonin all affect Ca^{++} binding. In a recent study of the action of adrenocorticotrophic hormone in isolated adrenal cells, it has been proposed (119) that the stimulus initiated by the hormone-receptor interaction and transmitted through the membrane to adenyl cyclase is Ca^{++}-dependent increasing in strength with increasing $[Ca^{++}_{EXT}]$. A regulatory influence of insulin, glucagon, hydrocortisone and epinephrine upon Ca^{++} binding to rat liver cell membranes has been shown by Shlatz and Marinetti (120); glucagon, epinephrine and hydrocortisone increasing and insulin decreasing Ca^{++} binding. It has been estimated for this system that one molecule of hydrocortisone initiates binding of 3,000 Ca^{++} ions thus suggesting that the hormone-receptor interaction leads to rather widespread membrane perturbations. Furthermore, there exists suggestive evidence to indicate that the prostaglandins, known to control the sensitivity of cellular systems towards other hormones and neurotransmitters, may achieve such regulation through manipulation of Ca^{++}_{MEM} levels (121).

Finally, we may note that Ca^{++} has been proposed to play a fundamental role in the primary process of visual excitation (122,123) whereby Ca^{++} flux, serving as a first-stage signal amplification, perhaps utilizing rhodopsin as a shuttle carrier, regulates Na^+ permeability.

From the examples quoted and from others known to be available (62) a reasonable case can be made that the fundamental control of modification of membrane function induced by a variety of stimuli is mediated through control of Ca^{++}_{MEM}.

Presented by D. J. Triggle.

References

1. Del Castillo, J. and B. Katz. On the localization of acetylcholine receptors. J. Physiol. London 128: 157-181 (1955).
2. Cuatrecasas, P. Interaction of insulin with the cell membrane: the primary action of insulin. Proc. Natl. Acad. Sci. U.S. 63: 450-457 (1969).
3. De Robertis, E. Molecular biology of synaptic receptors. Science 171: 963-971 (1971).
4. Kasai, M. and J. P. Changeux. In vitro excitation of purified membrane fragments by cholinergic agonists. I. Pharmacological properties of the excitable membrane fragments. J. Mem. Biol. 6: 1-23: (1971) [see also references to preceding work contained therein].
5. Richardson, M. C. and D. Schulster. β1-24-Adrenocorticotrophin diazotized to polyacrylamide: effects on isolated adrenal cells. Biochem. J. 125:60P (1971).
6. Krug, F., B. Debuquois and P. Cuatrecasas. Glucagon affinity absorbants: selective binding of receptors of liver cell membranes. Nature New Biol. 234: 268-270 (1971).
7. Hecht, J. P., J. M. Dellacha, J. A. Santome and A. C. Paladinc. Lipolytic activity of bovine growth hormone bound to sepharose beads. FEBS Letters 20: 83-86 (1972).
8. Johnson, C. B., M. Blecher and M. N. A. Giorgio. Activation of plasma membrane adenyl cyclase by agarose glucagon and agarose norepinephrine gels. Fed. Proc. Am. Soc. Exptl. Biol. 31: 439 (1972).
9. Cuatrecasas, P. Isolation of the insulin receptor of liver and fat cell membranes. Proc. Natl. Acad. Sci. U.S. 69: 318-322 (1972).
10. Heilbrunn, L. V. and F. J. Wiercinski. The action of various cations on muscle protoplasm. J. Cell Comp.

Physiol. 29: 15-32 (1947).

11. Ebashi, S., M. Endo and I. Ohtsuki. Control of muscle contraction. Quart. Rev. Biophys. 2: 351-384 (1969).

12. Triggle, D. J. Neurotransmitter-Receptor Interactions. Ch. VII. Academic Press, London and New York (1971).

13. Hill, A. V. The abrupt transition from rest to activity in muscle. Proc. Royal Society London. Ser. B 136: 399-420 (1949).

14. Sandow, A. Excitation-contraction coupling in skeletal muscle. Pharmacol. Rev. 17: 265-320 (1965).

15. Needham, D. M. and J. M. Williams. Proteins of the dilution precipitate obtained from salt extracts of pregnant and non-pregnant uterus. Biochem. J. 89: 534-545 (1963).

15a Somlyo, A. P., C. E. Devine, A. V. Somlyo and S. R. North. Sarcoplasmic reticulum and the temperature-dependent contraction of smooth muscle in calcium-free solutions. J. Cell. Biol. 51: 722-741 (1971).

15b Devine, C. E.,A. B. Somlyo and A. P. Somlyo. Sarco-plasmic reticulum and excitation-contraction coupling in mammalian smooth muscles. J. Cell. Biol. 52: 690-718 (1972).

16. Holman, M. E. Membrane potentials recorded with high-resistance microelectrodes and the effects of changes in ionic environment on the electrical and mechanical activity of the smooth muscle of the taenia coli of the guinea-pig. J. Physiol. London 141: 464-488 (1958).

17. Bülbring, E. and H. Kuriyama. Effects of changes in the external sodium and calcium concentrations on spontaneous electrical activity in smooth muscle of guinea-pig taenia coli. J. Physiol. London 166: 29-58 (1963).

18. Brading, A. F., E. Bülbring and T. Tomita. The effect of sodium and calcium on the action potential of the smooth muscle of the guinea-pig taenia coli. J. Physiol. London 200: 637-654 (1969).

19. Tomita, T. In: E. Bülbring, A. F. Brading, A. W. Jones and T. Tomita (Editors), Smooth Muscle, Williams and Wilkins, Co., Baltimore, Maryland (1970), p. 197.

20. Bülbring, E. and T. Tomita. In: A. W. Cuthbert (Editor), Calcium and Cellular Function, Macmillan Co., London (1970), p. 249.

21. Sakamoto, Y. Electrical activity of guinea-pig taenia-coli in calcium locke solution. Jap. J. Physiol 21: 295-306 (1971).

22. Nonomura, Y., Y. Hotta and H. Ohashi. Tetrodotoxin and manganese ions: effects on electrical activity and tension in taenia coli of guinea-pig. Science 152: 97-99 (1966).

23. Bülbring, E. and T. Tomita. Effect of calcium, barium and manganese on the action of adrenaline in the smooth muscle of the guinea-pig taenia coli. Proc. Roy. Soc. Lond. Ser. B 172: 121-136 (1969).

24. Kuriyama, H., T. Osa and N. Toida. Effects of tetrodotoxin on smooth muscle cells of the guinea-pig taenia coli. Brit. J. Pharmacol. Chemotherap. 27: 366-376 (1966).

25. Bülbring, E. and T. Tomita. Properties of the inhibitory potential of smooth muscle as observed in the response to field stimulation of the guinea-pig taenia coli. J. Physiol. London 189: 299-315 (1967).

26. Fatt, P. and B. L. Ginsborg. The ionic requirements for the production of action potentials in crustacean muscle fibres. J. Physiol. London 142: 516-543 (1958).

27. Hagiwara, S. and S. Nakajima. Differences in Na and Ca spikes as examined by application of tetrodotoxin, procaine and manganese ions. J. Gen. Physiol. 49: 793-806 (1966).

28. Hagiwara, S. and S. Nakajima. Effects of the intracellular Ca ion concentration upon the excitability of the muscle fiber membrane of a barnacle. J. Gen. Physiol. 49: 807-818 (1966).

29. Hagiwara, S. and K. Takahashi. Surface density of calcium ions and calcium spikes in the barnacle muscle fiber membrane. J. Gen. Physiol. 50: 583-601 (1967).

30. Washio, H. The ionic requirements for the initiation of action potentials in insect muscle fibers. J. Gen Physiol. 59: 121-134 (1972).

31. Ito, Y., H. Kuriyama and N. Tashiro. Effects of divalent cations on spike generation in the longitudinal somatic muscle of the earthworm. J. Exp. Biol. 52: 79-94 (1970).

32. Hagiwara, S. and Y. Kidokoro. Na and Ca components of action potential in amphioxus muscle cells. J. Physiol. Longon 219: 217-232 (1971).

33. Hagiwara, S., M. P. Henkart and Y. Kidokoro. Excitation-contraction coupling in amphioxus muscle cells. J. Physiol. London 219: 233-251 (1971).

34. Chapman, R. A. and R. Niedergerke. Interaction between heart rate and calcium concentration in the control of contractile strenth of the frog heart. J. Physiol.

London 211: 423-443 (1970).

35. Morad, M. and R. K. Orkand. Excitation-contraction coupling in frog ventricle: evidence from voltage clamp studies. J. Physiol. London 219: 167-189 (1971).

36. Douglas, W. W. Stimulus-secretion coupling: the concept and clues from chromaffin and other cells. Brit. J. Pharmacol. 34: 451-474 (1968).

37. Frankenhaeuser, B. and A. L. Hodgkin. The action of calcium on the electrical properties of squid axons. J. Physiol. London 137: 218-244 (1957).

38. Blaustein, M. P. and D. E. Goldman. The action of certain polyvalent cations on the voltage-clamped lobster axon. J. Gen. Physiol. 51: 279-291 (1958).

39. Hille, B. Charges and potentials at the nerve surface: divalent ions and pH. J. Gen. Physiol. 51: 221-236 (1968).

40. Koketsu, K. Calcium and the excitable membrane. Neuro-Sciences Res. 2: 2-41 (1969).

41. Shanes, A. M. Electrochemical aspects of physiological and pharmacological action in excitable cells. Pharmacol Rev. 10: 59-164 (1958).

42. Weidmann, S. Effects of calcium ions and local anesthetics on electrical properties of purkinje fibers. J. Physiol. London 129: 568-582 (1955).

43. Ishiko, N. and M. Sato. The effect of calcium ions on electrical properties of striated muscle fibers. Jap. J. Physiol. 7: 51-63 (1957).

44. Frankenhaeuser, B. The effects of calcium on the myelinated nerve fiber. J. Physiol. London 137: 245-260 (1957).

45. Lüttgau, H. C. The action of calcium ions on potassium contractions of single muscle fibres. J. Physiol. London 168: 679-697 (1963).

46. Aceves, J. and X. Machne. The action of calcium and of local anesthetics on nerve cells and their interaction during excitation. J. Pharmacol. Exptl. Therap. 140: 138-148 (1963).

47. Hodgkin, A. L., A. F. Huxley and B. Katz. Measurement of current voltage relations in the membrane of the giant axon of Loligo. J. Physiol. Lond. 116: 424-448 (1952).

48. Straub, R. Die wirkungen von veratridin und ionen auf das ruhe potential markhaltiger nervenfasern des frosches. Helv. Physiol. Acta 14: 1-28 (1956).

49. Niedergerke, R. Movements of Ca in frog heart ventricles

at rest and during contractures. J. Physiol. London
107: 515-550 (1963).

50. Somlyo, A. P. and A. V. Somlyo. Vascular Smooth Muscle.
I. Normal structure, pathology, biochemistry and biophysics. Pharmacol. Rev. 20: 197-272 (1968).

51. Hodgkin, A. L. and A. F. Huxley. A quantitative description of membrane current and its application to
conduction and excitation in nerve. J. Physiol. London
117: 500-544 (1952).

52. Elul, R. Fixed charge in the cell membrane. J. Physiol.
London 189: 351-365 (1967).

53. Segal, J. R. Surface charge of giant axons of squid
and lobster. Biophys. J. 8: 470-489 (1968).

54. Gilbert, D. L. and G. Ehrenstein. Effect of divalent
cations on potassium conductance of squid axons: determination of surface charge. Biophys. J. 9: 447-463
(1969).

55. McLaughlin, S. G. A., G. Szabo, G. Eisenman and S. M.
Ciani. Surface charge and the conductance of phospholipid membranes. Proc. Natl. Acad. Sci. U. S. 67: 1268-
1275 (1970).

56. Goodford, P. J. The calcium content of the smooth
muscle of the guinea-pig taenia coli. J. Physiol.
London 192: 145-157 (1967).

57. Goodford, P. J. In: E. Bülbring, A. F. Brading, A. W.
Jones and T. Tomita (Editors). Smooth Muscle, Williams
and Wilkins, Co., Baltimore, Maryland (1970), p. 100.

58. McLaughlin, S. G. A., G. Szabo and G. Eisenman. Divalent ions and the surface potential of charged phospholipid membranes. J. Gen. Physiol. 58:667-687 (1971).

59. Danielli, J. F. The biological actions of ions and the
concentrations of ions at surfaces. J. Exp. Biol. 20:
167-176 (1944).

60. Carvalho, A. P.,H. Sanui and N. Pace. Calcium and
magnesium binding properties of cell membrane materials.
J. Cell. Comp. Physiol. 37: 311-317 (1963).

61. Forstner, J. and J. F. Manery. Calcium binding by
human erythrocyte membranes. Biochem. J. 124: 563-571
(1971).

62. Triggle, D. J. Effect of calcium on excitable membranes
and neurotransmitter action. Adv. Surface and Membrane
Science 5: 267-331 (1972).

63. Baudouin, M., P. Meyer, S. Fermandjian and J. -L. Morgat,
Calcium release induced by interaction of angiotensin

with its receptors in smooth muscle cell microsomes. Nature, London 235: 336–338 (1972).

64. Gordon, H. T. and J. H. Welsh. The role of ions in axon surface reactions to toxic organic compounds. J. Cell Comp. Physiol. 31: 396–419 (1948).

65. Brink, F. Calcium ions and neural processes. Pharmacol. Revs. 6: 243–298 (1954).

66. Goldman, D. E. A molecular structural basis for the excitation properties of axons. Biophys. J. 4: 167–188 (1964).

67. Tasaki, I. Nerve excitation: a macromolecular approach. Thomas, Springfield, Illinois (1968).

68. Hotta, Y. and R. Tsukui. Effect on the guinea-pig taenia coli of the substitution of strontium or barium ions for calcium ions. Nature, London 217: 867–869 (1968).

69. Chang, K. -J. and D. J. Triggle. Calcium and the excitation of longitudinal smooth muscle by a series of muscarinic agonists: a quantitative approach to agonist-receptor interactions. Submitted to J. Theoret. Biol. (1972).

70. Brading, M. F., E. Bülbring and T. Tomita. The effect of temperature on the membrane conductance of the smooth muscle of the guinea-pig taenia coli. J. Physiol. London 200: 621–635 (1969).

71. Lüttgau, H. C. and R. Niedergerke. The antagonism between Ca and Na ions on the frog heart. J. Physiol. London 143: 486–505 (1958).

72. Niedergerke, R. and R. K. Orkand. The dependence of the action potential of the frog's heart on the external and intracellular sodium concentration. J. Physiol. London 184: 312–334 (1966).

73. Jahn, T. L. The mechanism of ciliary movement. II. Ion antagonism and ciliary reversal. J. Cell. Physiol. 60: 217–228 (1962).

74. Naitoh, Y. Ionic control of the reversal response of cilia in paramecium caudatum. A calcium hypothesis. J. Gen. Physiol. 51: 85–108 (1968).

75. Goodford, P. J. and M. W. Wolowyk. Counter-cation interaction at the smooth muscle cell membrane of guinea-pig taenia coli. J. Physiol. London 218: 36–37P. (1971).

76. Bülbring, E. and H. Kuriyama. Effects of changes in ionic environment on the action of acetylcholine and adrenaline on the smooth muscle cells of guinea-pig taenia coli. J. Physiol. London 166: 59–74 (1963).

77. Hubbard, J. I. Mechanism of transmitter release. Prog. Biophys. Mol. Biol. 21: 33-124 (1970).

78. Katz, B. and R. Miledi. Tetrodotoxin and neuromuscular transmission. Proc. Roy. Soc. London Ser. B 167: 8-22 (1967).

79. Katz, B. and R. Miledi. A study of synaptic transmission in the absence of nerve impulses. J. Physiol. London 192: 407-436 (1967).

80. Katz, B. and R. Miledi. Spontaneous and evoked activity of motor nerve endings in calcium ringer. J. Physiol. London 203: 689-706 (1969).

81. Kajimoto, N. and S. M. Kirkepar. Effect of manganese and lanthanum on spontaneous release of acetylcholine at frog motor nerve terminals. Nature New Biol. 235: 29-30 (1972).

82. Hubbard, J. I., S. F. Jones and E. M. Landau. On the mechanism by which calcium and magnesium affect the spontaneous release of transmitter from mammalian motor nerve terminals. J. Physiol. London 194: 355-380 (1968).

83. Hubbard, J. I., S. F. Jones and E. M. Landau. On the mechanism by which calcium and magnesium affect the release of transmitter by nerve impulses. J. Physiol. London 196: 75-86 (1968).

84. Katz, B. and R. Miledi. The timing of calcium action during neuromuscular transmission. J. Physiol. London 189: 535-544 (1967).

85. Rahamimoff, R. A. A dual effect of calcium ions on neuromuscular facilitation. J. Physiol. London 195: 471-480 (1968).

86. Katz, B. and R. Miledi. The role of calcium in neuromuscular facilitation. J. Physiol. London 195: 481-492 (1968).

87. Chapman, R. A. and R. Niedergerke. Interaction between heart rate and calcium concentration in the control of contractile strength of the frog heart. J. Physiol. London 211: 423-443 (1970).

88. Chapman, R. A. and J. Tunstall. The dependence of the contractile force generated by frog auricular trabeculae upon the external calcium concentration. J. Physiol. London 215: 139-162 (1971).

89. Jenkinson, D. H. The nature of the antagonism between calcium and magnesium ions at the neuromuscular junction. J. Physiol. London 138: 434-444 (1957).

90. Dodge, F. A. and R. Rahamimoff. Co-operative action of calcium ions in neurotransmitter release at the neuro-

muscular junction. J. Physiol. London 193: 419-432 (1967).

91. Katz, B. and R. Miledi. Further study of the role of calcium in synaptic transmission. J. Physiol. London 207: 789-801 (1970).

92. Belleau, B. and D. J. Triggle. Studies on the chemical basis for cholinomimetic and cholinolytic activity. Can. J. Chem. 40: 1201-1215 (1962).

93. Chang, K. J., R. C. Deth and D. J. Triggle. Structural parameters determining cholinergic and anticholinergic activities in a series of 1,3-dioxolanes. J. Med. Chem. 15: 243-247 (1972).

94. Chang, K. J. and D. J. Triggle. Papaverine and lanthanum inhibition of contractile response in the guinea-pig ileum. Submitted to J. Theoret. biol. (1972).

95. Daniel, E. E. Effect of drugs on contractions of vertebrate smooth muscle. Ann. Rev. Pharmacol. 4:189-222 (1964).

96. Simonis, A. M., E. J. Ariëns and J. J. W. Van den Broeke. Non-competitive spasmolytics as antagonists of Ca^{++}-induced smooth muscle contraction. J. Pharm. Pharmacol. 23: 107-110 (1971).

97. Imai, S. and K. Takeda. Effect of vasodilators upon the isolated taenia coli of the guinea-pig. J. Pharmacol. Exptl. Therap. 156: 557-564 (1967).

98. Ferrari, M. and F. Carpenedo. On the mechanism of action of some myolytic agents on depolarized guinea-pig taenia coli. Arch. int. Pharmacodyn. 174: 223-232 (1968).

99. Van Breemen, C. Permselectivity of a porous phospho-lipid-cholesterol artificial membrane. Calcium and lanthanum effects. Biochem. Biophys. Res. Comm. 32: 977-983 (1968).

100. Miledi, R. Lanthanum ions abolish the "calcium response" of nerve terminals. Nature 229: 410-411 (1971).

101. Goodman, F. R. and G. B. Weiss. Dissociation by lanthanum of smooth muscle responses to potassium and acetylcholine. Amer. J. Physiol. 220: 759-766 (1971).

102. Van Breemen, C., B.R. Farinas, P. Gerba and E. D. McNaughton. Excitation-contraction coupling in rabbit aorta studied by the lanthanum method for measuring cellular calcium influx. Circulation Res. 30: 44-54 (1972).

103. Hurwitz, L. and A. Suria. The link between agonist

action and response in smooth muscle. Ann. Rev.
Pharmacol. 11: 303-326 (1971).

104. Schirmer, R. H. Die besonderheiten des contractilen
proteins der arterien. Biochem. Zeit. 343: 269-282
(1965).

105. Schadler, M. Proportionale acktivierung von ATPase-
aktivitat und kontractionspannung durch calciumionen
in isolierten contractilen strukturen verschiedener
Muskelarten. Pflug. Arch. 296: 70-90 (1967).

106. Hellam, D. C. and R. J. Podolsky. Force measurements
in skinned muscle fibers. J. Physiol. London 200:
807-819 (1969).

107. Werman, R. The number of receptors for calcium ions
at the nerve terminals of one endplate. Comp. Gen.
Pharmacol. 2: 129-137 (1971).

108. Goodford, P. J. In: E.E. Bittar (Editor), Membranes
and Ion Transport. Vol. 2, Wiley & Sons, New York
(1970), pp. 33-74.

109. Paton, W. D. M. and H. P. Rang. The uptake of atropine
and related drugs by intestinal smooth muscle of the
guinea pig in relation to acetylcholine receptors.
Proc. Roy. Soc. London Ser. B 163: 1-44 (1965).

110. Lüllmann, H. and P. Mohns. The Ca^{++} metabolism of
intestinal smooth muscle during forced electrical
stimulation. Pflüg. Arch. ges. physiol. 308: 214-
224 (1969).

111. Katz, B. and S. Thesleff. A study of the "desensitization" produced by acetylcholine at the motor end-plate.
J. Physiol. London 138: 63-80 (1957).

112. Rang, H. P. and J. M. Ritter. The relationship between
desensitization and the metaphilic effect at cholinergic
receptors. Mol. Pharmacol. 6: 383-390 (1970).

113. Pöch, G. and W. R. Kukovetz. Papaverine-induced inhibition of phosphodiesterase activity in various mammalian
tissues. Life Sciences 10 (I): 133-142 (1971).

114. Triner, L., G. G. Nahas, Y. Vulliemoz, N. I. A. Overweg,
M. Verosky, D. V. Habif and S. H. Nagai. Cyclic AMP
and smooth muscle function. Ann. N. Y. Acad. Sci. 185:
458-476 (1971).

115. Tashiro, N. and T. Tomita. The effects of papaverine
on the electrical and mechanical activity of the guinea-
pig taenia coli. Brit. J. Pharmacol. 39: 608-618 (1970).

116. Krejií, I., I. Poláček and J. Rudinger. The action of
2-0-Methyltyrosine-oxytocin on the rat and rabbit uterus:

effect of some experimental conditions on change from agonism to antagonism. Brit. J. Pharmac. Chemother. 30: 506-517 (1967).

117. Kafka, M. S. and C. Y. C. Pak. Effects of polypeptide and protein hormones on lipid monolayers. I. Effect of insulin and parathyroid hormone on monomolecular films of monooctadecyl phosphate and stearic acid. J. Gen. Physiol. 54: 134-143 (1969).

118. Kafka, M. S. and C. Y. C. Pak. Effects of polypeptide hormones on lipid monolayers. II. On the effects of insulin analogs, vasopressin, oxytocin, thyrocalcitonin, adrenocorticotrophin and $3',5'$-cyclic AMP on the uptake of Ca^{2+} by monomolecular films of monooctadecyl phosphate. Biochim. Biophys. Acta 193: 117-123 (1969).

119. Sayers, G., R. J. Beall and S. Seelig. Isolated adrenal cells: adrenocorticotrophic hormone, calcium, steroidogenesis and cyclic adenosine monophosphate. Science, Washington 175: 1131-1133 (1972).

120. Shaltz, L. and G. V. Marinetti. Hormone-calcium interactions with the plasma membrane of rat liver cells. Science, Washington 175: 175-177 (1972).

121. Eagling, E. M., H. G. Lovell and V. R. Pickles. Interaction of prostaglandin E_1 and calcium in guinea-pig myometrium. Brit. J. Pharmacol. 44: 510-516 (1972).

122. Yoshikami, S. and W. A. Hagins. Light, calcium and the photo current of rods and cones. Biophys. J. 11: 47a (1971).

123. Cone, R. A. Rotational diffusion of rhodopsin in the visual receptor membrane. Nature New Biology 236: 39-43 (1972).

TABLE I

STRUCTURES, INTRINSIC ACTIVITIES (i.a.) AND AFFINITIES (pD$_2$)
OF CHOLINERGIC AGONISTS

*i.a. is measured by the ratio of the maximum response given
by an agonist relative to that produced by CD (cumulative
concentration-response curve) in normal Tyrode's solution;
pD$_2$ is a measure of the apparent affinity of the agonist and
is the negative logarithm of the molar concentration required
to produce 50% of the individual maximum response.*

R$_1$[a]	R$_2$[a]	i.a.	pD$_2$
Me	H	1.0	7.96 ± 0.01 (7)
Me	Me	1.0	5.05 ± 0.03 (6)
Et	Et	0.85	4.92 ± 0.02 (6)
Pr^i	Pr^i	0.78	4.64 ± 0.03 (4)

[a]

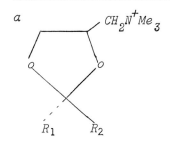

95

TABLE II

SLOPES OF DOUBLE LOGARITHMIC PLOTS FOR AGONIST-CONCENTRATION RESPONSE CURVES AT VARIOUS Ca_{EXT}^{++} LEVELS

[A] \ [Ca_{EXT}^{++}]	0.1mM	0.4mM	1.8mM
CD	5.62	2.71	1.07
DMD	4.90	2.94	1.39
DED	4.76	2.71	1.25
DPD	4.51	2.32	1.47

TABLE III

% INHIBITION BY PAPAVERINE OF PHASIC AND TONIC
COMPONENTS OF AGONIST-INDUCED CONTRACTIONS

To obtain the % inhibition, the control phasic and tonic components of each agonist have been set at 100% and the % inhibition for each component of each agonist with increasing papaverine concentration based on this figure.

Agonist	Papaverine Concentration, M		
	10^{-5}	2×10^{-5}	4×10^{-5}
Phasic, % inhibition			
CD	11.0	21.4	37.6
DMD	7.7	16.5	30.9
DED	13.5	26.9	48.4
DPD	17.0	43.2	60.0
Tonic, % inhibition			
CD	38.7	83.6	94.5
DMD	24.5	76.3	91.4
DED	12.6	70.9	94.3
DPD	6.4	51.8	92.4
Tonic/phasic ratio			
CD	3.5	3.9	2.5
DMD	3.2	4.6	3.0
DED	0.94	2.6	1.9
DPD	0.39	1.2	1.5

TABLE IV

EXPONENT VALUES OF AGONIST AND CALCIUM
CONCENTRATION-RESPONSE CURVES

A \ $[Ca^{++}]mM$	n.o exponent^a			n exponent^{2b}
	0.1	0.4	1.8	
CD	6	3	1	6
DMD	6	3	1	6
DED	6	3	1	6
DPD	6	2	1	6

[a] Determined from modified double reciprocal plots of response versus agonist concentration at the indicated $[Ca_{EXT}^{++}]$ levels (Fig. 8 c,d).

[b] Determined from modified double reciprocal plots of response versus calcium concentration at saturated agonist levels (Fig. 8a,b).

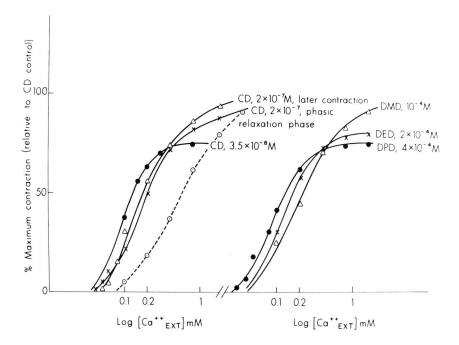

Fig. 1. *Concentration-response curves for Ca++ obtained in the presence of fixed concentrations of the dioxolane agonists.* For CD, at 2 x 10⁻⁷M, the contractions are measured separately for the initial phasic contraction, the intermediate relaxation phase and the later contraction. Only the initial contraction heights were measured for CD (3.5 x 10⁻⁸ M), DMD (10⁻⁴M), DED (2 x 10⁻⁴M) and DPD (4 x 10⁻⁴M). Each point is the mean of at least six preparations and all contractions are expressed relative to the maximum contraction obtained with CD in a cumulative concentration-response curve.

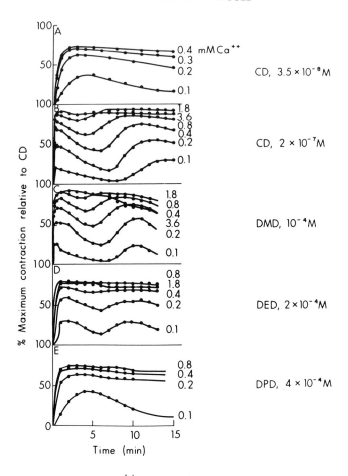

Fig. 2a. *Effect of* $[Ca_{EXT}^{++}]$ *on the time course of contraction induced by single doses of agonists at the concentrations shown in the figures.* The Ca^{++} ion was allowed to equilibrate 30 min with the tissue before the agonist was added. Each point represents the mean of a minimum of 6 preparations. The points on the experimental curves represent intervals of one minute. Contractile heights are shown relative to a reference of contraction obtained with CD in a cumulative concentration-response curve.

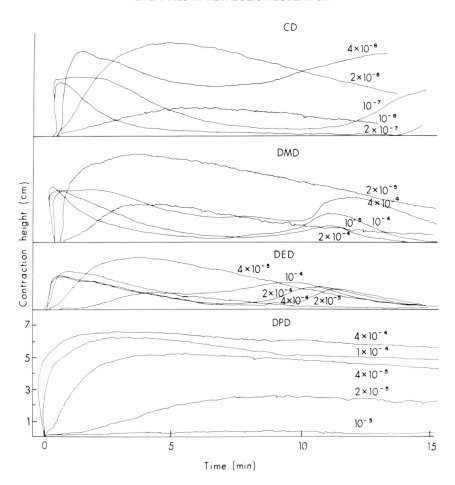

Fig. 2b. *Tracings of time courses of contractions induced by the indicated concentrations of agonists at low (0.1mM) levels of Ca_{EXT}^{++}.* The ordinate represents contraction height (cm) and the abscissa the time after addition of agonist (min).

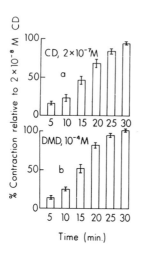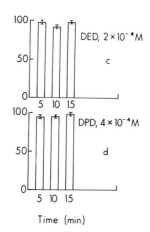

Fig. 3. *Graphical representation of the extent of and re-covery from desensitization by maximum doses of the four agonists to a standard submaximal concentation of CD (2 x $10^{-8}M$).* Tissues were incubated in normal Tyrodes solution with the maximum agonist concentration for 5 min, washed and the responses to CD exposure (2 x 10^{-8} M/1 min) were measured at 5 min intervals. Contractile responses are expressed as a percentage of the control response to CD (2 x 10^{-8}M). Each bar represents an average of a minimum of 8 preparations ± S.E.M.

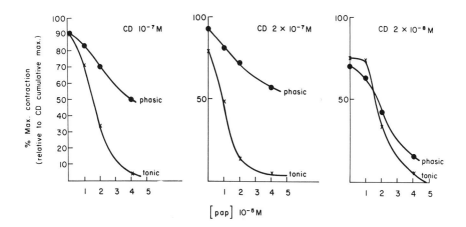

Fig. 4. *The inhibitory effects of papaverine (1-5 x 10⁻⁵M) on the phasic and tonic components of contraction induced by three concentrations of CD.* Note that the selectivity of papaverine for the phasic component of contraction increases with increasing CD concentration.

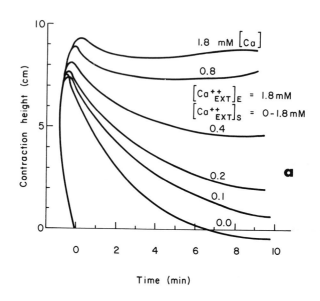

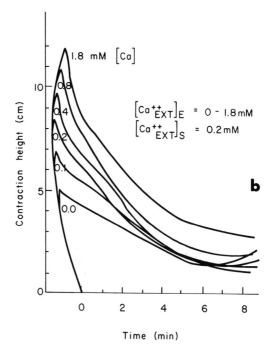

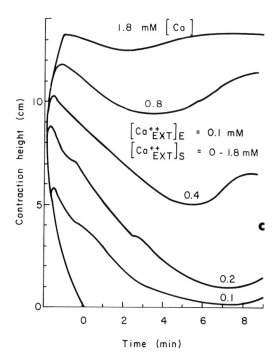

Figs 5a-c. *Superimposed tracings of time courses of con-*
tractions showing the effects of different Ca^{++} concentra-
tions for equilibration, $[Ca^{++}_{EXT}]_E$, and stimulus, $[Ca^{++}_{EXT}]_S$,
during excitation by CD (single dose, $2 \times 10^{-7} M$). a. Equilibrating concentrations of Ca^{++} maintained at 1.8 mM and
stimulating concentration varied between 0 and 1.8 mM.
b. Equilibrating concentrations of Ca^{++} varied between 0
and 1.8 mM and stimulating concentration maintained at 0.2
mM. c. Equilibrating concentration of Ca^{++} maintained at
0.1 mM and stimulating concentration varied between 0 and
1.8 mM.

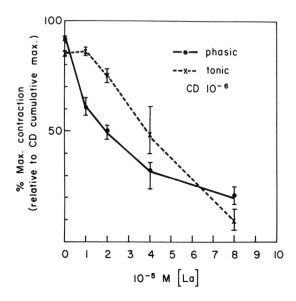

Fig. 6. *Effect of La^{+++} on the phasic and tonic concentrations produced by a single concentration of CD ($10^{-6}M$).* The results are expressed as a percentage of reference maximum (CD cumulative). Each point represents the mean of 6 preparations ± S.E.M.

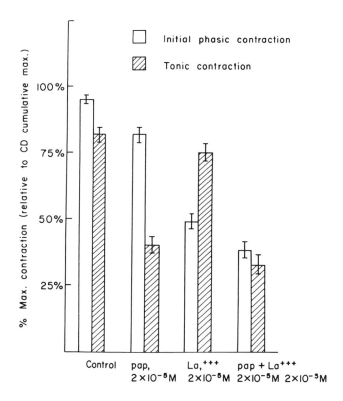

Fig. 7. *The additive effects of papaverine (2 x $10^{-5}M$) and La^{+++} (2 x $10^{-5}M$) on the phasic and tonic contractions produced by a single concentration of CD ($10^{-6}M$).* The results are expressed as a percentage of the reference maximum (CD cumulative). Each bar represents an average of 6 preparations ± S.E.M.

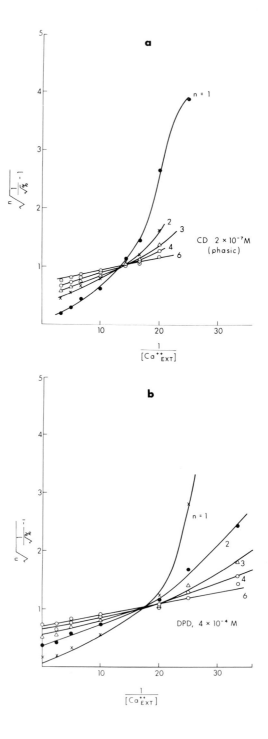

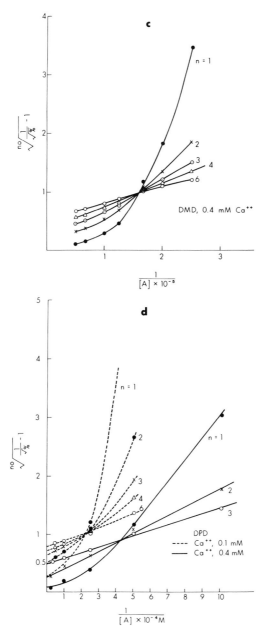

Figs. 8a–d. *Modified reciprocal plots of the experimentally observed relationship between* [Ca_{EXT}^{++}] *and response at maximum (indicated) concentrations of CD and DPD (a,b) and* [A] *and response at the indicated concentrations of* Ca_{EXT}^{++} *(c,d).* Ca_{EXT}^{++} concentrations expressed as mM.

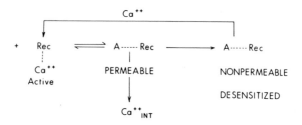

Fig. 9. *Schematic representation of the activation and desensitization of the acetylcholine receptor in guinea pig ileal longitudinal muscle.* The active state of the receptor is represented as a Ca^{++}-associated state which upon activation by A (agonist) is converted to a Ca^{++}-dissociated permeable state. In the presence of high concentrations of full agonists this can be converted to a nonpermeable desensitized state from which a Ca^{++}-dependent recovery to the active state can take place.

ANTIBIOTIC A23187 AS A PROBE FOR THE STUDY OF CALCIUM AND MAGNESIUM FUNCTION IN BIOLOGICAL SYSTEMS

Peter W. Reed and Henry A. Lardy

Introduction

Certain toxic antibiotics are useful tools for the study of metabolic reactions (1,2). Investigation of mitochondrial function has been aided by antibiotics which inhibit electron transfer, adenine nucleotide translocation and the ATPase enzyme (2). The ionophorous antibiotics (3) produce alkali metal cation uptake or exchange across several types of membranes (3-6) and have been important tools in the study of mitochondrial and chloroplast function (7, 8). Recently (9), we described the effects on mitochondria exerted by a new ionophorous antibiotic, A23187, which specifically binds divalent cations at neutral pH. While antibiotic X537A also binds alkaline earth cations (10,11), it complexes a variety of monovalent cations as well (4,6). Thus, A23187 appeared to be a unique probe for the study of divalent cation function in mitochondria and other systems.

A23187 is a monocarboxylic acid (m.w. 523) which transfers calcium and magnesium, but not potassium, from an aqueous medium at pH 7.4 into a bulk organic phase (12). The A23187-Me^{2+} complex appears to be a neutral, 2:1 species since the amount of divalent cation transported by the antibiotic approaches half the molar amount of A23187 and the organo-soluble thiocyanate anion does not facilitate cation transfer. The affinity of A23187 for various divalent cations as detected by alterations in the absorption spectrum of the antibiotic in an aqueous medium is $Mn^{2+} \gg Ca^{2+} \simeq Mg^{2+} > Sr^{2+} > Ba^{2+}$ (9,12). A23187 discharges endogenous calcium and magnesium from rat liver mitochondria and produces simultaneous uncoupling of oxidative phosphorylation and inhibition of ATPase (9,12). This report extends these earlier observations and describes effects of the antibiotic on erythrocytes and spermatozoa. The data indicate that

A23187 can be used to alter divalent cation distribution across several types of membranes and this markedly affects certain functions of cells and organelles.

Methods

Mitochondria were prepared by the method of Johnson and Lardy (13). In some cases, EDTA was omitted from the homogenizing medium in order to produce elevated mitochondrial calcium and in other instances, 1 mM EGTA was present during all steps of preparation (6) except final suspension in 250 mM mannitol, 70 mM sucrose. Rat erythrocytes were prepared from blood collected into an equal volume of 150 mM choline chloride + 5 mM Tris-Cl, pH 7.4 (6), containing approximately 60 U.S.P. units of heparin/ml. After filtration through cheesecloth and gentle centrifugation at room temperature, plasma and leukocytes were removed by aspiration and erythrocytes were washed once in a large volume of the above medium, with heparin omitted. Bovine epididymal spermatozoa were collected by the method of Henle [*c.f.* (14)] with 250 mM sucrose + 5 mM TEA-Cl, pH 7.4, as the perfusion medium. Incubations were carried out at 30° with mitochondria, 25° with red cells and 37° with sperm.

The procedures for measuring oxidative phosphorylation, ATPase, cation content of mitochondrial pellets, inorganic phosphate, protein, cation fluxes with ion-specific glass electrodes, and polarigraphic measurement of respiration were described previously (12). All nucleotides, substrates, EGTA and EDTA were brought to pH 7.4 with triethanolamine base or HCl before use.

Results

Mitochondria

When rat liver mitochondria are incubated in the presence of EDTA to bind discharged divalent cations, A23187 produces a large efflux of endogenous calcium and magnesium which is maximal after 30 seconds of incubation (12). Figure 1 shows that, under these conditions, half maximal release of mitochondrial calcium and magnesium occurs at a concentration of approximately 0.1 nmole A23187/mg protein.

In the absence of EDTA, low concentrations of A23187 produce a time-dependent efflux of endogenous magnesium while
mitochondrial calcium content remains largely unchanged
(12). Since rat liver mitochondria actively take up calcium, but not magnesium (15-17), calcium discharged by
A23187 may be reaccumulated whereas magnesium may not.

A23187 had variable effects on oxidative phosphorylation by mitochondria prepared by different methods. Low
concentrations of the antibiotic uncoupled mitochondria with
elevated calcium content (15 to 20 nmole Ca^{2+}/mg protein)
more effectively, whereas A23187 often failed to uncouple
mitochondria prepared with 1 mM EGTA or EDTA present during
all washings (Fig. 2). Addition of low concentrations of
calcium chloride, which alone had no appreciable effect on
coupling, restored the ability of A23187 to uncouple these
latter mitochondria (Fig. 2). Since the calcium and magnesium content of mitochondria washed in the presence of
1 mM EGTA was the same as that of mitochondria washed in
the absence of chelator, it appeared that low concentrations
of EGTA adhering to the mitochondria (18) might be preventing uncoupling by A23187. Figure 3 shows that release of
state 4 succinate oxidation by A23187 was inhibited by low
concentrations of added EGTA or EDTA and exogenous calcium
reversed this inhibition.

Although incubation with A23187 (0.3 nmole/mg protein)
plus EDTA decreased magnesium to 2-3 nmole/mg protein in
less than 30 seconds, mitochondria remained coupled and
able to phosphorylate ADP at 70 to 80% of control rate with
succinate or β-hydroxybutyrate as substrate (12). In contrast, the marked inhibition of mitochondrial ATPase by
A23187 was not prevented by EDTA but high concentrations of
magnesium chloride in the incubating medium were able to
reverse partially this inhibition (Fig. 4). Thus, uncoupling by A23187 was not simply due to magnesium loss and required free calcium while inhibition of ATPase appeared to
result from antibiotic-mediated magnesium efflux.

A23187 produced a slow efflux of endogenous mitochondrial potassium when EDTA was present in the incubating
medium (Fig. 5) and the loss of calcium and magnesium was
very rapid and large (Fig. 1). Figure 6B shows that A23187
produced a rapid, partial reversal of potassium uptake by
mitochondria incubated with valinomycin although it was
unable to stimulate succinate oxidation itself unless calcium was added to the medium (Fig. 6A ①). Addition of

calcium prior to A23187 allowed the carboxylic acid to produce a slightly greater potassium release (Fig. 6C) and A23187 was still able to partially prevent valinomycin-induced potassium accumulation when uncoupling by the carboxylic acid was prevented by 0.1 mM EGTA (Fig. 6A(2)). Since A23187 failed to transfer potassium from a pH 7.4 aqueous medium into an organic phase, mitochondrial potassium loss in the absence of uncoupling appeared to be secondary to effects of the antibiotic on divalent cations.

Erythrocytes

Erythrocytes bind calcium (19) and, in contrast to mitochondria, actively extrude intraerythrocytic calcium by an energy dependent process (20,21). Figure 7A shows that addition of a high concentration of A23187 to rat erythrocytes incubated in a medium containing 2 mM calcium chloride produces uptake of calcium by red cells with a rapid release of protons and potassium to the external medium. When proton efflux is complete, calcium uptake appears to cease but potassium loss continues. No additional hemolysis or change in light scattering (600 nm) occurs during these ion exchanges whereas addition of azalomycin F (22) produces complete hemolysis and release of potassium, protons and accumulated calcium (Fig. 7A). Both calcium uptake and proton release by erythrocytes incubated with A23187 depend on the concentration of external calcium at high levels of the antibiotic (Fig. 8A) and on antibiotic concentration in the presence of 2 mM added calcium chloride (Fig. 8B). At the point of maximal proton release, the $\Delta H^+/\Delta Ca^{2+}$ ratio equals 0.8 to 1.3.

While low concentrations of A23187 (0.1 µM or less) were unable to produce a measurable Ca^{2+}/H^+ exchange by erythrocytes incubated in the presence of 2 mM calcium chloride (Fig. 8B), they still caused a rapid and large efflux of potassium from red cells accompanied by a delayed proton uptake (or hydroxyl release) (Fig. 7B). Subsequent addition of a higher concentration of A23187 produced a proton efflux typical of that seen during calcium accumulation and no further potassium release (Fig. 7B). Release of erythrocyte potassium by low concentrations of A23187 increased as the calcium content of the incubation medium was elevated (Fig. 9A).

114

In the absence of added calcium chloride, increasing concentrations of A23187 produced a progressively greater potassium loss and increased light scattering (shrinkage) (Fig. 9B) which depended on calcium bound to erythrocytes or present as a contaminant in the choline chloride. Thus, low concentrations of EGTA rapidly inhibited the potassium efflux produced by A23187 alone (Fig. 10A) and small amounts of calcium restored the potassium loss. Low concentrations of lanthanum did not affect potassium loss produced by the antibiotic alone, but relatively high concentrations of magnesium inhibited the potassium efflux (Fig. 10B). Intermediate concentrations of A23187 produced a limited efflux of potassium from erythrocytes and the subsequent addition of 2 mM calcium, strontium or manganese produced varying rates of potassium loss (Fig. 9B). While barium and magnesium did not allow A23187 to produce a potassium loss under these conditions, neither did they markedly affect the ability of 2 mM calcium to subsequently allow potassium efflux (Fig. 9B).

Spermatozoa

Figure 11A shows that A23187 can mediate a calcium/ proton exchange across the membranes of bovine epididymal sperm and this is accompanied by a slow loss of intracellular potassium. With caffeine present in the incubation medium, epididymal sperm show unusually vigorous progressive motility (14) and this is observed even in the presence of high concentrations of calcium chloride (arrow 1, Fig. 11A). As calcium uptake induced by A23187 proceeds, motility becomes depressed (arrow 2, Fig. 11A) and finally arrested (arrow 3, Fig. 11A). Nigericin produces a potassium/proton exchange across sperm membranes (Fig. 11B) with a subsequent loss of motility (arrow 1, Fig. 11B) but the addition of caffeine restores and maintains motility. Inhibition of motility by A23187 under these conditions, therefore, is apparently due to calcium uptake or internal alkalinization rather than potassium loss. A23187 produces a typical calcium/proton exchange even after sperm are depleted of potassium (Fig. 11B) similar to that which occurs with erythrocytes (Fig. 7B).

Discussion

A23187 apparently acts as a freely mobile carrier a-
cross membranes to catalyze equilibration of divalent cations between external medium and organelle or cell interior. Thus, the antibiotic produces calcium uptake by erythrocytes, sperm and non-respiring mitochondria (23) incubated with high concentrations of calcium chloride. Similarly, A23187 produces magnesium accumulation and proton
release by erythrocytes incubated in 2 mM magnesium chloride and magnesium uptake by depleted mitochondria (23). In
the absence of exogenous divalent cations and presence of
EDTA, A23187 releases endogenous calcium and magnesium from
mitochondria, erythrocytes and sperm.

Uncoupling of mitochondria and potassium loss from
erythrocytes due to A23187 are both dependent on free calcium whereas inhibition of mitochondrial ATPase results
from magnesium depletion by the antibiotic. EGTA inhibits
both the former effects of A23187 and ATPase inhibition is
reversed only by conditions which prevent antibiotic-mediated magnesium loss, *i.e.*, incubation in high concentrations of magnesium chloride. Release of endogenous
magnesium would be expected to severely diminish intramitochondrial $MgATP^{2-}$ concentrations and lead to inhibition of
the ATPase by free ATP^{4-}. Low concentrations of lanthanum
chloride and ruthenium red inhibit energy-dependent uptake
of calcium by mitochondria (17,24,25) and uncoupling by
A23187 (9,12). These observations suggest that uncoupling
produced by A23187 may result from an energy dissipating
flux of calcium across the inner mitochondrial membrane
established by antibiotic-mediated release in concert with
energy-dependent reaccumulation of calcium on the high
affinity divalent cation carrier (12).

Potassium loss produced by A23187 appears to be secondary to effects of the antibiotic on divalent cations,
for A23187 is not a potassium ionophore in bulk phase experiments at pH 7.4 (12). Release of endogenous mitochondrial potassium by the antibiotic is appreciable only
in the presence of EDTA when calcium and magnesium loss are
rapid and A23187 is inhibited from uncoupling. The rapid
release by A23187 of potassium accumulated by mitochondia
incubated with valinomycin may result from the increased
potassium permeability already established by valinomycin
(26). Increased permeability to potassium is observed in

mitochondria deficient in magnesium (18,26,27) or calcium (27). Finally, in contrast to the effects of other carboxylic acid antibiotics (3,6,8), A23187 does not produce a K^+/H^+ exchange across membranes of mitochondria, red cells or sperm.

The calcium-dependent, potassium efflux from rat erythrocytes incubated with A23187 is similar in some respects to the increased potassium loss from energy-depleted red cells (28-31) or ghosts (32) with elevated internal calcium. Both types of potassium loss are prevented by EGTA or EDTA (29,30,32) and partially inhibited by oligomycin (23,29, 32). Potassium loss due to A23187, however, contrasts to that produced by elevated intraerythrocytic calcium since the former is extremely rapid, is inhibited by magnesium and is insensitive to ouabain (23,29). Magnesium most likely prevents the potassium efflux by binding to A23187.

Calcium may alter erythrocyte permeability to potassium through a direct inhibition of the $Na^+ + K^+ + Mg^{2+}$-ATPase (32,33) or as a result of the complex interrelationship of the $Ca^{2+} + Mg^{2+}$-ATPase (20,34,35), $Na^+ + K^+ + Mg^{2+}$-ATPase and intracellular ATP concentrations (29-31). A23187 might effectively deliver calcium to an inhibitory site on the membrane-bound $Na^+ + K^+ + Mg^{2+}$-ATPase. Alternatively, transport by A23187 of small amounts of calcium into the erythrocyte interior might activate the $Ca^{2+} + Mg^{2+}$-ATPase to extrude the calcium (20,21,35) and establish an energy-dissipating, cyclic flux of calcium across the red cell membrane. Experiments designed to investigate these possibilities as well as the relationship of internal divalent cations to ATP concentrations and potassium permeability of erythrocytes are currently in progress. It is unlikely that the red cell membrane modifies antibiotic specificity to allow a Me^{2+}/K^+ exchange , since magnesium is transported into erythrocytes by A23187 but prevents the potassium efflux

Summary

A23187 is a divalent cation ionophore which acts as a freely mobile carrier to equilibrate calcium and magnesium across various membranes. The antibiotic induces calcium uptake and proton release by sperm and erythrocytes incubated in the presence of high concentrations of calcium chloride. Calcium loading of sperm by A23187 produces a complete inhibition of motility. The antibiotic produces a calcium-dependent, potassium efflux from red cells. A23187 inhibits mitochondrial ATPase by releasing endogenous magnesium while uncoupling oxidative phosphorylation by a calcium-requiring mechanism. The carboxylic acid produces potassium loss from mitochondria apparently secondary to its release of endogenous divalent cations. Since calcium and magnesium are essential components of many diverse biological systems, A23187 should be a useful probe to study the function of these divalent cations.

Presented by Peter W. Reed

References

1. Lardy, H.A., D. Johnson, and W.C. McMurray, Antibiotics as tools for metabolic studies. I. A survey of toxic antibiotics in respiratory, phosphorylative and glycolytic systems. Arch. Biochem. Biophys. 78:587-597 (1958).
2. Henderson, P.J.F. and H.A. Lardy. Antibiotic inhibition of mitochondrial energy-transfer reactions. Antimicrob. Agents Chemother. 18-27 (1969).
3. Pressman, B.C., E.J. Harris, W.S. Jagger, and J.H. Johnson. Antibiotic-mediated transport of alkali ions across lipid barriers. Proc. Nat. Acad. Sci. USA. 58:1949-1956 (1967).
4. Lardy, H.A., S.N. Graven, and S. Estrada-O. Specific induction and inhibition of cation and anion transport in mitochondria. Fed. Proc. 26:1355-1360 (1967).
5. Pressman, B.C. Mechanism of action of transport-mediating antibiotics. Ann. N.Y. Acad. Sci. 147:829-841 (1969).
6. Henderson, P.J.F., J.D. McGivan, and J.B. Chappell. The action of certain antibiotics on mitochondrial, erythrocyte and artifical phospholipid membranes. Biochem. J. 111:521-535 (1969).
7. Mitchell, P. In: Chemiosmotic coupling and energy transduction, 111 pp., Glynn Research Ltd., Bodmin, England.

8. Henderson, P.J.F. Ion transport by energy-conserving biological membranes. Ann. Rev. Microbiol. 25: 393-428 (1971).

9. Reed, P.W. A23187: A divalent cation ionophore. Fed. Proc. 31:432 (1972).

10. Johnson, S.M., J. Herrin, S.J. Liu and I.C. Paul. The crystal and molecular structure of the barium salt of an antibiotic containing a high proportion of oxygen. J. Amer. Chem. Soc. 92:4428-4435 (1970).

11. Pressman, B.C. Properties of ionophores with broad range cation selectivity. Fed. Proc. 31: in press.

12. Reed, P.W. and H.A. Lardy. A23187: A divalent cation ionophore. Submitted for publication.

13. Johnson, D. and H.A. Lardy. Isolation of liver or kidney mitochondria. In: R.W. Estabrook and M.E. Pullman (Editors), Methods in Enzymology, Vol. X, Academic Press, New York (1967), pp. 94-96.

14. Garbers, D.L., W.D. Lust, N.L. First, and H.A. Lardy. Effects of phosphodiesterase inhibitors and cyclic nucleotides on sperm respiration and motility. Biochemistry 10:1825-1831 (1971).

15. Lehninger, A.L., E. Carafoli, and C.S. Rossi. Energy-linked ion movements in mitochondrial systems. Adv. Enzymol. 29:259-320 (1967).

16. Drahota, Z., P. Gazzotti, E. Carafoli, and C.S. Rossi. A comparison of the effects of different divalent cations on a number of mitochondrial reactions linked to ion translocation. Arch. Biochem. Biophys. 130:267-273 (1969).

17. Vainio, H., L. Mela, and B. Chance. Energy dependent bivalent cation translocation in rat liver mitochondria. Eur. J. Biochem. 12:387-391 (1970).

18. Settlemire, C.T., G.R. Hunter, and G.P. Brierley. Ion transport in heart mitochondria. XIII. The effect of ethylenediaminetetraacetate on monovalent ion uptake. Biochim. Biophys. Acta 162:487-499 (1969).

19. Long, C. and B. Mouat. The binding of calcium ions by erythrocytes and "ghosts"-cell membranes. Biochem. J. 123:829-836 (1971).

20. Schatzmann, H.J. and F.F. Vincenzi. Calcium movements across the membrane of human red cells. J. Physiol. 201:369-395 (1969).

21. Lee, K.S. and B.C. Shin. Studies on the active transport of calcium in human red cells. J. Gen. Physiol. 54:713-729 (1969).

22. Arai, M. Azalomycin F, an antibiotic against fungi and Trichomonas. Arzneimittel Forsch. 18:1396-1399 (1968).
23. Reed, P.W., unpublished observations.
24. Mela, L. Interactions of La^{3+} and local anesthetic drugs with mitochondrial Ca^{2+} and Mn^{2+} uptake. Arch. Biochem. Biophys. 123:286-293 (1968).
25. Moore, C.L. Specific inhibition of mitochondrial Ca^{2+} transport by ruthenium red. Biochem. Biophys. Res. Commun. 42:298-305 (1971).
26. Harris, E.J., G. Catlin, and B.C. Pressman. Effect of transport-inducing antibiotics and other agents on potassium flux in mitochondria. Biochemistry 6:1360-1370 (1967).
27. Lee, N.M., I. Wiedemann, and E. Kun. Control of cation movements in liver mitochondria by a cytoplasmic factor. Biochem. Biophys. Res. Commun. 42:1030-1034 (1971).
28. Gardos, G. The role of calcium in the potassium permeability of human erythrocytes. Acta Physiol. Hung. 15:121-125 (1959).
29. Hoffman, J.F. The red cell membrane and the transport of sodium and potassium. Amer. J. Med. 41:666-680 (1966).
30. Romero, P.J. and R. Whittam. The control by internal calcium of membrane permeability to sodium and potassium. J. Physiol. 214:481-507 (1971).
31. Lew, V.L. On the ATP dependence of the Ca^{2+}-induced increase in K^+ permeability observed in human red cells. Biochim. Biophys. Acta 233:827-830 (1971).
32. Blum, R.M. and J.F. Hoffman. Ca-induced K transport in human red cells: localization of the Ca-sensitive site to the inside of the membrane. Biochem. Biophys. Res. Commun. 46:1146-1152 (1972).
33. Skou, J.C. Enzymatic basis for active transport of Na^+ and K^+ across cell membrane. Physiol. Rev. 45:596-616 (1965).
34. Dunham, E.T. and I.M. Glynn. Adenosinetriphosphatase activity and the active movements of alkali metal ions. J. Physiol. 156:274-293 (1961).
35. Schatzmann, H.J. and G.L. Rossi. $(Ca^{2+} + Mg^{2+})$-activated membrane ATPases in human red cells and their possible relations to cation transport. Biochim. Biophys. Acta 241:379-392 (1971).

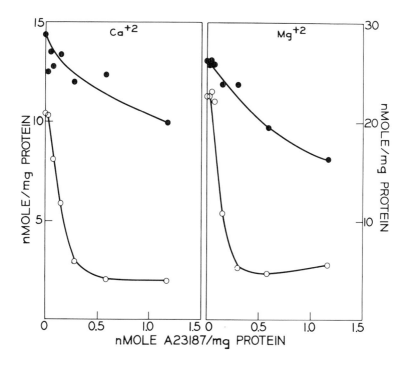

Fig. 1. *Calcium and magnesium efflux from mitochondria incubated with A23187 in the presence and absence of EDTA.* Mitochondria prepared in the absence of EDTA were added (32 mg) to polyethylene tubes containing medium and various concentrations of A23187, mixed and immediately sedimented (*ca.* 30 sec.). The medium contained 4 mM Cl-(TEA) (pH 7.4), 8 mM succinate, 1.5 µM rotenone, 7 mM KCl, 133 mM sucrose and 121 mM mannitol. ● , no EDTA; ○ , 0.6 mM EDTA.

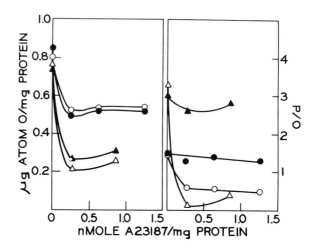

Fig. 2. *Calcium dependent uncoupling of oxidative phosphorylation by A23187.* Mitochondria were prepared as described
in Methods with 1 mM EDTA present only during initial homo-
genation ($\bigcirc$) or with 1 mM EGTA present during homogeniza-
tion of liver *and* all washings of mitochondria ($\bullet$, $\blacktriangle$, $\triangle$).
The incubation medium contained 13 mM PO$_4$-(TEA) (pH 7.4), 15
mM KCl, 2 mM ATP, 42 mM mannitol, 132 mM sucrose and 10-15
mg protein of mitochondria. Glucose (final concentration
18 mM), hexokinase (2 mg), substrate and A23187 were added
after a 10 min thermal equilibration and the incubation was
continued for 10 min. $\bullet$, $\bigcirc$, 10 mM succinate plus 1 µM
rotenone; $\blacktriangle$, $\triangle$, 5 mM glutamate plus 5 mM malate; $\triangle$, 25
µM CaCl$_2$.

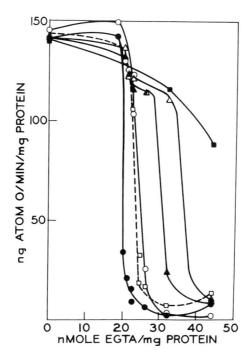

Fig. 3. *Inhibition by EGTA or EDTA of A23187-stimulated
succinate oxidation.* Mitochondria (1 mg protein) were incubated in 2.3 ml of a medium containing 4 mM Cl-(TEA) (pH 7.4),
8 mM succinate plus 1.3 μM rotenone, 7 mM KCl, 220 mM sucrose
and various concentrations of EGTA or EDTA (□, dashed line).
Respiration was measured polarigraphically. ● □ , no added
CaCl₂; ○, 5 nmole; ▲, 10 nmole; △, 15 nmole; and ■ , 20
nmole CaCl₂.

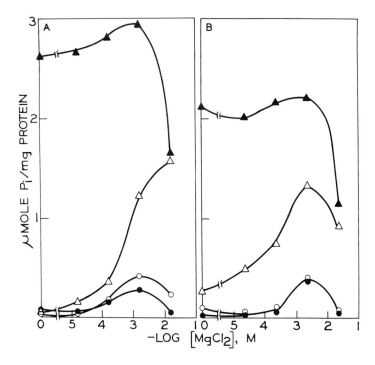

Fig. 4. *Prevention by magnesium chloride of ATPase inhibition by A23187.* Mitochondria (1-2 mg protein) were incubated for 10 min in 1 ml of a medium which contained 6 mM ATP, 10 mM Cl-(TEA), pH 7.4, 30 mM KCl, 96 mM sucrose, 75 mM mannitol and various concentrations of MgCl$_2$. ●, no further additions; ○, A23187, 2.2 nmole/mg in A, 0.5 nmole/mg in B; ▲, inducer, 2 μM monazomycin in A, 0.1 mM 2,4-dinitrophenol in B; △, inducer plus A23187.

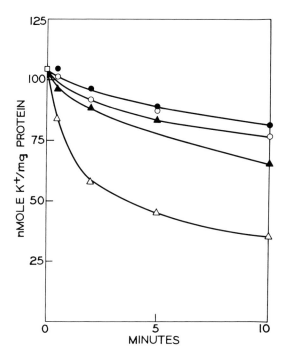

Fig. 5. *Effect of A23187 on mitochondrial potassium content.*
Mitochondria (21 mg protein) were incubated in the medium
described in the legend to Fig. 1 except that KCl was omitted.
●, no further additions; ○, 0.6 mM EDTA; ▲, 0.3 nmole
A23187/mg protein and △, A23187 plus EDTA.

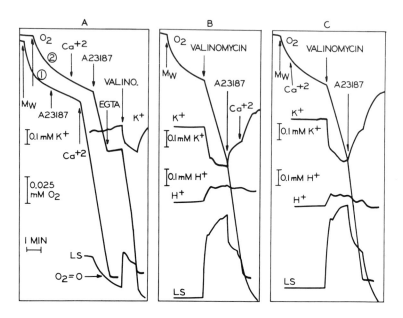

Fig. 6. *Reversal by A23187 of potassium uptake by mitochondria incubated with valinomycin.* Mitochondria were prepared with 1 mM EGTA present in all solutions except the final suspending medium. The incubation medium contained 4 mM Cl-(TEA) (pH 7.4), 2 mM PO₄-(Tris) (pH 7.4), 12 mM succinate plus 0.7 μM rotenone, 6 mM KCl, 212 mM sucrose, 10 mM mannitol and 7 mg protein of mitochondria. A23187, 0.8 μM (0.5 nmole/mg protein), valinomycin, 0.1 μM, CaCl₂, 20 μM and EGTA, 0.1 mM were added as indicated. A downward deflection of the oxygen, potassium or hydrogen ion electrode trace represents a decrease in the medium and an upward deflection of the light scattering trace indicates a decrease in absorbance (mitochondrial swelling).

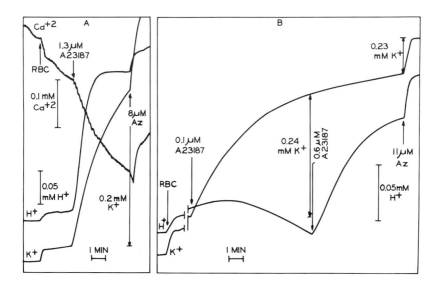

Fig. 7. *The effect of A23187 on ion content of erythrocytes incubated with calcium chloride.* Rat erythrocytes (94 mg protein in <u>A</u>, 106 mg protein in <u>B</u>) were added to 15 ml of a medium which contained 5 mM Tris-Cl (pH 7.4), 2 mM $CaCl_2$, 0.1 mM KCl and 150 mM choline chloride. AZ is azalomycin F (Lilly A17178). A downward deflection of the calcium, potassium or hydrogen ion electrode trace represents a decreased concentration in the medium.

127

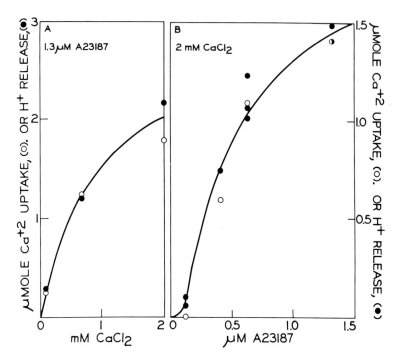

Fig. 8. *Calcium/proton exchange in erythrocytes incubated with A23187.* Erythrocytes (123 mg protein in A, 105 mg protein in B) were incubated in the medium described in the legend to Fig. 7 except that calcium chloride concentration was varied in the experiment described in panel A. Calcium uptake and proton release were measured at the point of maximal hydrogen ion exchange.

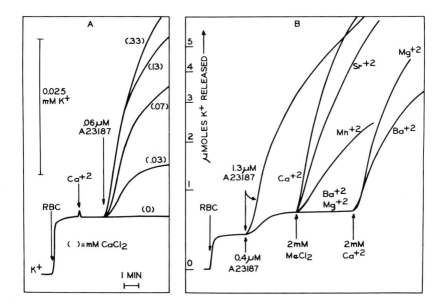

Fig. 9. *Potassium efflux from erythrocytes incubated with A23187 ± divalent cations.* Erythrocytes (23 mg protein in A, 95 mg protein in B) were added to a medium which contained 5 mM Tris-Cl (pH 7.4), 0.1 mM KCl, 150 mM choline chloride and other additions as indicated.

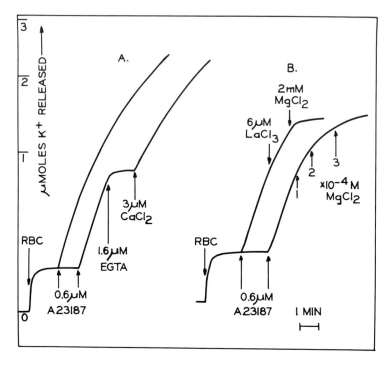

Fig. 10. *The effect of EGTA, lanthanum chloride and magnesium chloride on the potassium release from erythrocytes incubated with A23187.* Erythrocytes (33 mg protein) were incubated in the medium described in the legend to Fig. 9 with additions as indicated.

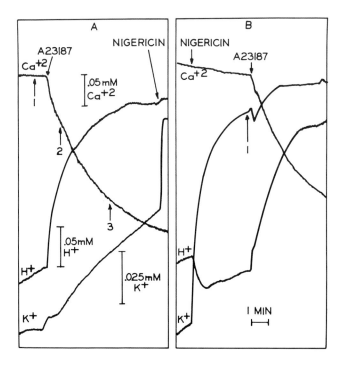

Fig. 11. *The effect of A23187 on ion movements in sperma-*
tozoa incubated with calcium chloride. Sperm (7.3 x 10^8)
were incubated in 12 ml of a medium which contained 4 mM
Cl-(TEA) (pH 7.4), 4 mM acetate-(TEA) (pH 7.4), 2.5 mM CaCl2,
0.8 mM KCl and 209 mM sucrose. In the experiment described
in panel A, 1.7 mM caffeine was present. A23187, 4 μM and
nigericin, 0.3 μM were added as indicated.

REGULATION OF GLUCOSE TRANSPORT IN HEART MUSCLE AND ERYTHROCYTES

Howard E. Morgan, Carol F. Whitfield and James R. Neely

Introduction

Sugar transport in muscle, adipose tissue, and erythrocytes is regulated by both hormonal and metabolic factors. The transport process involves the combination of sugar with a site within the membrane, referred to as a carrier, followed by the translocation of sugar into the cell. Kinetics of sugar transport have been studied in greatest detail in human and rabbit erythrocytes, but transport in these cells has not been found to be regulated by either hormonal or metabolic factors (1,2).

Detailed studies of kinetics of regulated transport have been hampered by a variety of factors. 1) Transport regulation occurs most commonly in cells that are organized into tissues. Studies of transport in tissues requires either that the tissue be perfused or be sufficiently thin to minimize restriction of access of sugar to the cells in the preparation. 2) Studies of the kinetics of glucose efflux have been among the most helpful in characterizing transport in human and rabbit erythrocytes. Since regulated transport is often a major restraint to glucose utilization, intracellular glucose accumulates to only low levels in the absence of an acceleratory factor. These low levels of intracellular glucose prevent efflux measurements. Even in the presence of such factors, transport often remains slow relative to the rate of glucose phosphorylation and only low levels of intracellular glucose are found. 3) An ideal non-metabolized glucose analog is not available. 3-0-methyl glucose, the most commonly employed analog, has high affinity for the carrier, but has the disadvantage that a significant fraction of its membrane penetration may be by simple diffusion. All other non-metabolized glucose analogs have relatively low affinity for the carrier. As a result, sufficiently high concentrations often cannot be achieved to adequately characterized the kinetic constants. Since these limitations have prevented detailed kinetic studies, regulated transport has been dealt with thus far on the basis of a simple carrier model.

Experiments that are reported in this paper will focus on non-hormonal factors regulating transport in heart muscle and avian erythrocytes. *In vitro* preparations of heart muscle that were perfused and physiologically active were employed for these studies. Avian erythrocytes were investigated since they represent a free cell that can be obtained in large numbers and possess a regulated transport system.

Methods

Isolated rat hearts were perfused either by the classical Langendorff technique or in an apparatus designed to permit varying degrees of heart work (3,4). In the Langendorff preparation, Krebs-Henseleit bicarbonate buffer, gassed with either $O_2:CO_2$ (95:5%) or $N_2:CO_2$ was introduced into the aorta and passed through the coronary vessels. Perfusion pressure was generated by a peristaltic pump. Ventricular pressure development in this preparation could be varied by increasing perfusion pressure.

In working preparations, buffer was introduced into the left atrium from a reservoir whose position above the heart could be varied to change left atrial filling pressure. The left ventricle pumped the fluid into a pressure chamber which was 1/3 filled with air to provide elasticity to the system. Fluid was pumped from this chamber to a height of 70 cm where it flowed back into the apparatus. Pressure development by the heart was varied by changing left atrial filling pressure.

At the end of perfusion, hearts were frozen while still being perfused by clamping the tissue between blocks of aluminum cooled to the temperature of liquid nitrogen (5). The tissue was powdered in a percussion mortar that was also maintained at the temperature of liquid nitrogen. Aliquots of the powder were used for estimation of sugar and extracellular spaces and dry weight (6). Utilization of glucose was estimated by measuring disappearance of sugar from the perfusate.

Red cells were obtained from domestic geese and washed with Krebs-imidazole glycylglycine buffer containing 0.2% bovine serum albumin (7). White cells were removed during the washing procedure. Cells were incubated at 37° in tissue culture roller bottles and the suspensions were gassed with O_2 or N_2. In some experiments, glucose utilization was estimated by following its disappearance from the extracellular medium. In other experiments, ^{14}C-3-0-methyl glucose was added to give a final concentration of 12.5 mM and its rate of entry was followed over the next 30 min.

Results and Discussion

Regulation of Sugar Transport in Heart Muscle.

Glucose transport is the major reaction regulating consumption of exogenous glucose by the perfused heart. As seen in Table I, aerobic hearts had a low rate of glucose uptake and intracellular glucose levels that were too low to be detected. These findings indicated that phosphorylation was able to dispose of the glucose as rapidly as it entered the cell and that transport restricted the overall rate of glucose utilization (8). Insulin increased the rate of glucose uptake and led to accumulation of free intracellular glucose. These findings indicated that the hormone had accelerated transport to the extent that the capacity of glucose phosphorylation was exceeded (8-10). Anoxia markedly accelerated transport as indicated by a large increase in glucose uptake and by accumulation of free intracellular glucose (11,12). These studies indicated that sugar transport was a major rate-limiting step for glucose utilization in heart muscle and that this step was markedly accelerated by insulin and anoxia.

Increased ventricular pressure development in hearts perfused with left atrial filling pressures of 10 or 20 mm Hg accelerated glucose uptake (6). Free intracellular glucose was not detected at any of these levels of filling pressure indicating that glucose phosphorylation was able to keep pace with entry under all of these conditions. These data also indicated that membrane transport was accelerated as the work and pressure development of the heart was increased.

In other experiments, acceleration of sugar transport by insulin, increased ventricular pressure development, and

anoxia was confirmed by measuring the accumulation of non-
metabolized glucose analogs, L-arabinose and 3-0-methyl
glucose. In earlier experiments, L-arabinose, 3-0-methyl
glucose, and glucose were shown to share the same transport
system by demonstrations of counterflow and competitive
inhibition (13). The fraction of intracellular water equilibrated with L- arabinose in a period of 10 min was increased
from 1 to 29% by insulin, to 19% by raising left atrial
pressure to 10 mm Hg, and to 28% by anoxia. These studies
confirmed the conclusion based on measurements of glucose
uptake that these factors accelerated glucose transport.

Following the observation of Shipp *et al.* (14) that
long chain fatty acid would inhibit glucose uptake by muscle, the role of fatty substrates in regulating various
steps in the uptake process was extensively investigated.
Williamson and Krebs (15) found that ketone bodies would
inhibit uptake and Randle *et al.* (16) localized the effects
of these substrates to transport and phosphofructokinase.
The effect of fatty acids on transport that was identified
by these workers involved an inhibition of the insulin
stimulation. In addition, fatty acids had a powerful inhibitory effect on the stimulation of glucose transport
that was associated with increased ventricular pressure
development (17). When pressure development was increased
by raising left atrial filling pressure to 10 mm Hg, glucose
uptake increased approximately 3 fold (Table I). Addition
of 1.6 mM palmitate bound to 3% albumin had little effect
at 0 mm Hg left atrial filling pressure but completely
blocked the increased glucose utilization seen at the higher
filling pressure. Under all of these conditions, intracellular free glucose remained below the level of detection
indicating that transport remained the major limiting step.
In other experiments, an effect of fatty acid on transport
was confirmed by studying the entry of 3-0-methyl glucose
into the heart. Addition of palmitate reduced methyl glucose entry slightly in hearts developing low levels of
ventricular pressure, but completely inhibited the rise
in transport associated with development of higher levels
of ventricular pressure. β-hydroxybutyrate and acetate
were also able to block the rise in transport associated
with increased pressure development. These results indicate
that either long or short chain fatty acids would inhibit
sugar transport.

In summary, the major non-hormal factors affecting
transport in heart muscle were absence of oxidative metabol-

ism, increased pressure development by the ventricle, and availability of fatty substrates. Insulin exerted the major hormonal control. These factors, as well as others, interacted to give a fine control of transport rate. Although large effects of hormonal and metabolic factors could be demonstrated in the perfused heart, the complexity of the tissue made studies of the mechanisms difficult. As a result, studies of a simpler system, the avian erythrocyte, in which transport regulation occurred was undertaken.

Regulation of Sugar Transport in Avian Erythrocytes.

In 1925, Negelein (18) observed that uptake of glucose by nucleated, respiring erythrocytes of geese was stimulated by cyanide poisoning. Since, in most non-primate erythrocytes, transport is rate-limiting for glucose utilization, these results suggested that avian erythrocytes might be a useful model for study of the mechanism of the anaerobic stimulation of transport. As seen in Table II, an accelerated rate of glucose uptake was found in the anaerobic cells that was due to a 3 fold increase in maximal transport rate. In these studies, intracellular glucose levels were below the level of detection indicating that glucose transport was a major rate-limiting step for glucose utilization in avian erythrocytes and that this step was facilitated by anoxia.

In other experiments, the conclusion that sugar transport was accelerated in anaerobic cells was confirmed by measuring entry of 3-0-methyl glucose, L-glucose, and D-sorbitol into avian erythrocytes that were incubated in an atmosphere of either oxygen or nitrogen. After 1 hour of incubation, 6% of the intracellular water was equilibrated with L-glucose in either aerobic or anaerobic cells. Under similar conditions, 8% of the intracellular water was equilibrated with D-sorbitol. On the other hand, 36% of the intracellular water was equilibrated with 3-0-methyl glucose in aerobic cells and 60% in anaerobic suspensions. These studies indicated that the stereospecific sugar transport system had been accelerated rather than a diffusion pathway that served L-glucose and D-sorbitol.

The magnitude and reversibility of the effect of anoxia on 3-0-methyl glucose transport was also investigated. Cell suspensions that were pre-incubated for 1 hour under aerobic conditions had a half-time for 3-0-methyl glucose entry of

60 min. In this system 30–45 min of anoxia were required
for a significant stimulation of transport. After 1 hour
of preincubation under anaerobic conditions, half-time for
3-0-methyl glucose entry was 25 min. If the gas phase was
switched from N_2 to O_2 after 60 min of incubation, transport rate reverted to the aerobic rate with a T 1/2 of
67 min, indicating that the anoxic effect on sugar transport
was reversible.

Aerobic restraint of transport was lost in red cells
that had been subjected to reversible hemolysis (7). In
the experiments presented in Table III, cells were rapidly
suspended in buffers containing ^{14}C-3-0-methyl glucose and
^{3}H-sorbitol at the osmolality that is indicated. After 1
min of exposure to this osmolality, sufficient 2.5 M KCl
was added to restore osmolality to 300 milliosmoles/l. The
cells were washed three times and suspended in buffer for
measurement of exit of 3-0-methyl glucose and D-sorbitol.
The aerobic restraint of sugar transport was lost when the
osmolality of the lysing solution was below 100 millios-
moles/l. In association with the increase in transport,
both hemoglobin and acid-soluble material absorbing at
260 nm were lost. In contrast, membrane permeability of
D-sorbitol remained low indicating that the membranes had
resealed and were selectively permeable. The maximal effect
was achieved when the osmolality of the lysing solution was
25 milliosmoles.

The aerobic restraint on transport also depended upon
the presence of sulfhydryl groups (7). Addition of a
variety of sulfhydryl blocking agents including iodoacetate,
n-ethylmaleimide, or mercuric chloride markedly accelerated
entry of 3-0-methyl glucose into the cells. The effect of
treatment with mercuric chloride was greater than the effect
of cyanide. The sulfhydryl blocking agents appeared to
affect the carrier-mediated entry of 3-0-methyl glucose
since this entry was competitively inhibited by glucose.
In addition, the effects of mercuric chloride on the rate
of sugar entry was rapidly reversed by addition of dithiothreitol. These experiments indicated that the aerobic
restraint on transport depended upon the presence of sulfhydryl groups. Addition of blocking agents removed this
restraint and allowed transport rate to increase approximately 5-fold.

The anaerobic effect on sugar transport in avian
erythrocytes did not depend upon the ionic composition of
the buffer. An anaerobic stimulation of transport was seen

in Na-free, K-free, Mg-free, Mg and Ca-free buffer, and in buffer containing ouabain.

The properties of transport regulation that have been described thus far are consistent with a model of transport control that was originally suggested by Randle and Smith (19). In this model, the sugar carrier in the membrane is considered to be a protein with hydroxyl groups, such as those on serine residues, exposed to the inside of the cell and available for phosphorylation. In the phosphorylated form, the carrier would be immobile, but when dephosphorylated it would change configuration to allow transport. Phosphorylation could be regulated either by changing the activity of a protein kinase or a phosphatase. The enzyme activities could be controlled by the levels of high and low energy intermediates such as ATP, AMP, and inorganic phosphate. In aerobic cells in which ATP levels are high and AMP and P_i levels are low, the carrier is assumed to be in the phosphorylated form. In the anaerobic state, the carrier would be dephosphorylated and, therefore, mobile. In this model, reversible hemolysis could be envisioned to stimulate transport either by loss of ATP or of the protein kinase. The stimulatory effect of sulfhydryl blocking agents could be accounted for by inhibition of the kinase. The first step in testing this model was to relate changes in the levels of nucleotide triphosphates and P_i to the onset of the anoxic effect on sugar transport.

When avian erythrocytes were incubated in substrate-free buffer, intracellular nucleotide triphosphate concentration was maintained at about 3.5 mM for 40 min in anoxic cells, but then fell rapidly (Table IV). Nucleotide triphosphate declined more slowly in aerobic cells. Transport stimulation began when nucleotide triphosphate levels started to fall, but transport stimulation was well-developed before nucleotide triphosphate loss was extensive. It should be noted that aerobic cells incubated for 180 min had the same nucleotide triphosphate level as anoxic cells that were incubated for 60 min but the anaerobic rate of transport was 2-3 times the aerobic rate.

The inorganic phosphate content of the cells varied inversely with the level of nucleotide triphosphate (Table IV). In aerobic cells, P_i either decreased slightly or remained the same. While in anaerobic cells, P_i increased to 7.5 mM. P_i began to rise before a loss of nucleotide triphosphate could be detected. In both aerobic and anoxic

139

cells, P_i was released from the cells into the medium along its concentration gradient. In suspensions of anoxic cells, the increase in P_i in the medium plus the intracellular water corresponded to a gain of 3 phosphates for each nucleotide triphosphate lost. Nucleotide triphosphate levels and 3-0-methyl glucose transport were inversely related. When nucleotide triphosphate concentrations were between 1.0 and 3 mM, a decrease of 0.5 mM was associated with approximately a 50% increase in transport rate. From these results, it appeared that extensive depletion of nucleotide triphosphate was not required for the initial stimulation of sugar transport but was coincident with maximal transport rate.

The time course of changes in P_i would suggest that it could be a candidate for a transport stimulator since it increased significantly before transport was accelerated. To test the effect of a change in intracellular P_i on the rate of transport, cells were incubated in buffer with increasing concentrations of P_i and 3-0-methyl glucose entry and intracellular P_i were measured. Incubation in 10 mM P_i, increased intracellular P_i to the same extent as occurred during anoxia, but had no effect on the transport of 3-0-methyl glucose. This would indicate that an increase in P_i alone was not responsible for initiation of the anoxic effect.

The role of adenine nucleotides as modulators of the anoxic effect has been explored by incubating cells in buffers containing a range of these compounds from adenine to ATP, and measuring the rate of 3-0-methyl glucose entry. ATP (5 mM) consistently stimulated entry of sugar into aerobic cells, decreasing the half-time of entry from 70 to 41 min. Addition of UTP or GTP had no effect on transport rate. On the other hand, adenine (3 mM) inhibited the anaerobic stimulation of transport, increasing half-time from 20 to 32 min. Adenosine, AMP, ADP, or mixtures of AMP or ADP and P_i had no effect. When ATP was added to the extracellular medium it was broken down to AMP and a small amount of IMP within 10 min. When the effects of anoxia and ATP were compared, both factors produced about the same changes in cell levels of P_i, but extracellular ATP had a smaller effect to accelerate the rate of 3-0-methyl glucose transport. Anoxia reduced the half-time of 3-0-methyl glucose entry from 81 to 35 min while extracellular ATP reduced the half-time to only 54 min. These studies reinforced the suggestion that anoxia was affecting the rate of sugar transport by mechanisms other than increasing intracellular inorganic phosphate.

Summary

Membrane transport in muscle was accelerated by insulin, anoxia, and increased rates of ventricular pressure development. Fatty substrates effectively antagonized the stimulation of transport associated with increased pressure development. Anoxia also stimulated stereospecific sugar entry into avian erythrocytes. The aerobic restraint was lost if the red cells were reversibly hemolyzed or exposed to sulfhydryl blocking agents. Acceleration of sugar transport in avian erythrocytes began as nucleotide triphosphate levels started to fall. However, addition of ATP to the extracellular phase stimulated entry of 3-0-methyl glucose. Inorganic phosphate did not appear to be primarily responsible for regulating transport rate. These findings are consistent with a phosphorylation-dephosphorylation model of transport regulation.

Presented by Howard E. Morgan. Supported by NIH Grant No. HL-13029-03

References

1. Wilbrandt, W. and T. Rosenberg. The concept of carrier transport and its corollaries in pharmacology. Pharm. Rev. 13: 109 (1961).
2. Regen, D. M. and H. E. Morgan. Studies of the glucose-transport system in the rabbit erythrocyte. Biochim. Biophys. Acta 79: 151 (1964).
3. Morgan, H. E., J. R. Neely, R. E. Wood, C. Liebecq, H. Liebermeister and C. R. Park. Factors affecting glucose transport in heart muscle and erythrocytes. Fed. Proc. 24: 1040 (1965).
4. Neely, J. R., H. Liebermeister, E. J. Battersby and H. E. Morgan. Effect of pressure development on oxygen consumption by the isolated rat heart. Amer. J. Physiol. 212: 804 (1967a).
5. Wollenberger, A., O. Ristau and G. Schoffa. A simple

technic for extremely rapid freezing of large pieces of tissue. Pflueger Arch. Ges. Physiol. 270: 399 (1960).

6. Neely, J. R., H. Liebermeister and H. E. Morgan. Effect of pressure development on membrane transport of glucose in isolated rat heart. Amer. J. Physiol. 212: 815 (1967b).

7. Wood, R. E. and H. E. Morgan. Regulation of sugar transport in avian erythrocytes. J. Biol. Chem. 244: 1451 (1969).

8. Morgan, H. E., M. J. Henderson, D. M. Regen and C. R. Park. Regulation of glucose uptake in muscle. The effects of insulin and anoxia on glucose transport and phosphorylation in the isolated, perfused heart of normal rats. J. Biol. Chem. 236: 253 (1961).

9. Lundsgaard, E. On the mode of action of insulin. Uppsala Läkareforen Förh. 45: 143 (1939).

10. Park, C. R., J. Bornstein and R. L. Post. Effect of insulin on free glucose content of rat diaphragm *in vitro*. Amer. J. Physiol 182: 12 (1955).

11. Randle, P. J. and G. H. Smith. Regulation of glucose uptake by muscle. The effects of insulin, anaerobiosis and cell poisons on the uptake of glucose and release of potassium by isolated rat diaphragm. Biochem. J. 70: 490 (1958).

12. Morgan, H. E., P. J. Randle and D. M. Regen. Regulation of glucose uptake by muscle. The effects of insulin, anoxia, salicylate and 2:4-dinitrophenol on membrane transport and intracellular phosphorylation of glucose in the isolated rat heart. Biochem. J. 73: 573 (1959).

13. Morgan, H. E., D. M. Regen and C. R. Park. Identification of a mobile carrier-mediated sugar transport system in muscle. J. Biol. Chem. 239: 369 (1964).

14. Shipp, J. C., L. H. Opie and D. Challoner. Fatty acid and glucose metabolism in the perfused heart. Nature 189: 1018 (1961).

15. Williamson, J. R. and H. A. Krebs. Acetoacetate as fuel of respiration in the perfused rat heart. Biochem. J. 80: 540 (1961).

16. Randle, P. J., E. A. Newsholme and P. B. Garland. Regulation of glucose uptake by muscle. Effects of fatty acids, ketone bodies and pyruvate and of alloxan diabetes and starvation, on the uptake and metabolic fate of glucose in rat heart and diaphragm muscle. Biochem. J. 93: 652 (1964).

17. Neely, J. R., R. H. Bowman and H. E. Morgan. Effects of

ventricular pressure development and palmitate on glucose transport. Amer. J. Physiol. 216: 804 (1969).

18. Negelein, D. Versuche über glykolyse. Biochem. Z. 158: 121 (1925).

19. Randle, P. J. and G. H. Smith. Mechanism of action of insulin. In: F. G. Young, W. A. Broom and W. F. Wolff (Editor), Mechanism of action of insulin. Oxford Press, London (1960), pp. 65-76.

20. Neely, J. R., C. F. Whitfield and H. E. Morgan. Regulation of glycogenolysis in hearts; effects of pressure development, glucose and FFA. Amer. J. Physiol. 219: 1083 (1970).

TABLE I

REGULATION OF GLUCOSE TRANSPORT IN THE PERFUSED RAT HEART

Uptake was measured over a period of 1 hour following a preliminary perfusion of 10 min. Perfusate glucose was 16 mM. The concentration of insulin was 0.5 µg/ml; the palmitate was 1.6 mM.

Left Atrial Filling Pressure	Gas Phase	Insulin	Palmitate	Glucose Uptake	Intracellular Glucose
mm Hg				*µmoles/g/hr*	*mM*
0	$O_2:CO_2$	0	0	76 ± 29^a	N.D.^{b}
0	$O_2:CO_2$	+	0	373 ± 17	5.9 ± 0.8
0	$N_2:CO_2$	0	0	638 ± 39	2.7 ± 0.7
0	$O_2:CO_2$	0	+	58 ± 10	N.D.
10	$O_2:CO_2$	0	0	219 ± 40	N.D.
10	$O_2:CO_2$	0	+	35 ± 7	N.D.
20	$O_2:CO_2$	0	0	378 ± 53	N.D.

[a] *Data are expressed as Mean±SEM*

[b] *N.D. - none detected*

TABLE II

EFFECT OF INHIBITION OF OXIDATIVE METABOLISM
ON GLUCOSE TRANSPORT IN AVIAN ERYTHROCYTES

*Goose red cells were incubated as described in Experimental
Procedure. Data from Wood and Morgan (7).*

Condition	V_{max}	K_m
	μmoles/g/hr	*mM*
Aerobic	1.04	0.35
Cyanide-treated	3.36	0.80

TABLE III

EFFECT OF REVERSIBLE HEMOLYSIS ON EXIT OF
3-0-METHYL GLUCOSE AND D-SORBITOL FROM GOOSE ERYTHROCYTES

The experiment is described in the text. Data from Wood and Morgan (7).

Conditions of incubation	Osmolality of lysing solution, *milliosmoles/l*			
	25	50	100	300
% equilibrium/min				
Aerobic				
3-0-methyl glucose	2.8	‾2.4	0.7	0.7
D-sorbitol	0.2	0.3	0.3	---
Cyanide-treated	---	3.2	2.8	2.7

TABLE IV

EFFECT OF ANOXIA ON INTRACELLULAR LEVELS OF ATP AND INORGANIC
PHOSPHATE IN GOOSE ERYTHROCYTES.

*Suspensions of goose erythrocytes were incubated for the periods that are indicated.
Nucleotide triphosphate and P_i were measured in perchloric acid extracts as described
earlier (20).*

Metabolite	Gas Phase	Period of incubation, min				
		0	20	40	60	80
Nucleotide triphosphate, mM	O_2	3.5 ± 0.2[a]	3.5 ± 0.2	3.4 ± 0.2	----	2.8 ± 0.2
	N_2	3.5 ± 0.2	3.4 ± 0.2	3.4 ± 0.1	2.0 ± 0.1	0.7 ± 0.1
P_i, mM	O_2	3.8 ± 0.1	3.6 ± 0.6	2.9 ± 0.5	2.6 ± 0.2	2.1 ± 0.2
	N_2	3.8 ± 0.2	3.8 ± 0.6	5.3 ± 0.5	7.1 ± 0.5	7.3 ± 0.7

[a]*Data are expressed as Mean ± SEM*

CARBOXYLIC IONOPHORES AS MOBILE CARRIERS FOR DIVALENT IONS

Berton C. Pressman

Despite its simplicity of structure, ionic Ca^{++} is one
of the most important mediators of membrane-related phenomena
in biology. This ion plays a key role in muscular contraction, both in the coupling of neural excitation to the
contractile process and in the mechanism of contraction at
the molecular level (1). In nerves Ca^{++} is involved in
determining the firing threshold and has been implicated in
the propagation of the action potential (2). It is required
for the function of secretory granules in synaptic transmission as well as the neural release of catacholamines from the
adrenal (3). Its removal is required for the formation of
high permeability cellular junctions which have been implicated in the regulation of cell growth via contact inhibition
(4). This list is by no means complete.

All these processes are subject to regulation by the
level of available Ca^{++}, which, in turn, is a function of
the active and passive transport of Ca^{++} across membranes.
A variety of substances is known which inhibit the Ca^{++}
permeability of membranes thereby producing a multitude of
profound *in vitro* and *in vivo* effects. Among these are
local anaesthetic amines (5), La^{+++} (5) and ruthenium red
(6). As a corollary, agents which could increase the permeability of membranes would be expected to exert equally profound effects.

The class of antibiotics known as ionophores take their
name from their ability to carry ions across membranes (7).
The structure of the first member of this class recognized,
valinomycin (8), is illustrated in Fig. 1 (9). It forms
lipid soluble complexes with alkali ions by enfolding them
in a cage which focuses the polar liganding oxygens about the
cation within the center of a cylinder, the alkyl groups
orienting about the exterior. This complex can easily
traverse the low polarity interior barrier of biological
membranes by simple diffusion. This, in conjunction with

rapid complexation-decomplexation capability at the polar membrane interfaces, adequately explains the ion carrier capacity of ionophores.

The neutral ionophores form complexes analagous to those of valinomycin, which display a net charge arising from the complexed ion. Nigericin (Fig. 2) illustrates a second class of ionophores which feature a highly assymetric chain of heterocyclic rings containing a terminal carboxyl (10). Since the carboxyl must be deprotonated when the cation complexes are formed, the latter are electrically neutral zwitterions; differences in response to a trans-membrane potential between the charged complexes of neutral ionophores and the neutral complexes of carboxylic ionophores account for the former acting as electrophoretic carriers while the carboxylic ionophores behave as neutral, exchange diffusion carriers (7).

The larger energies of desolvation required for dehydra-tion of divalent cations had suggested that they would not be efficient complexations substrates for ionophores and hence in earlier work little attention was given to the possibility of divalent cation complexes of ionophores. The published X-ray crystallographic structure of X-537A however suggested to us that ionophore-mediated divalent cation trans-port is indeed feasible (11). We had previously established the affinity monovalent cation selectivity pattern of X-537A by means of equilibrium two phase association complex deter-minations ($Cs^+>Rb^+ = K^+>Na^+>Li^+$), and the kinetic function, the rate of release of alkali cations from resealed human erythrocytes ($Cs^+>Rb^+>K^+>Na^+>Li^+$) (12). By analagous pro-cedures we have been able to establish the existence of lipid soluble divalent cation complexes of X-537A. Table I gives the divalent cation association complexes of X-537A ($Ba^{++}>Sr^{++}>Ca^{++}>Mg^{++}$) as determined by two phase distribution studies.

Although the ability to form a complex with a given cation is a prerequisite for ionophore mediated transport, the fulfilling of this criterion does not necessarily guar-antee that complexation-decomplexation kinetics will favor efficient transport of a given cation by a given ionophore. Figure 3 established experimentally that X-537A does indeed transport Ca^{++}, as well as K^+, across a low polarity bulk solvent.

Figure 4 provides a formal representation of the molec-ular features of X-537A as revealed by X-ray crystallography

150

of its Ba^{++}salt (11). One ionophore moiety of the 2:1 complex, termed the *unprimed* ionophore, ligands to the cation via two ether oxygens, two hydroxyls, a ketonic carboxyl and a carboxyl oxygen (Fig. 4). These six ligands create a configuration not too dissimilar to that known for the silver complexes of other carboxylic ionophores (*c.f.* Fig. 2) and indicate a likely structure for X-537A in monovalent cation complexes. The second for *primed* ionophore (Fig. 5) has an entirely different configuration, liganding by the carboxyl, a hydroxyl at the other end of the molecule, and a water molecule held to the ionophore backbone by hydrogen bonds. The two ionophore moieties ligand to the Ba^{++} by a total nine oxygens, the largest number of ligands yet reported in an ionophore complex.

A space filling model of X-537A, constructed according to the configurations indicated by X-ray crystallography, differs significantly from that of nigericin in the orientation of the liganding oxygens. Whereas those of nigericin form a buckled plane with the oxygens focused toward the center, in X-537A the liganding oxygens all orient toward the same side of the ring. This implies that while nigericin engulfs its complexed cation equitorially, X-537A prefers to offer cations a polar platform to sit on. The fact that the size fit required to sit on a platform is less demanding than that required for a cation inserting itself within the plane of the ring may explain the relatively low degree of monovalent cation selectivity of X-537A as compared to nigericin.

In complexes of X-537A one side of the complexed cation is relatively unhindered by ligands to the platform-forming ionophore. In the case of divalent cations, which have a strong positive charge, a second ionophore ligands to this side. Since its access to the cation is evidently impeded by the first ionophore, fewer ligands are formed to the second ionophore.

The chromophores of X-537A, the aromatic system which absorbs at 245 and 310 nm, and the ketonic carbonyl absorbing at 290 nm offer a convenient conformational probe in solution via circular dichroism measurements. The elipticity of the ketonic carbonyl is not altered markedly during complexation, however the elipticity of the 245 nm spectral band varies greatly depending on the cationic species complexed, indicative of conformational distinctions between different ionophore complexes. Moreover, the monovalent cation complexes of X-537A as a group differ qualitatively in conformation from those of the divalent cations. Molecular models suggest that in monovalent complexes the

151

carboxyl is flexible enough to ligand to the side opposite
the platform thereby wedging the cation into a sandwich; in
the divalent cation complexes the equivalent sandwich is
formed by two ionophore moieties. Thus the tendency to
form platforms, with the oxygens available for liganding
all oriented towards the same side, may account for the
divalent ion affinity of X-537A (13).

In the course of studies of the osmotic effects of
ionophore-induced permeability in chloroplasts and erythrocytes, it became apparent that X-537A is not only able to
transport alkali and alkaline earth cations, but also the
Tris buffer cation as well. Further study revealed that
X-537A is an excellent complexing agent for primary amines
in general, having progressively less affinity for the
increasingly hindered nitrogens of secondary and tertiary
amines, and virtually no affinity for quaternary amines,
e.g. tetraalkylammonium ions.

Since the aromatic ring of X-537A is particularly
amenable for derivatizing, it was possible to obtain an
extensive series of derivatives in which the ring was
substituted at position "X" (Fig. 4) by electronegative
groups or the phenolic hydroxyl was acylated by various
groups. All derivatives of this type tested formed lipid
soluble cation complexes.

If one grants as reasonable that the substituents on
the phenolic ring do not affect the ionophore conformation
directly, but only indirectly primarily by their inductive
effect on the liganding carboxyl, it then becomes possible
to examine the effects on complexation of progressively
reducing the charge on the carboxylate group. The inductive
effects of the various substituents can in turn be calibrated
by determining the carboxyl pK_a by titration with a non
complexing base (Table II). It can be seen that the rank
order of electronegativity is $NO_2 > I > Br > Cl$. Acetylation of
the phenolic hydroxyl raises the pK_a above that of the parent ionophore. In this case however there may be some more
direct effect on conformation since the hydrogen bond to the
carboxylic oxygen is eliminated. As can be seen in Table I,
lowering the pK_a raises the complexing affinity for divalent
ions (according to other experiments, monovalent ions as
well). This indicates that reducing the carboxylic negative
charge by pulling its electrons through the aromatic ring
into the substuent group actually increases complexation
affinity for cations, an unexpected relationship the explanation of which is not obvious.

The biological implications of the ability of X-537A and its derivatives to complex amines were explored by testing its ability to form complexes with catacholamines. In Table III we see that X-537A, better than any of the other tested ionophores, is able to form complexes with norepinephrine and its parent compound ethanolamine. As implied above, the hindering effect of the N-methyl group of epinephrine is strongly evident. The relative proclivity of X-537A for forming primary amine complexes is perhaps best dramatized by comparing the ratio of its K_A for ethanolamine to that of nigericin (360:1), with the relative K_A's of these ionophores for K^+ (1:90). In line with previous considerations this might be interpreted in terms of the platform structure of X-537A providing less opportunity for hinderance by the alcoholic group of ethanolamine than does the open hole structure of nigericin. Thus, the ability to complex divalent ions and primary amines probably both depend on the same molecular feature, orientation of the liganding oxygens to the same side of the plane of the complex. In this light it is interesting to note that dianemycin, which is the ionophore second best to X-537A in divalent complex formation, is also runner up in primary amine complexation.

These data indicate not only that ionophores, particularly X-537A, have the physiologically important capability of altering the intra- and intercellular distribution of biologically active amines, but that they also offer a model for adrenergetic receptors, possessing the molecular requisites for sharp discrimination between norepinephrine and epinephrine.

We shall now examine what effects these ionophores produce on actual biological preparations. Despite the ease with which the distinguishing chemical and physical properties of ionophores can be observed in retrospect, historically it was the effect of ionophores on mitochondrial energy-linked K^+ transport which led to their recognition (8). Some of the effects of the divalent ionophore A23187, which is highly selective for divalent over monovalent ions on mitochondria, erythrocytes and sperm, have been reported by Reed and Lardy at this conference (14).

We chose to examine the effects of the divalent ionophore on the smooth muscle of the aorta because this preparation is thin, readily permeated by external agents, and well characterized pharmacologically. In Fig. 6 we see that X-537A is able to induce a contraction of aortic rings similar to that of a subsequent addition of norepinephrine.

In view of the previously described properties of X-537A the contraction could have been due to one of three possibilities: availability to the myofibrils of Ca^{++} permeating from the exterior; availability to the myofibrils of Ca^{++} relocated from interior sites; or direct mobilization of intracellular catacholamines followed by a secondary release of intracellular Ca^{++} (8). Contemplated experiments in which Ca^{++} fluxes will be isotopically monitored ought to resolve these possibilities.

Although the contraction of aortic strips induced by A23187 (Fig. 7) is not as dramatic as that produced by X-537A, its interpretation is less ambiguous. The contraction in the bathing medium containing 1.5 mM Ca^{++} is just barely discernable. However, when the external Ca^{++} is raised to 10 mM a slow but definite contraction is obtained. Control strips showed no response to the elevated Ca^{++} alone. Moreover A23187 does not show any marked ability to complex norepinephrine or alkali ions. In this case the contraction appears to be unambiguously due to the entry of Ca^{++} into the strip under the combined influence of the Ca^{++} gradient and the ionophore-induced permeability of the plasmalemma.

The vesicular preparations derived from the sarcoplasmic reticulum of skeletal or cardiac muscle also responds to divalent ionophores (15,16). These vesicles are derived from the cisternae of the sarcoplasmic reticulum, which is the principle reservoir for the Ca^{++} released on neural excitation to effect contraction. The fluorescent probe technique of Caswell and Warren (17), which monitors intravesicular Ca^{++}, has been used to follow the ionophore-induced release of accumulated Ca^{++}. By this technique A23187 is sixty fold more potent than X-537A in transporting Ca^{++} across the membrane of the vesicles even though the Ca^{++} affinity of A23187 is one hundreth that of X-537A as determined by the two phase toluene-butanol water cation distribution technique (18).

Among the known ionophores, A23187 and X-537A are uniquely fluorescent, and the quenching of this electronic function upon complexation offers a means for determining the cationic K_A in a single polar phase. The Ca^{++}-A23187 K_A measured in this fashion in 80% ethanol is fifty fold greater that that of the Ca^{++}-X-537A K_A, in line with their respective abilities to transport Ca^{++} across the sarcoplasmic reticulum(18). Two important conclusions may be drawn from this data.

The rate-limiting reaction of ionophore-mediated Ca^{++} transport across the sarcoplasmic reticulum vesicles occurs in a polar environment and is therefore likely to be complexation between the intramembranal ionophore and extramembranal Ca^{++} at the interface; since the ionophore mediates a passive transport of Ca^{++} down its concentration gradient, the free concentration of Ca^{++} accumulated within the vesicles is higher than that of the medium. This latter conclusion is incompatible with suggested mechanisms of intravesicular ion accumulation driven by a simple membrane-binding process (18).

The heart has even more options of response to ionophores since it combines systems for electrical pacemaking, impulse conduction, chemoreception and muscular contraction. In Fig. 8 we see that X-537A can increase both the strength of contraction (positive ionotropic effect) and the rate of contraction. X-537A is also able to increase the contractility of electrically paced atrial strips.

Determination of the membrane potential of the isolated Purkinje fiber indicate that X-537A hyperpolarizes this intracardiac conductive element thereby lowering its excitability. This latter effect has salutary implications for the control of cardiac arrythmias while the contractile effects of X-537A may suggest a new agent for stimulating the output of the failing heart.

The recent discovery of ionophores which can transport divalent ions indicate that we may not have a definitive picture of all possible patterns of ionophore behavior. Thus X-537A not only forms complexes ($Ba^{++}>Sr^{++}>Ca^{++}>Mg^{++}$) and transports ($Sr^{++}>Ca^{++}>Mg^{++}>Ba^{++}$) divalent cations but alkali ions and organic amines as well. A23187 on the other hand is highly selective for divalent ions ($Ca^{++}>Mg^{++}>Sr^{++}>Ba^{++}$) (14) having little tendency to interact with alkali ions and organic amines. The fluorescent properties of these ionophore species have also opened up new approaches for elucidation of their molecular properties and may provide a sensitive enough means for observing them directly while functioning within membranes. The ionophores described here increase the experimental tools at our disposal for perturbing biological systems in order to uncover new details of their component mechanisms. Ultimately it may be possible to harness the properties of ionophores so as to provide new therapeutic agents for the pharmacolocical alleviation of pathological conditions.

Presented by Berton C. Pressman. The author wishes to thank Robert Adair, Frank Lattanzio, Virginia Posey, Peggy Gerba and Drs. Kenneth Lasseter, Anthony H. Caswell, Norberto T. de Guzman and Sigma R. Alpha who contributed to various phases of this work. The work was supported by grants from NIH (HE-14434) and the Florida Heart Association (71-A6-36) and gifts from Eli Lilly and Hoffman-LaRoche. He is also indebted to the latter two companies for the antibiotics used in these studies.

References

1. Harris, P. and L. H. Opie (Editors), Calcium and the Heart (several articles containing both new and review material on the role of Ca^{++} in muscle contraction may be found in this publication), (1971) Academic Press, New York.
2. Shanes, A. M. Electrochemical aspects of physiological and pharmacological action in excitable cells. Pharmacol. Rev. 10: 59 (1958).
3. Douglas, W. W. and R. P. Rubin. The mechanism of catecholamine release from the adrenal medulla and the role of calcium in stimulus-secretion coupling. J. Physiol. (London) 167: 288 (1963).
4. Loewenstein, W. R. Permeability of membrane junctions. Ann. N.Y. Acad. Sci. 137: 441 (1966).
5. Mela, L. Inhibition and activation of calcium transport in mitochondria. Effect of Lanthanides and local anesthetic drugs. Biochemistry 8: 2481 (1969).
6. Moore, C. L. Specific inhibition of mitochondrial Ca^{++} transport by ruthenium red. Biochem. Biophys. Res. Commun. 42: 298 (1971).
7. Pressman, B. C., E. J. Harris, W. S. Jagger, and J. H. Johnson. Antibotic mediated transport of alkali ions across lipid barriers. Proc. Natl. Acad. Sci. 58: 1949 (1967).
8. Moore, C. and B. C. Pressman. Mechanism of action of valinomycin on mitochondria. Biochem. Biophys. Res. Commun. 15: 562 (1964).
9. Shemyakin, M. M., N. A. Aldanova, E. I. Vinogradova, and M. Yu. Fiegina. The structure and total synthesis of valinomycin. Tetrahedron Letters 1921 (1963).

10. Steinrauf, L. K. and M. Pinkerton. The structure of nigericin. Biochem. Biophys. Res. Commun. 33: 29 (1968).
11. Johnson, S. M., J. Herrin, S. J. Liu, and I. C. Paul. The crystal and molecular structure of the barium salt of an antibiotic containing a high proportion of oxygen. J. Am. Chem. Soc. 92: 4428 (1970).
12. Pressman, B. C. and M. J. Heeb. In: D. Vasquez (Editor), Symposium on Molecular Mechanisms of Antibiotic Action on Protein Synthesis and Membranes, Amsterdam: Elsevier. In press.
13. Alpha, S. R. and B. C. Pressman. Manuscript in preparation.
14. Reed, P. W. and H. A. Lardy, Chapter 4, this conference.
15. Scarpa, A. and G. Inesi. Ionophore mediated equilibration of calcium ion gradients in fragmented sarcoplasmic reticulum. FEBS Letters 22: 273 (1972).
16. Entman, M. L., P. C. Gillette, E. T. Wallick, B. C. Pressman, and A. Schwartz. Biochem. Biophys. Res. Commun. In press (1972).
17. Caswell, A. S. and S. Warren. Observation of calcium uptake by isolated sarcoplasmic reticulum employing a fluorescent chelate probe. Biochem. Biophys. Res. Commun. 46: 1757 (1972).
18. Caswell, A. S. and B. C. Pressman. Manuscript submitted for publication.

TABLE I

RELATIVE AFFINITIES OF X-537A AND DERIVATIVES FOR DIVALENT IONS

Complex formation was determined as the migration upon shaking of the test cation from an aqueous Tricine buffer (pH 9.0) into an organic phase consisting of 70% toluene and 30% n-butanol in which the test ionophore was dissolved. Cation concentrations in each phase were determined by either atomic absorption (Mg^{++}) or radioisotope techniques ($^{45}Ca^{++}$, $^{89}Sr^{++}$, $^{133}Ba^{++}$). The ionophore was held constant at 5×10^{-4} M and the two phase complexation K_A calculated from the average value obtained over a range of aqueous cation concentrations according to the equation:

$$K_A = \frac{M^{++}I_2^{-}{}_{org}}{M^{++}_{H_2O} \cdot \left(I_{org}\right)^2} = \frac{M^{++}_{org}}{M^{++}_{org} \cdot \left(I_i - \dfrac{M^{++}_{org}}{2}\right)^2}$$

where M^{++}_{org} is the concentration of radioactive cation measured in the organic phase (indicative of $M^{++}I_2$ formation), $M^{++}_{H_2O}$ is the concentration of radioactive cation in water, I_i the concentration of ionophore initially added to the organic phase and $\dfrac{M^{++}_{org}}{2}$ the amount of I_i complexed as $M^{++}I_2$.

All values obtained were divided through by the K_A for the Ca – X-537A complex.

	Ac-537A	X-537A	Br-537A
Mg^{++}	0.26	0.38	0.54
Ca^{++}	0.29	1	2.8
Sr^{++}	1.8	8.5	18
Ba^{++}	72	2600	5600

TABLE II

pK_a OF X-537A AND RELATED COMPOUNDS

Acetyl - X-537A	6.30
X-537A	5.80
Cl - X-537A	5.35
Br - X-537A	4.95
I - X-537A	4.75
NO_2- X-537A	4.20
Nigericin	8.45
Salicylic Acid	5.05

pK_a was determined by titrating in 90% ehtanol at 30° with tetramethylammonium hydroxide.

TABLE III

AFFINITIES OF ORGANIC AMINES FOR CARBOXYLIC IONOPHORES

The procedure employed was the same as described in Table II except that ^{14}C-labeled ethanolamine and D,L-epinephrine and ^{3}H-D,L-norepinephrine were used in place of the test cations. K_A were calculated as:

$$K_A = \frac{M^+I^-_{org}}{M^+_{H_2O} \cdot I_{org}} = \frac{RNH_3^+{}_{org}}{\left(RNH_2 + RNH_3^+\right)_{H_2O} \cdot \left(I_i - RNH_3^+\right)_{org}}$$

where $RNH_3^+{}_{org}$ is the concentration of radioactive amine in the organic phase, $(RNH_2 + RNH_3^+)_{H_2O}$ is the concentration of radioactive amine in the water phase, I_i the initial concentration of ionophore in the organic phase and $(I_i - RNH_3^+)_{org}$ the concentration of uncomplexed I in the organic phase.

IONOPHORE	ETHANOLAMINE	NOREPINEPH.	EPINEPH.
X-537A	415	163	5.8
Dianemycin	65	31	4.2
Monensin	3	9	0.9
Nigericin	1.2	5	1.8

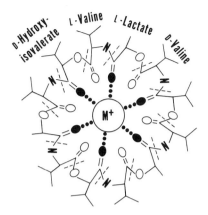

Fig. 1. *Formal structure of ionophore complexes of valinomycin.* The filled in oxygens are those which are involved in cation liganding according to X-ray crystallography.

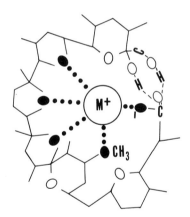

Fig. 2. *Formal structure of ionophore complexes of nigericin.* The liganding oxygens are filled in; hydrogen bonds are indicated by dashed lines.

161

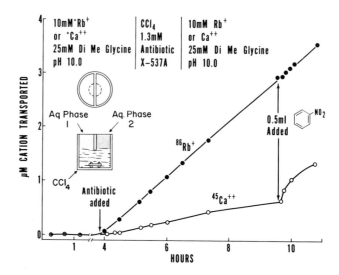

Fig. 3.   *X-537A mediated bulk phase transport of* $^{86}Rb^+$ *and* $^{45}Ca^{++}$.   The construction of the experimental vessel is indicated in the insert.   At t=0, $^{86}Rb^+$ or $^{45}Ca^{++}$ was placed in one aqueous compartment and its appearance in the oppo- site compartment monitored by periodic sampling.   No detect- ible radioactivity traversed the CCl$_4$ layer prior to the addition of ionophore.   Addition of nitrobenzene after 9 hours, which raised the polarity of the organic phase, stimulated $^{45}Ca^{++}$ transport but not that of $^{86}Rb^+$.

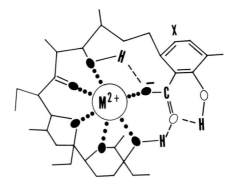

Fig. 4.   *Formal structure of the "unprimed" ionophore moiety of the barium complex of X-537A.*

162

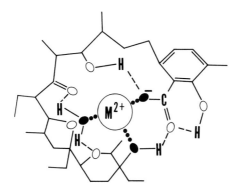

Fig. 5. *Formal structure of "primed" ionophore moiety of the barium complex of X-537A.*

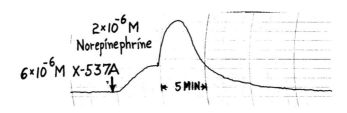

Fig. 6. *X-537A Induced contraction of rabbit aortic ring.*
The ring was mounted to a tension transducer in an isotonic
medium buffered with Tris and containing 1.5 mM Ca^{++}. After
the ring had completed its response to X-537A addition of
norepinephrine produced a further contraction.

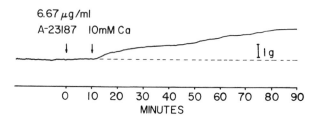

Fig. 7. *Ca⁺⁺ induced contraction of rabbit aortic ring
pretreated with A23187.* The barely discernable contraction
induced by A23187 is augmented by raising the Ca^{++} content
of the Tris buffer medium from 1.5 mM to 10 mM.

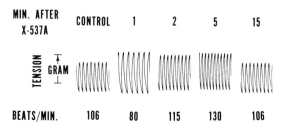

Fig. 8. *Effect of X-537A on the contraction of the perfused
rabbit heart.* The isolated heart was perfused with Tyrode's
solution containing 1.5 mM Ca^{++} and the contractions recorded
isometrically. A single dose of 8×10^{-8} moles of X-537A
produced an immediate increase in contractile force of 43%
and a decrease in beat frequency. Beat frequency then
increased to a maximum 5 min after the addition accompanied
by a slow decrease in contractile force. After 15 min the
heart had returned to its control beat frequency and tension.

REGULATION OF THE TRANSLOCATION OF ADENINE NUCLEOTIDES ACROSS THE INNER MITOCHONDRIAL MEMBRANE BY LONG CHAIN ACYL COA ESTERS

Earl Shrago, Austin Shug, Charles Elson and Edith Lerner

Introduction

It is now recognized that the translocation of adenine nucleotides, *i.e.* ADP and ATP, across the inner mitochondrial membrane constitutes a key role in energy linked respiration. The translocase enzyme or carrier, though not solubilized or purified, has been studied extensively, and the considerable amount of experimental data suggest a close relationship between adenine nucleotide translocation and oxidative phosphorylation. The ADP specificity of oxidative phosphorylation results from the nucleotide specificity of the adenine nucleotide translocase (1); the number of adenine nucleotide binding sites equals the number of cytochrome oxidase molecules (2); and in the steady state of phosphorylation the rate of ATP formation inside the mitochondria equals the rate of ATP transport out of the mitochondria (3). Because of the central role of adenine nucleotide transport in mitochondrial metabolism, any natural inhibitors would serve as potential physiological regulators. Atractyloside (4) and bonkreckic acid (5) inhibit adenine nucleotide translocation; however, these compounds are not normally found in animal tissues.

More recently, it has been shown that long chain acyl CoA esters, normal constituents of animal tissues, can act as natural *in vivo* inhibitors of the adenine nucleotide translocase (6). This inhibition, which is reversible, can effectively control State3-State4 respiration and perform a physiological role in the regulation of mitochondrial metabolism. Long chain acyl CoA esters, which accumulate in the liver of diabetic and fasting animals, are associated with alterations in the adenine nucleotide ratio and redox state of the cell (7). The direct *in vivo* observation of an inhibited adenine nucleotide translocase in diabetes (6) suggests a casual relationship of translocation to the altered pyridine and adenine nucleotide levels found in the diabetic liver.

Methods

Experimental details for the translocation studies are given in a previous publication (6). Carnitine acyltransferase was assayed according to the procedure of Bremer (8) as modified by Hoppel and Tomec (9). The assay measures the formation of radioactive palmityl carnitine from palmityl CoA and labeled carnitine.

Results and Discussion

There is considerable evidence that at relatively high concentrations, long chain fatty acids stimulate ATPase activity (10) and uncouple oxidative phosphorylation (11). The isolation of an endogenous uncoupling and swelling agent with the properties of oleic acid (12) and the ability of albumin to reverse the uncoupling effect of fatty acids (11), suggest their possible physiological role in the regulation of oxidative metabolism. Alternatively, the specificity and significance of these effects have been questioned because of the general detergent like properties of long chain fatty acids. Falcone and Mao (13) observed that certain long chain saturated and unsaturated fatty acids at concentrations too low to cause uncoupling or stimulate ATPase activity inhibit the $^{32}P_i$-ATP exchange activity in rat liver mitochondria. The effectiveness of the saturated fatty acids were directly proportional to chain length up to C-16. These results were compatible with previous observations of Pressman and Lardy, who first described the stimulation of endogenous ATPase activity by long chain fatty acids (10). Effects of fatty acids on mitochondrial metabolism are shown in Table I. Inhibition of $^{32}P_i$-ATP exchange activity is only apparent when oxidation of the fatty acids is blocked by KCN. Exchange activity, which measures a partial reaction of oxidative phosphorylation, is dependent upon penetration of ATP through the inner mitochondrial membrane. More direct experiments of nucleotide transport using ^{14}C ADP indicate translocation is inhibited by the long chain fatty acids plus KCN.

Myristic acid was the most potent inhibitor of the saturated fatty acids. Oleic acid but not its trans isomer, eleidic acid, produced marked inhibition. Substitution of a bromine for a hydrogen atom in the α position *eliminated* the inhibitory effect of myristic acid. Pande *et al.* (14) have shown that α-bromopalmitate inhibits the activation of long chain fatty acids by rat liver preparations.

Wojtczak and Zaluska (15) have shown a direct effect of oleic acid on adenine nucleotide translocation. The requirement for KCN in our studies suggested that a metabolic intermediate, most likely the acyl CoA derivative of the fatty acid, was the actual inhibitory agent. Studies using the CoA esters rather than the fatty acids themselves gave more clear cut results and support this hypothesis. Strong inhibition of adenine nucleotide translocation was observed particularly with myristoyl CoA, palmityl CoA, and oleoyl CoA (Table II). This inhibition could be reversed by simultaneous addition of carnitine. It seems likely that carnitine permits further metabolism of the CoA derivative by the carnitine acyltransferase enzyme.

Long chain acyl CoA esters have demonstrable effects on respiratory control (Fig. 1). Mitochondria incubated with succinate show a sharp increase in State 3 respiration upon addition of ADP. Prior addition of oleoyl CoA inhibits penetration of ADP and stimulation of respiration. Addition of uncouplers of oxidative phosphorylation (salicylanilide XIII) bypasses the poor penetration of ADP and restores respiration by uncoupling it from endogenous phosphorylation.

Long chain fatty acids and their CoA esters are elevated in liver during those physiological (hibernation) and pathophysiological (diabetes) conditions associated with increased fatty acid oxidation (16,17). In comparison to control animals, respiration by mitochondria from diabetic rats and hibernating ground squirrels, prepared with minimal washing in order not to remove endogenous lipid (Fig. 2), was slow and only minimally stimulated by ADP. Again, addition of salicylanilide XIII increased respiration by uncoupling endogenous oxidative phosphorylation. When penetration of adenine nucleotides was measured directly with ^{14}C–ADP, considerably lower values than normal were obtained (Table III). Normalization of translocation could be achieved by addition of carnitine or albumin to stimulate further metabolism of the acyl CoA ester and complex the fatty acids.

These *in vivo* observations substantiate the *in vitro* results and give strong indication that a reversible in-

hibition of adenine nucleotide translocation constitutes
an important regulatory mechanism in cell metabolism.
Although fatty acid stimulation of gluconeogenesis in rat
liver is well documented, postulated mechanisms of action
which include an effect on the oxidation-reduction state
of the cell (18) and provision of excess acetyl CoA to
inhibit pyruvate oxidase and stimulate pyruvate carboxylase
(19) are still incomplete. It has been suggested that
elevated levels of long chain free fatty acids in liver
could enhance gluconeogenesis from certain amino and keto
acids by partially uncoupling oxidative phosphorylation
(20). A subsequent increase in the rate of flow of inter-
mediates to oxalacetate and stimulation of GTP production
would result from substrate level phosphorylation coupled
to oxidation of ketoglutarate. The majority of reducing
equivalents in rat liver mitochondria for reduction of
oxalacetate to malate could be supplied by the oxidation of
fatty acids, either directly or possibly through an energy
linked reversal of electron transport (21). Long chain
acyl CoA esters may, by inhibiting adenine nucleotide translocation and inducing a transition from State 3 to State 4
respiration, serve in this capacity. This metabolic condi-
tion would be particularly effective in regulating the
ADP/ATP ratio and in generating reducing equivalents through
reverse electron transfer. Figure 3 represents the proposed
mechanism of action of the long chain acyl CoA ester on the
translocase site as compared to the inhibitors atractyloside
and bongkreckic acid. It appears logical to assume that the
ADP moiety of the CoA derivative displaces the free nucleotide or competitively competes for the binding site on the
translocase. Chain length of the CoA ester is important
since neither the shorter chain esters nor CoA itself are
inhibitory.

The accumulation of the long chain acyl CoA ester
necessary to inhibit the adenine nucleotide translocase is
naturally dependent upon its synthesis and subsequent metabolism. It may be significant that the rate limiting step
for fatty acid oxidation is the transport of the long chain
acyl CoA through the inner mitochondrial membrane as an
acyl carnitine intermediate (22). A schematic representation illustrates the sequence of reactions which effects
the transfer of long chain fatty acids across the inner
mitochondrial membrane to their site of oxidation inside
the mitochondria (Fig. 4). It is now known that there are
two long chain carnitine acyltransferase enzymes located on

the inner mitochondrial membrane, one more tightly bound
than the other (9). Transport across the inner mitochondrial membrane is thus the major site of regulation for
penetration of both adenine nucleotides and long chain acyl
CoA esters. It might be speculated, therefore, that the
juxtaposition of the adenine nucleotide translocase and
carnitine acyltransferase may be such as to permit an inter-
dependent regulation of their enzymatic activities.

The potential significance of reversible inhibition of
adenine nucleotide translocation in the control of intermediary metabolism is particularly apparent in the rat (6).
The potent stimulus for gluconeogenesis by fatty acid
oxidation may be the result of a transition from State 3
to State 4 respiration with a concomitant reversal of
electron transfer. This would alter the DPN/DPNH and
ATP/ADP ratios to favor gluconeogenesis. However, in some
animals, particularly the guinea pig, long chain fatty
acids are ineffective and even inhibitory to gluconeogenesis
(23). Differences between the rat and the guinea pig might
be explicable on the basis of the sensitivity of the adenine
nucleotide translocase to long chain acyl CoA esters, or the
metabolism of the esters via the carnitine acyltransferase.
Table IV shows that when KCN is omitted, $^{32}P_i$-ATP exchange
activity in guinea pig liver mitochondria is more susceptible to oleoyl CoA than is rat mitochondria. In Table V,
comparison of the carnitine acyltransferase enzymes in the
two animals indicates that guinea pig liver mitochondria
contains considerably less enzyme than the rat, under both
normal and fasting conditions. These conditions might
predispose to an inhibited translocase in the guinea pig,
not freely reversible, and place a severe drain on ATP
synthesis necessary for gluconeogenesis. This data is as
yet too incomplete, however, to be anything more than suggestive.

Respiratory control and adenine nucleotide translocation in rat heart as well as liver mitochondria are sensitive to long chain acyl CoA esters (Tables VI and VII).
The heart preferentially utilizes fatty acids over glucose
for energy purposes (24). There is a growing body of evidence to indicate that under anoxic conditions, fatty acids
can be deleterious to myocardial function, and they have
been incriminated as causative factors leading to severe
arrhythmias and sudden death following myocardial infarction (25). Impaired circulation of the heart might mimic
the experimental system shown here with KCN and anaerobiasis

(Table VIII).Inability to metabolize the fatty acids normally could lead to irreversible inhibition of adenine nucleotide translocation which would be incompatible with life.

It is likely that a number of drugs, many of clinical significance, can act similar to long chain acyl CoA esters as effectors of adenine nucleotide translocation. It is of interest that atractyloside, a potent glycoside inhibitor of adenine nucleotide translocation, was originally studied when it was found to possess toxic properties producing fatal hypoglycemia (26).

Summary

The importance of adenine nucleotide translocation in the regulation of energy linked mitochondrial respiration was implied from the elegant studies carried out by many investigators in this area of research (1-5). It is now apparent that the levels of the long chain acyl CoA esters can act as natural effectors in this process. The exact regulatory mechanism, however, is yet to be defined. A pulsatile process might be envisioned in which the level of long chain acyl CoA esters is controlled at the inner mitochondrial membrane by the carnitine acyltransferase enzymes. Since the activation of the fatty acid to the acyl CoA ester is not rate limiting, momentary accumulation could occur under conditions of high rates of lipolytic activity and fatty acid oxidation. Alternate metabolic pathways, such as transacylation of the CoA ester to tri-glyceride and phospholipids, would also contribute to the existing concentration of the long chain CoA ester at the inhibitory site.

Presented by Earl Shrago

References

1. Souverijn, J. H. M., P. T. Weijers, G. S. P. Groot and A. Kemp, Jr. The adenine nucleotide translocator and the nucleotide specificity of oxidative phosphorylation. Biochim. Biophys. Acta 223: 31 (1970).

2. Weidemann, N. J., H. Erdelt and M. Klingenberg. The elucidation of a carrier site for adenine nucleotide translocation in mitochondria with the help of atractyloside. In: T. Bücher and H. Sies (Editors), Inhibitors-tools in cell research, Springer - Verlag, Heidelberg (1969), p. 324.

3. Heldt, H. W. Analysis of phosphorylation of edogenous ADP and of translocation yielding the overall reaction of oxidative phosphorylation. FEBS Symp. 17: 93 (1969).

4. Bruni, A., S. Luciani and C. Bortignon. Competitive reversal by adenine nucleotides of atractyloside effect on mitochondrial energy transfer. Biochim. Biophys. Acta 97: 434 (1965).

5. Henderson, P. J. F. and H. A. Lardy. Bongkrekic acid. An inhibitor of the adenine nucleotide translocator of mitochondria. J. Biol. Chem. 245: 1319 (1970).

6. Lerner, E., A. L. Shug, C. Elson and E. Shrago. Reversible inhibition of adenine nucleotide translocation by long chain fatty acyl coenzyme A esters in liver mitochondria of diabetic and hibernating animals. J. Biol. Chem. 247: 1513 (1972).

7. McLean, P., K. A. Gumma and A. L. Greenbaum. Long chain acyl CoA, adenine nucleotide translocation and the coordination of the cytosolic and mitochondrial compartments. FEBS Lett. 17: 345 (1971).

8. Bremer, J. Carnitine in intermediary metabolism. The biosynthesis of palmityl carnitine by cell subfractions. J. Biol. Chem. 238: 2774 (1963).

9. Hoppel, C. L. and R. J. Tomec. Carnitine palmityl transferase. Location of two enzymatic activities in rat liver mitochondria. J. Biol. Chem. 247: 832 (1972).

10. Pressman, B. C. and H. A. Lardy. Effect of surface active agents on the latent ATPase of mitochondria. Biochim. Biophys. Acta 21: 458 (1956).

11. Borst, P., O. A. Loos, E. O. Christ, E. C. Slater. Uncoupling activity of long chain fatty acids. Biochim. Biophys. Acta 62: 509 (1962).

12. Lehninger, A. L. and L. F. Remmert. An endogenous uncoupling and swelling agent in liver mitochondria and its enzymic formation. J. Biol. Chem. 234: 2459 (1959).

13. Falcone, A. B. and R. L. Mao. The effect of long chain fatty acids on orthophosphate-adenosine 5'-triphosphate exchange activity associated with oxidative phosphorylation. Biochim. Biophys. Acta 105: 233 (1965).

14. Pande, S. V., A. W. Siddiqui and A. Gattereau. Inhibi-

tion of long chain fatty acid activation by bromopalmitate and phytanate. Biochim. Biophys. Acta 248: 156 (1971).

15. Wojtczek, L. and H. Zaluska. The inhibition of translocation of adenine nucleotides through mitochondrial membranes by oleate. Biochem. Biophys. Res. Commun. 28: 76 (1967).

16. South, F. E. and W. A. House. Energy metabolism in hibernation. In: K. C. Fisher, A. R. Dawe, C. P. Lyman, E. Schonbaum and F. E. South (Editors), Mammaliam hibernation III. Elsevier, New York (1967), p. 305.

17. Wieland, O. Ketogenesis, gluconeogenesis and lipogenesis in diabetes mellitus and related states. In: J. Ostman and R. D. G. Milner (Editors) Diabetes, supplement. Excerpta Medical Foundation, Amsterdam (1969), p. 14.

18. Williamson, J. R. Interrelationships between fatty acid oxidation and the control of gluconeogenesis in perfused rat liver. Adv. in Enzyme Regul. 6: 67 (1968).

19. Tuefel, H., L. A. Menahan, J. C. Shiff, S. Bonig and O. Wieland. Effect of oleic acid on oxidation and gluconeogenesis from pyruvate $1-^{14}C$ in the perfused rat liver. Eur. J. Biochem. 2: 182 (1967).

20. Davis, E. J. and D. M. Gibson. Regulation of the metabolism of rabbit liver mitochondria by long chain fatty acids and other uncouplers of oxidative phosphorylation. J. Biol. Chem. 244: 161 (1969).

21. Walter, P., V. Paetkau and H. A. Lardy. Paths of carbon in gluconeogenesis and lipogenesis III. The role and regulation of mitochondrial processes involved in supplying precursors of phosphoenolpyruvate. J. Biol. Chem. 241: 2523 (1966).

22. Fritz, I. B. The metabolic consequences of the effects of carnitine on long chain fatty acid oxidation. FEBS Symp. 4: 39 (1968).

23. Söling, H. D., B. Willms, J. Kleineke and N. Gehloff. Regulation of gluconeogenesis in the guinea pig liver. Eur. J. Biochem. 16: 289 (1970).

24. Paul, O. Myocardial infarction and sudden death. Hosp. Pract. 6: 91 (1971).

25. Shipp, J. C., L. H. Opie and D. Challoner. Fatty acid and glucose metabolism in the perfused heart. Nature 189: 1018 (1961).

26. Bruni, A., H. R. Contessa and S. Luciani. Atractyloside as inhibitor of energy-transfer reactions in

liver mitochondria.   Biocheim. Biophys. Acta 60: 301
(1962).

TABLE I

EFFECT OF FATTY ACIDS ON $^{32}P_i$.–ATP EXCHANGE AND
^{14}C–ADP TRANSLOCATION IN RAT LIVER MITOCHONDRIA

*The basic incubation mixture for the exchange activity
contained 10 mM ATP, 10 mM $^{32}P_i$. (20,000 cpm), 75 mM Tris-
HCl (pH 7.0), and 45 mM sucrose in a volume of 1.0 ml.
The reaction was initiated with 2.5 mg of mitochondrial
protein and incubated at 20° for 15 min.   The basic
reaction mixture for ^{14}C ADP translocation of 40 mM Tris-
HCl (pH 7.4), 100 mM KCl, 1.0 mM MgCl$_2$, and 2.5 mg of
mitochondrial protein in a volume of 1.0 ml was incubated
for 4 min at 25°.   The reaction was then initiated by the
addition of 0.08 mM ^{14}C ADP (40,000 cpm).   After 2 min,
the reaction was terminated with atractyloside.*

Fatty Acid	KCN	Exchange Activity	Translocase Activity
0.03 mM	*1.0 mM*	*cpm/μmole ATP*	*cpm/pellet x 10^{-2}*
–	–	474	286
–	+	341	261
Butyric	–	455	283
Butyric	+	331	265
Octanoic	–	464	–
Octanoic	+	330	–
Myristic	–	425	286
Myristic	+	103	140
αBr Myristic	–	440	–
αBr Myristic	+	318	–
Palmitate	–	456	280
Palmitate	+	250	97
Stearic	–	460	289
Stearic	+	331	265
Oleic	–	418	292
Oleic	+	98	139
Elaidic	–	436	289
Elaidic	+	301	201

TABLE II

REVERSAL OF ACYL–CoA ESTER INHIBITION OF ^{32}P.–ATP
EXCHANGE ACTIVITY AND ^{14}C ADP TRANSLOCATION IN
RAT LIVER MITOCHONDRIA BY CARNITINE

Additions	Acyl–CoA	Exchange activity	Translocase activity
	μM	*cpm/μmole ATP*	*cpm/pellet x 10*$^{-2}$
None		452	145
Butyroyl–CoA	30	401	141
Stearoyl–CoA	3		139
Stearoyl–CoA	30	393	39
Stearoyl–CoA + Carnitine	30	440	141
Myristoyl–CoA	3		78
Myristoyl–CoA	30	78	11
Myristoyl–CoA + Carnitine	30	399	132
Palmitoyl–CoA	3		136
Palmitoyl–CoA	30	170	30
Palmitoyl–CoA + Carnitine	30	390	131
Oleoyl–CoA	3		77
Oleoyl–CoA	30	51	11
Oleoyl–CoA + Carnitine	30	376	127

TABLE III

(^{14}C)ADP TRANSLOCATION IN LIVER MITOCHONDRIA OF NORMAL AND
DIABETIC ANIMALS AND HIBERNATING GROUND SQUIRRELS

cpm/pellet x 10^{-2}

Additions	Rat		Monkey		Ground Squirrel	
	Normal	Diabetic	Normal	Diabetic	Active	Hibernator
None	282 ± 6.7[a]	157 ± 21.4	263 ± 18.6	85 ± 9.5	267 ± 4.6	27 ± 1.8
DL-Carnitine, 5mM	280 ± 2.0	255 ± 9.5	258 ± 17.1	168 ± 14.1	265 ± 4.2	55 ± 9.1
Albumin, 15 mg	279 ± 2.3	228 ± 10.4	261 ± 8.5	134 ± 17.1	266 ± 3.7	52 ± 1.7

[a]*Standard error (five to six animals in each group).*

TABLE IV

COMPARISON OF INHIBITION OF $^{32}P_i$-ATP EXCHANGE ACTIVITY BY
OLEIC ACID IN RAT AND GUINEA PIG LIVER MITOCHONDRIA

*Additions were KCN, 1.0 mM; CoA, 1.0 mM; and oleic acid
0.03 mM.*

Additions	Exchange Activity
	cpm/μmole ATP
Rat	
None	399
KCN	350
CoA	380
Oleic Acid	389
Oleic Acid + KCN	100
Oleic Acid + CoA	95
Guinea Pig	
None	360
KCN	295
CoA	315
Oleic Acid	210
Oleic Acid + KCN	85
Oleic Acid + CoA	60

TABLE V

COMPARISON OF LONG CHAIN CARNITINE ACYLTRANSFERASE
ENZYME ACTIVITY IN RAT AND GUINEA PIG LIVER MITOCHONDRIA

The incubation mixture contained 100 μmoles morpholinopro-
pane (pH 7.3), 0.4 μmole palmityl CoA, 4.0 μmoles D,L-
carnitine, 0.1 μCi D,L-(Me-^{14}C) carnitine, 160 μmoles KCl,
2.0 mg fatty acid poor albumin and 0.25-0.5 mg protein in
a total volume of 2 ml. The reaction was carried out for
5 min at 37°.

Parameters Examined	Rat	Guinea Pig
	μmoles/min/mg protein	
Liver		
normal	6.45 ± 4.8[a]	2.35 ± 0.3
fasted 48 hrs.	13.35 ± 2.0	3.73 ± 0.1
refed 48 hrs.	3.63 ± 0.3	3.40 ± 0.5
Heart		
normal	3.73[b]	3.25

[a]*Standard error for five animals in each group.*

[b]*Average of two experiments. Four heart combined in each*
experiment.

TABLE VI

ADENINE NUCLEOTIDE TRANSLOCASE ACTIVITY IN RAT HEART MITOCHONDRIA

Additions were at 0.03 mM.

Additions	Translocase Activity
	$cpm/pellet \times 10^{-2}$
None	609
Palmitic Acid	663
Oleic Acid	458
Palmityl CoA	49
Oleoyl CoA	36

TABLE VII

INHIBITION OF STATE 3 RESPIRATION IN HEART AND LIVER MITOCHONDRIA BY OLEOYL COA AND ITS REVERSAL BY CARNITINE

Additions were oleoyl CoA, 0.03 mM; thenoyltrifluroacetone 0.3 µM; and D,L-Carnitine, 5.0 mM. Experiments carried out as in Fig. 1.

Additions	O_2 Uptake	
	Heart	Liver
	µmoles/hr/mg protein	
None	4.75	1.30
Oleoyl CoA	1.45	0.71
Thenoyltrifluoroacetone	4.48	1.26
D,L Carnitine	4.63	1.38
Oleoyl CoA + D, L Carnitine	4.61	1.33

TABLE VIII

$^{32}P_i$-ATP EXCHANGE IN RAT HEART MITOCHONDRIA UNDER
ANOXIC CONDITIONS

KCN, 1.0 mM; Oleic acid, 0.03 mM; Nitrogen, 1.0 Atmosphere

Additions	Exchange Activity
	cpm/μmole ATP
None	325
KCN	297
KCN + Oleic Acid	145
Nitrogen	268
Nitrogen + Oleic Acid	98

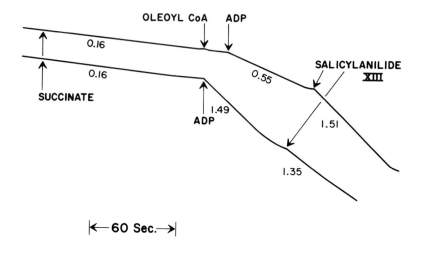

Fig. 1. *Control of respiration and response to oleoyl CoA by rat liver mitochondria.* Liver mitochondria (7.0 mg protein) was added to 2.0 ml reaction mixture containing 20 mM KCl, 225 mM sucrose, 10 mM KH_2PO_4, 5 mM $MgCl_2$ and 20 mM triethanolamine-HCl (pH 7.4). At the points indicated, 2.0 mM succinate was added followed by additions of 0.03 mM oleoyl CoA, 0.35 mM ADP, and 0.2 µM salicylanilide XIII. The numbers in the O_2 tracing represent the respiration rate expressed in µmoles of oxygen/mg protein/hour.

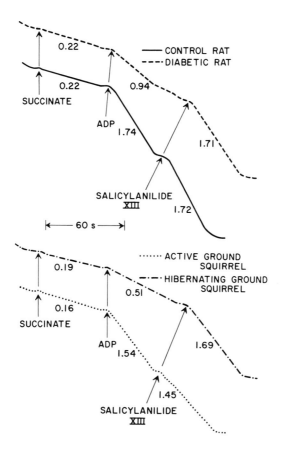

Fig. 2. *Respiratory control and response to salicylanilide XIII by liver mitochondria from normal and diabetic rats and active and hibernating ground squirrels.* Experiments carried out as in Fig. 1.

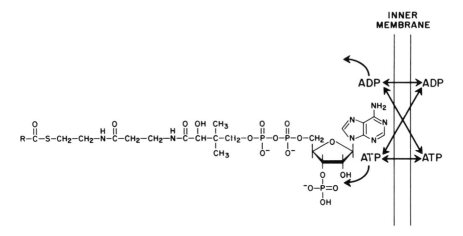

Fig. 3. *Schematic representation of how the long chain acyl CoA ester might inhibit translocation of adenine nucleotides across the inner mitochondrial membrane.* The adenine moiety of the CoA might effectively compete with the free nucleotide for the binding site on the translocase.

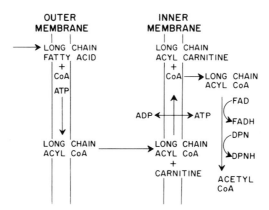

Fig. 4. *Metabolic pathway for the oxidation of long chain fatty acids.* Both long chain acyl CoA esters and adenine nucleotides (ADP and ATP) must be translocated across the inner mitochondrial membrane by specific enzymes. Interrelated activities of the long chain carnitine acyltransferase and adenine nucleotide translocase could affect the coordination of the ATP/ADP and DPN/DPNH ratios in the cell.

NAD$^+$ REDOX STATE AS RELATED TO MITOCHONDRIAL AND CELL MEMBRANES

Richard B. Tobin

Introduction

The redox state of NAD and NAD-linked substrates of different cellular compartments has been studied by a number of investigators (1-5). Their work indicates clearly that the redox ratios of free NAD associated with various dehydrogenase reactions in the cytoplams and in mitochondria are different. These references describe the relations between substrate concentrations and the redox state of NAD as well as the use of substrate assay to calculate NADH/NAD$^+$ ratios in cytoplasm and mitochondria.

We have for some time been interested in the effects of hydrogen ions on cellular metabolism, and through *in vitro* studies have made observations that shed light on the functioning of the plasma membrane and the mitochondrial membrane of liver cells.

The lactic dehydrogenase enzyme is located exclusively in the cytoplasm and the reaction is believed to be near equilibrium in living cells. Oxidized and reduced NAD$^+$ are cofactors in the reaction, and the redox ratio of lactate/pyruvate reflects directly the redox ratio of free cytoplasmic NAD (4). Similarly the enzyme β-hydroxybutyrate dehydrogenase is located exclusively in mitochondrial cristae and the redox state of its substrates β-hydroxybutyrate and acetoacetate reflect the redox ratio of intra-mitochondrial NADH and NAD$^+$. This enzyme reaction also takes place at or near equilibrium in cells. Williamson, *et al*. (4) showed that the NADH/NAD$^+$ ratio calculated from the β-hydroxybutyrate and acetoacetate is essentially the same as that calculated from α-ketoglutarate dehydrogenase substrates and products. α-Ketoglutarate dehydrogenase is located in the mitochondrial matrix, but apparently the NAD$^+$ associated with the enzyme in the cristae is in equilibrium with the matrix enzyme and either reaction can be utilized to evaluate the redox state of intramitochondrial NAD^+.

In evaluating these dehydrogenase reactions, people often overlook the fact that reduction of NAD from NAD^+ to NADH involves the dissociation of a proton. For example, lactate + $NAD^+ \rightleftharpoons$ pyruvate + NADH + H^+. References previously cited relate to studies performed with pH carefully controlled at or near 7. The effects of pH upon the redox state of NAD linked reactions are clearly demonstrable in systems *in vitro*, and we have studied the effects of pH changes upon the redox state of cytoplasmic and mitochondrial substrates that are in equilibrium with compartmental NAD of cells.

W. Mansfield Clark (6) has set forth a complete oxidation potential equation for lactate and pyruvate which is the following:

$$E_h = E_o + \frac{RT}{2F} \ln \frac{Pyruvate}{Lactate} + \frac{RT}{2F} \ln \frac{K'_L + [H^+]}{K'_p + [H^+]} + \frac{RT}{2F} hr [H^+]^2$$

Pyruvate and lactate are the total content of salt and undissociated acid. K'_L and K'_p are dissociation constants for lactic and pyruvic acids.

The measurable oxidation potential is related to the midpoint potential of the lactate and pyruvate system and to the total concentration of pyruvate and lactate. It is also related to the dissociation constants of these strong organic acids and to the hydrogen ion activity of the media. In living mammalian tissue the corrections for the undissociated forms of the two acids is small and at physiological pH values the redox formula may be simplified to the following equation:

$$E_h = E_m' - .03 \log_{10} \frac{[lactate]}{[pyruvate]} - .06 \text{ pH} \quad (7)$$

If one assumes that the oxidation potential of a system remains constant, one can calculate the effects of changes in pH upon the ratio of lactate/pyruvate from the above formula. Figure 1 shows a graph of the lactate/pyruvate ratio calculated in this manner as a function of pH. The E_m' for the reaction was taken as +.288 volts and E_h as -.185 volts, as has been measured at pH 7. This figure illustrates what we will call a theoretical plot of lactate/pyruvate

184

ratio versus pH. One can plot a similar theoretical β-hydroxybutyrate/acetoacetate ratio versus pH utilizing the measured $E_h = -.284$ at pH 7 and $E_o = .136$.

Methods

Free-hand cut rat liver slices were incubated in Krebs-Ringer-Phosphate with either 10 mM glucose or 10 mM pyruvate added as substrate. The pH of the preparations were measured after all components were added. Flasks were gassed with oxygen and incubated at 37° in a shaking water bath. Flasks were then placed on ice and aliquots of the media precipitated with perchloric acid. Lactate and pyruvate were assayed enzymatically (8,9). Acetoacetate and β-hydroxybutyrate were analyzed by the method of Mellanby and Williamson (10, 11).

Mitochondria were isolated by the method of Johnson and Lardy (12) and were incubated in a media containing 1 mM EDTA, 55 mM KCl, 5 mM magnesium chloride, 15 mM K_2HPO_4, 25 mM sucrose, and 25 mM TRIS. Ten millimolar β-hydroxybutyrate was added as substrate. Mitochondria were added and the flasks were gassed with oxygen and incubated at 25° for 30 min. The reaction was terminated by addition of 30% perchloric acid, and the β-hydroxybutyrate and acetoacetate content of the mitochondria were assayed as described above.

Liver homogenates were prepared with glass and teflon mortar and pestles. The homogenate was shaken and incubated in a well oxygenated media, gassed with 100% oxygen, and incubated at 37° for 30 min. An aliquot of the preparation was assayed for protein by biuret method and the remainder of the solution was precipitated with perchloric acid and assayed for lactate and pyruvate by the methods described above.

Direct assays of NAD^+ and NADH were made by the method of Van Dam (13).

Results and Discussion

Figure 2 shows the lactate and pyruvate contents and the lactate to pyruvate ratio of liver slices incubated at 37° for 1 hour. The content of both lactate and pyruvate have increased in the more alkaline media. This is the consequence of increased glycolytic rates in the more alka-

line media and also the result of trapping of organic acids
by the media. More interesting is the lactate/pyruvate
ratio which has increased in media with pH above 8. It is
readily apparent that this curve is completely different
from the theoretical lactate/pyruvate versus pH curve
presented in Fig. 1.

We have assumed in these studies that the oxidation
potential remains constant because of gassing of the flasks
with oxygen before and during the experimental procedure.
Since these are *in vitro* studies with liver slices, there
is no problem of pH altering perfusion of the tissue and we
have presumed that there is constant oxygen diffusion to
the cells of the slices. Study of oxygen consumption by
liver slices in Krebs Ringers Phosphate media shows that
the rate changes from 2.5 μM of oxygen/g dry weight/min at
pH 6 to a maximum of 3.5 at pH 8.5. Because oxygen consumption has increased in more alkaline media, the oxygen
requirement of these tissues is somewhat greater. The
slices were quite thin (approximately 0.3 mm in thickness)
and in the presence of high concentrations of oxygen,
diffusing of oxygen into the slice should not have been
rate limiting.

Because the cytoplasmic redox couplet was not in equilibrium with theoretically predicted values, we looked next
at the redox ratio of mitochondrial NAD by assay of the
β-hydroxybutyrate and acetoacetate couplet. Results of
these studies are shown in Fig. 3, and these data with ketone bodies parallel rather closely the results of studies
of lactate and pyruvate. The content of ketone body in the
media increased as the pH of the media increased. In a
manner very similar to the lactate/pyruvate ratio the β-
hydroxybutyrate to acetoacetate ratio increased as pH
increased thus differing from the theoretically predicted
curve.

Since neither cytoplasmic nor mitochondrial redox
couplets of NAD linked reactions were influenced by pH of
the media in a manner predicted from a redox equation, we
considered next the role of the plasma membrane as a
barrier to pH effects. Figure 4 presents the results of
experiments with liver homogenates. In this case the content of the lactate and pyruvate was relatively constant
at pH above 7, but significantly lower at pH 6. The lactate/
pyruvate ratio of the homogenates much more closely approxi-
mates a theoretical ratio. The calculated lactate/pyruvate
ratios however were not identical with theoretical values

at any pH, and at pH's greater than 7.4 the measured ratios
tended to rise. It is clear from these experiments that
disrupting the plasma membrane by homogenizing the liver
preparations permits the lactate/pyruvate redox ratio of
the preparation to come much more closely into accord with
the theoretical equilibrium values.

To gain further insight into the nature of membranes
of a subcellular particle we carried out studies of pH
effects upon the β-hydroxybutyrate to acetoacetate ratio of
isolated rat liver mitochondria. Results of these studies
are presented in Fig. 5. The acetoacetate content tended
to increase from pH 5 to 7 and remain constant at pH greater
than 7. The β-hydroxybutyrate content decreased markedly
from pH 5 to 6.5 and tended to remain constant at pH's
greater than 6.5. The ratio paralleled the β-hydroxybutyrate content and is fairly similar to the theoretically
predicted ratio. These studies show that the pH of the
incubating media has marked influence upon the redox ratio
of β-hydroxybutyrate/acetoacetate in a manner that is quite
similar to the theoretically predicted influence. This is
in contrast to the studies with the liver slices wherein
both lactate/pyruvate ratio and β-hydroxybutyrate to acetoacetate ratio are quite different from the theoretically
predicted values. Thus, it appears that the mitochondrial
membranes offers no major barrier to pH influence since in
the incubated slices the β-hydroxybutyrate to acetoacetate
ratio was very similar to the lactate to pyruvate ratio
and in isolated rat liver mitochondria the pH effect upon
the β-hydroxybutyrate to acetoacetate ratio was quite
similar to the theoretically predicted value. It appears
then that cytoplasmic mechanisms are the primary determinants
of the redox state of these substrates of dehydrogenase
reactions linked to NAD. Our findings also indicate that
there is no major pH gradient between cytoplasm and mitochondria in the relatively intact cells and do not support
the chemiosmotic theory of oxidative phosphorylation.

Since our data suggest that cytoplasmic processes are
responsible for setting the redox state of the NAD linked
substrates and since these studies do not pinpoint the primary site of determination of redox ratio, we next looked
at the total NAD^+ and NADH content of rat liver slices incubated *in vitro*. The free cellular NAD participating in
the lactic dehydrogenase and β-hydroxybutyrate dehydrogenase
reaction represents a small portion of the total cellular
NAD. The majority of NAD appears to be bound to cell pro-

187

teins, but the bound NAD must be in some sort of equilibrium or steady state relation to the free-NAD. We questioned if we could evaluate potential control of the NAD redox state through study of the total NAD rather than through study of the small fraction of free NAD associated with the two dehydrogenases in question.

The results of these studies are shown in Fig. 6 which graphs the NADH to NAD^+ ratio versus pH at the media. In this case, flasks were incubated for 30 min at 37° and the media contained 40 mM niacin. The sum of NAD^+ + NADH was the same at all pH's. The ratio with pyruvate as a sub-strate was constant whereas the ratio with glucose as sub-strate increased significantly at pH's above 6. This was due largely to the decrease in the NAD^+ content with a slight increase in NADH. The finding of constant total NADH to NAD^+ ratio versus pH with pyruvate as substrate and in-creasing ratio with glucose as substrate suggests to us that glycolytic mechanisms were responsible for these findings. We postulate that pyruvate participated as a metabolic sub-strate, bypassing the glycolytic system, and entered the TCA cycle and electron transport chain directly. Glucose, however, prior to entry to the TCA cycle, traversed the entire glycolytic chain. We feel that glycolysis is pH sensitive and that it is the determinant of the NAD redox ratios in these experiments and probably the determinant of the free NAD redox ratio as assayed by lactate/pyruvate and β-hydroxybutyrate/acetoacetate. We feel that greater rates of glycolysis at higher pH has led to reduction of cytoplas-mic NAD occuring in the reactions catalyzed by glyceraldehyde phosphate dehydrogenase or possibly D-glyceraldehyde dehydro-genase.

These data are quite consistent with work of Veech, *et al*. (14) who have shown that the redox state of the NAD^+/NADH in the cytoplasm is at least partially controlled by the phosphorylation state of adenine nucleotides. This relation is mediated through the glyceraldehyde 3-phosphate dehydrogenase and the 3-phosphoglycerate kinase reactions. Their formula interrelating these parameters is the follow-ing:

$$\frac{[NAD^+]}{[NADH]} = \frac{1}{K} \cdot \frac{[3\text{-Phosphoglycerate}]}{[Glyceraldehyde\ 3\text{-Phosphate}]} \cdot \frac{[ATP]}{[ADP]\ [HPO_4^{-2}]}$$

They found that the capacity of the enzymes involved are relatively high and they expect that the reactants of the system are at or near equilibrium *in vivo*. The agreement between measured and predicted adenine nucleotide values justify their assumption that in rat liver the two enzyme reactions control the redox state of NAD in the cytoplasm. Their studies were done with freeze clamped liver and work was done with pH controlled at neutrality.

Our finding of pH influence on the total NAD redox state in the presence of glucose substrate but not in the presence of pyruvate substrate is quite consistent with the concept of Veech, *et al*. (14) of the primary site of regulation of redox state of intracellular NAD. At more alkaline pH's, greater traffic over the glycolytic system leads to increased reduction of NAD causing the rise in redox ratio of both total NAD and of the free NAD linked substrates lactate and pyruvate.

Our conclusion from these studies is that the primary controlling point for setting the redox ratio of NAD and the substrates for which reduced and oxidized NAD are cofactors appears to be in the cytoplasm and is likely to be in the glyceraldehyde phosphate dehydrogenase and 3-phosphoglycerate kinase steps. Although the plasma membrane is an effective barrier to pH equilibrium of NAD linked reactions, it appears that the mitochondrial membrane offers no significant barrier to pH effects upon intramitochondrial NAD redox state.

Presented by Richard B. Tobin. Figures 1, 2, and 4 are reproduced by permission of the American Physiological Society and are from the American Journal of Physiology, 221: 1151-1155 (Oct. 1971).

References

1. Bücher, Th. and M. Klingenberg. Wege des Wasserstoffs in der lebendigen Organisation. Angew. Chem. 70: 552-570 (1958).
2. Jedeikin, L., A. J. Thomas and S. Weinhouse. Metabolism of neoplastic tissue. X. Diphosphopyridine nucleotide levels during azo dye hepatocarcinogenesis. Cancer Research. 16: 867-872 (1956).
3. Hohorst, H. J., F. H. Kreutz and M. Reim. Steady state

equilibria of some DPN-linked reactions and the oxidation/reduction state of the DPN/DPNH system in the cytoplasmic compartment of liver cells *in vivo*. Biochem. Biophys. Res. Comm. 4: 159-162 (1961).

4. Williamson, D. H., P. Lund and H. A. Krebs. The redox state of free nicotinamide-adenine dinucleotide in the cytoplasm and mitochondria of rat liver. Biochem. J. 103: 514-527 (1967).

5. Hohorst, H. J., F. H. Kreutz and Th. Bücher. Über metabolitgehalte und metabolit-konzentrationen in der leber der ratte. Biochem. Zeit. 332: 18-46 (1959).

6. Clark, W. M. In: Topics in Physical Chemistry. Baltimore, Williams and Wilkins, Co. (1958), p. 481.

7. Tobin, R. B. *In vivo* influences of hydrogen ions on lactate and pyruvate blood. Am. J. Physiol. 207: 601-605 (1964).

8. Hohorst, H. J. Enzymatische Bestimmung von L-(+)-Milchsaure. Biochem. Zeit. 328: 509-521 (1957).

9. Ochoa, S., A. H. Mehler and A. Kornberg. Biosynthesis of dicarboxylic acids by carbon dioxide fixation. 1. Isolation and properties of an enzyme from pigeon liver catalyzing the reversible oxidative decarboxylation of L-malic acid. J. Biol. Chem. 174: 979-1000 (1948).

10. Mellanby J. and D. H. Williamson. Acetoacetate. In: H. U. Bergmeyer (Editor), Methods of Enzymatic Analysis, Verlag-Academic (1965), p. 454-458.

11. Williamson, D. H. and J. Mellanby. D-(-)-β-hydroxy-butyrate. In: H. U. Bergmeyer (Editor), Methods of Enzymatic Analysis, Verlag-Academic (1965), p. 459-461.

12. Johnson, D. and H. Lardy. Isolation of liver or kidney mitochondria. In: R. W. Estabrook and M. E. Pullman (Editors), Methods in Enzymology, Vol. X, Academic Press, New York (1967), p. 94-96.

13. Van Dam, K. Nicotinamide-adenine dinucleotide en de adenhalingsketenfosforylering. Ph.D. Thesis, published by J. Van Campen Press, Amsterdam (1966).

14. Veech, R. L., L. Raijman and H. A. Krebs. Equilibrium relations between the cytoplasmic adenine nucleotide system and nicotinamide-adenine nucleotide system in rat liver. Biochem. J. 117: 499-503 (1970).

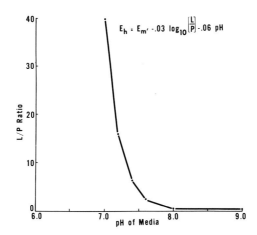

Fig. 1. *Theoretical lactate to pyruvate ratio vs. pH of media, based on oxidation potential equation for lactate and pyruvate.* E_h = measurable oxidation potential and is assumed to be -.185 v. E_m' = midpoint potential characteristic of the lactate and pyruvate system which is +.288 v.

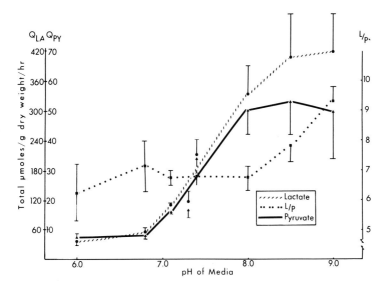

Fig. 2. *Net lactate and pyruvate production and L/P ratio of incubated liver slices plotted vs. pH of the media.* Ten millimolar glucose substrate was added to Krebs-Ringers phosphate media. Points indicate mean values of 10 or more determinations and vertical lines the SEM. Left ordinate shows the quantity of lactate and pyruvate measured expressed as μmoles/g dry wt/hr. The right ordinate shows L/P ratio.

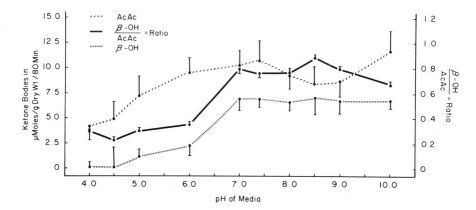

Fig. 3. *Acetoacetate and β-hydroxybutyrate content of liver slices and β-OH/AcAc ratio plotted vs. pH.* Ten millimolar glucose substrate in Krebs Ringers phosphate media was used. The left ordinate shows quantities of ketones produced expressed as μmoles/g dry wt/80 min. Right ordinate expresses the ratio. Points are mean values of 10 or more determinations and vertical bars show the SEM.

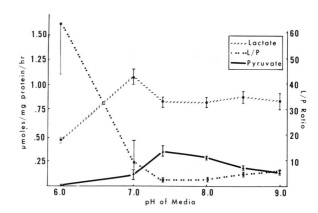

Fig. 4. *Lactate and pyruvate production and L/P ratio of liver homogenate.* See Fig. 2 for details.

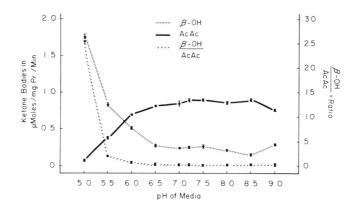

Fig. 5. *Acetoacetate and β-hydroxybutyrate content of rat liver mitochondria incubated with 10 mM β-hydroxybutyrate substrate for 30 min.* Left ordinate shows ketone body content/mg mitochondrial protein/min and right ordinate shows β-OH/AcAc ratio.

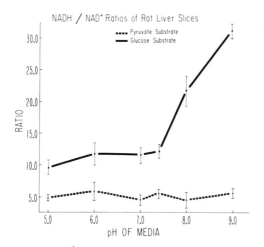

Fig. 6. *NADH to NAD^{+} ratio vs. pH of rat liver slices incubated 30 min in Krebs-Ringers Phosphate media with either 10 mM glucose or 10 mM pyruvate added as substrate.* Points show mean values of 10 or more slices and vertical bars express the SEM.

193

AFFINITY CHROMATOGRAPHIC STUDIES OF THE INSULIN RECEPTIVITY
ASSOCIATED WITH INTACT FAT CELLS, THEIR MEMBRANES AND
SOLUBILIZED EXTRACTS

Howard M. Katzen and Denis D. Soderman

Introduction

Earlier studies on the insulin receptor-like binding
properties of the cell membrane (1-8), as well as more recent attempts at solubilization and isolation of the receptor
(9,10), have extensively employed [131]I- or ^{125}I-labeled iodinated insulin as marker in the assays of binding. During
the latter part of this period, the use of biologically active protein ligands immobilized by covalent attachment to
insoluble polymeric carriers in isolation and purification
procedures (11-19) has become increasingly popular. Sur-
prisingly, despite the recent published reports demonstrating the retention of hormonal activity of insulin after
immobilizing it to Sepharose (20-22), the use of immobilized
insulin in the study or affinity chromatographic isolation
and purification of the insulin receptor has, until very recently (23), not been reported. The results of that preliminary study from our laboratory (23), formed the basis for
this Symposium report.

The objective of this study is to demonstrate the ability of insulin-Sepharose to bind firmly and selectively to
insulin-sensitive fat cells and their membrane "ghosts" in
order to provide a basis for utilizing the immobilized hormone in the affinity chromatographic isolation and purification of the insulin receptor. By selecting with affinity
chromatography the specific insulin receptor from various
possible fractions capable of binding insulin and ^{125}I-insu-
lin, it is hoped that the nagging questions that may per-
sist concerning the biological activity and specificity of
radioiodinated insulin may be obviated.

Until very recently, the notion that the firm binding of insulin to its receptor was the primary event required to initiate the hormone's biological actions on the cell has been generally accepted. However, as a result of the recent study by Oka and Topper [see Chapter 16; also (22)], this dogma may be subjected to question. Since they could find no actual binding of insulin-Sepharose to mammary epithelial cells that were sensitive to the immobilized but not the free hormone, they suggested that the collision with - or detachment of the hormone from - the cell rather than a firm binding is required for the biological response. Thus, from this mechanistic point of view, some new importance may be attached to the ability of insulin-Sepharose to bind to the insulin-sensitive cell. The studies reported here are also intended to shed some light on this question.

Methods

Male Charles River CD (Caesarean-delivered, pathogen-free) albino rats were obtained from the Charles River Breeding Company and allowed free access to Purina laboratory chow. Rats weighing between 140 and 180 g were used.

Sepharose 4B (agarose) and Sephadex G-100 were obtained from Pharmacia Fine Chemicals, Triton X-100 was obtained from Calbiochem, and fraction V, bovine plasma albumin, from the Sylvana Company. Crude collagenase and trypsin were products of Worthington Biochemicals. Insulin, recrystallized (25.9 U/mg) and the ^{14}C-algal protein hydrolysate (100 μCi/ml) were from Schwarz/Mann Laboratories. Guinea pig anti-bovine insulin serum (lyophilized powder; 1 μl of standard reconstituted solution neutralizes 1.53 mU insulin) was a product of Miles Laboratories. During the early experiments, ^{125}I-insulin was obtained (with less than one atom of ^{125}I per 6000 molecular weight) from Abbott Labs, dialyzed overnight before use, and used within 7 days of shipment and before less than 97 per cent of the radioactivity was trichloroacetic acid (TCA) precipitable. In later experiments, the ^{125}I-insulin was prepared fresh weekly in our laboratory according to the procedure of Greenwood et al. (24) as modified for insulin by Gavin et al. (25). This material was no less than 98 per cent TCA precipitable during its use. Other materials were obtained from routine commercial sources.

Isolated free fat cells and fat cell "ghosts" (plasma membrane preparation) were prepared essentially by the procedures of Rodbell (26, 27), and were derived from the distal half of the epididymal adipose tissue. "Lysing" and "wash" solutions for preparation of the ghosts (27) contained 1 mM $KHCO_3$ (pH 7.2), 2.5 mM $MgCl_2$ and 0.1 mM $CaCl_2$. When insoluble plasma membrane preparations were used, the ghost pellets prepared according to Rodbell (27) were washed twice in the "wash" solution using 900 x g centrifugations for 15 min each, and finally suspended in the designated buffer. For solubilized plasma membrane preparations, the ghosts were washed once by centrifugation for 30 min at 45,000 x g and the resultant pellet was mixed well with 0.5 % Triton X-100 in Krebs-Ringer buffer, as designated, for 15 min at 25°C.

The various insulin-Sepharoses[1] were prepared according to the general procedures described by Cuatrecasas and Anfinsen (19) and were extensively washed for periods of up to 7 days with buffer, 6M guanidine-HCl, 0.05N NaOH, 0.1N HCl and, finally, again the suspending buffer at pH 7.4, until protein [according to micro-biuret and Lowry *et al.* (28) protein assays and amidoblack staining on polyacrylamide gel disc electrophoresis] and radioactivity [from tracer amounts of ^{125}I-insulin coupled with native insulin to Sepharose] were no longer detectable in the washings. The amounts of insulin coupled to Sepharose were determined by amino acid analysis in the Beckman Model 120C amino acid analyzer after acid hydrolysis, and by isotopic dilution measurements of the ^{125}I-insulin with the unlabeled hormone

---

[1]*The abbreviations used are:*

ins-lys-S or ins-phe-S. Either the lysine (lys) or the N-terminal phenylalanine (phe) of the β-chain of insulin (ins) coupled directly to cyanogen bromide-activated Sepharose (S). (see Methods).

ins-lys-pent-S or ins-phe-pent-S. Insulin (as above) coupled to bromacetyl-activated 5-carbon diamine in turn coupled to cyanogen bromide-activated Sepharose (see Methods).

insulin-Sepharose or insulin-S. General terms designating insulin coupled to Sepharose as described in any of the above examples except without specifying the particular type of covalent bonds involved, but only referring specifically to the relevant preparations under immediate discussion.

AIS. Anti-insulin serum.

coupled to the Sepharose. The two methods yielded comparable results.

Preparation of ^{14}C-labeled ghosts.

^{14}C-labeled fat cell ghosts were prepared after incubation of intact fat cells for 90 min at 37°C in Krebs-Ringer phosphate buffer (pH 7.4), containing 4% albumin, 3 μmoles of glucose/ml, 0.125 μCi/ml of ^{14}C-algal protein hydrolysate and $10^{-5}M$ of a ^{12}C-amino acid mixture. Resultant cells were washed (about 4 times) with K-R albumin buffer until washings were essentially free of radioactivity. ^{14}C-ghosts prepared from these cells were washed (about 6 times) using centrifugations at 1500 x g for 15 min each time until washings were very low and constant in ^{14}C. Actinomycin, when used to inhibit incorporation of ^{14}C, was incubated at 9 μg/ml with cells for 15 min at 37°C, prior to addition of ^{14}C and ^{12}C amino acids. It was found to inhibit by 65%.

Affinity chromatographic procedure.

Siliconized glass columns, 6 mm x 105 mm, each containing 2 ml of settled Sepharose beads (or as designated), supported on a small glass wool wad, were used. To demonstrate that physical entrapment or retardation of insoluble membranes was not occurring as a consequence of packing on narrow columns in those experiments where ghost preparations were washed through, 11 mm x 30 mm columns with coarse sintered glass filters were occasionally tested. Use of these columns did not alter binding results. In addition, at the conclusion of the collected and measured washings, the narrow columns were repeatedly inverted to mix thoroughly the contents. These mixings did not lead to the reappearance of membranes in the subsequent washings.

Buoyant density fat cell: insulin-Sepharose binding procedure.

To 5 ml calibrated polypropylene test tubes (12 x 75 mm) were added, typically, in sequence: (a) 0.75 ml of a stock suspension of Sepharose or insulin-S, containing 2 volumes of settled beads per volume of K-R bicarbonate buffer (pH 7.4) and albumin at concentrations of up to 4%

(usually 0.1%); (b) 0.45 ml of buffer (for a final volume of 1.5 ml) in the presence or absence of designated test supplements; and (c) 0.3 ml of a fat cell suspension containing one volume of buffer per 2 volumes of packed cells. After gentle but thorough mixing of the final suspension, using a Vortex mixer, the resultant mixture was allowed to separate undisturbed at a constant temperature between 25° and 37° (routinely 30°) until buoyant equilibrium was reached (approximately 20 minutes). Measurements of cpm of ^{125}I-insulin-labeled insulin-Sepharose, ^{14}C-labeled Sepharose (20), lipid content of cells, or simply, volumes of the resultant layers of cells, beads, and infranatant, were made, as convenient, and compared with the control Sepharose-cell separation or other desired control. Depending on the requirements of the test system, cell:bead complexes could be made to sink or float by arbitrarily adjusting the cell to bead volume-ratio which, in turn, was found to determine the number of cells available to bind each bead.

Other assay procedures.

Native insulin and insulin-Sepharoses were assayed for *in vitro* hormonal activity by measurement of the two-hour oxidation of glucose-1-^{14}C to [14]CO$_2$ in isolated fat cells essentially according to the method of Rodbell (26). In the trypsin experiments *(see Results),* incubations were conducted for one instead of two hours to avoid appreciable "restoration" (7, 29) of insulin receptor-like binding.

Plasma membrane-bound hexokinase was determined by the nitroblue-tetrazolium (NBT): glucose-6-phosphate dehydrogenase coupled staining procedure previously described (30, 31). The intensities of the blue membrane-associated color resulting from this reaction were estimated visually and found to require glucose, ATP and Mg^{++}. According to the studies of Rodbell (27), 15% of the total cellular hexokinase is distributed in fractionated ghost preparations in proportions similar to those of the plasma membrane marker enzyme adenyl cyclase.

Turbidity measurements of diluted samples or fractions applied to,and eluted or washed off of, the insulin-S affinity columns were made at 280 nm or 450 nm in the Gilford 2000 spectrophotometer. Final total optical density readings ("O.D. turbidity") were calculated from dilution factors. ^{125}I-insulin measurements were made in the Packard

Model B-5219 Automatic Gamma Scintillation Spectrometer.

Results

Although general procedures for covalent attachment of ligands to several different polymeric supporting materials have been developed (14-19), it remains to be determined in each circumstance whether the ligand retains its biological activity and specificity after immobilization. It had been shown previously that insulin, coupled directly *via* its N-terminal phenylalanine or β-chain ε amino of lysine to cyanogen bromide-activated agarose (14, 15, 18), retained its hormonal activity (20). In the present study we have confirmed this, but, in addition, have tested their binding specificities and prepared and studied insulin-Sepharoses with varying hydrocarbon extensions interposed between the insulin ligand and Sepharose backbone.

In Fig. 1 is an example of the biological activity exhibited by our most frequently used preparation (see below). With a 5-carbon length hydrocarbon extension [called an "arm" (19)] interposed between insulin and the Sepharose, the resultant insulin-Sepharose beads were capable of stimulating the oxidation of ^{14}C-glucose to $^{14}CO_2$ in isolated fat cells in a manner characteristic of the native hormone. Although the insulin-Sepharose preparations stimulated the cells to the same maximum degree as the free hormone, they were only about 10% as active based on the full amount of insulin immobilized. Inasmuch as only a limited number of cells could be shown to crowd around each insulin-Sepharose bead (see below), and since some of the immobilized insulin molecules may be buried within the agarose matrix, these hormone molecules likely would be inaccessible to the available fat cells. On this basis, we were not surprised to find that the immobilized insulin appeared less potent than equimolar amounts of free insulin. To insure that no insulin was reversibly adsorbed to the Sepharose, all insulin-Sepharose preparations used in this study were extensively washed with 6 M guanidine·HCl, acidic and alkaline solutions, and finally, Krebs-Ringer bicarbonate buffers. Additionally, to ensure that no bound insulin was enzymatically or otherwise released as active free insulin from the Sepharose beads during the 2 hr incubation with the fat cells in the assay, protein assays as well as radioactivity measurements of the washings and incubation media containing insulin-

Sepharose with I^{125}-insulin covalently coupled as radioactive tracer, were run. All of these studies showed that no
detectable bound insulin was released as free insulin under
any of these conditions, and no detectable degradation of
the immobilized insulin by the intact fat cells occurred.
Clearly, the degree of biological activity associated with
the immobilized insulin could not be accounted for by the
insignificant amount of radioactivity occasionally found
associated with cells washed free of insulin-S. All of the
slight amount of soluble radioactivity detected in the ^{125}I
insulin-Sepharose incubation medium was found to be TCA-
soluble and shown not to be due to the presence of the fat
cells. Finally, other studies showed the time-course of the
insulin-stimulated oxidation of glucose-1-^{14}C to be identical to that stimulated by immobilized hormone (32). This
would be inconsistent with a time-required release of free
insulin from the Sepharose-bound state.

Binding of plasma membranes to affinity columns.

The isolated fat cells used in this study were found
to be highly sensitive to insulin. Stimulations by insulin
of from 15 to 20 fold over baseline could be obtained consistently (not shown). To examine the ability of immobilized insulin to bind to receptor-containing plasma membranes
derived from these cells, affinity chromatographic columns
that contained insulin coupled directly to Sepharose (ins-
lys-S and ins-phe-S) were studied. Fat cell ghosts, shown
by Rodbell to be in themselves insulin sensitive (33), were
applied to these columns, and measurements were made of the
membranes washed through in the collected fractions. It was
clear from these studies that the insulin-Sepharose columns
consistently retained a significant portion of the membranes
despite extensive washings, while all of the membranes passed unretarded through the control columns.

As seen in Fig. 2, the bulk of the unretained membranes
passed unretarded through all of the columns immediately
after the void volume (fractions 2 and 3). Although identical amounts of membranes were applied to each column,
significantly less could be found in these as well as in
the remaining fractions from the two insulin-Sepharose columns than from the control column. As also seen in Table I
(part A), the differences between the amounts applied and
those washed through represent the membranes retained on

(bound to) the columns. The maximum capacity of these preparations to bind membranes was reached at a concentration
of about 2.6 mg of insulin coupled per ml of settled Sepharose. At this concentration, about 2 "O.D. turbidity units",
or 25 to 30% of the membranes were retained (Fig. 2). That
a significant amount of turbidity passed unretarded through
the insulin-S columns would be expected in view of the significant amount of free nuclei and other non-plasma membrane
particulates (non-insulin receptor containing) contaminating
the "ghost preparation" (27).

It can also be seen in Table I that when the membranes
were measured using membrane-bound hexokinase (31) as a marker, according to enzyme-coupled nitro-blue tetrazolium staining, results similar to those seen in Fig. 2 were obtained.
Moreover, the hexokinase activity associated with the insulin-Sepharose beads themselves, after extensive washings of
the beads, corresponded well with that amount of membranes
absent from the collected washings (Table I, B). Extensive
mixing of the insulin-Sepharose beads by a batch procedure,
rather than this column method, confirmed the strong binding
to the beads.

Elution of membranes from affinity columns.

In attempts to elute the membranes from the affinity
columns, it was found that 1 M NaCl, 0.05 N acetic acid,
and 0.05 N NaOH were ineffective. However, 6 M guanidine·HCl
readily eluted off virtually all of the membranes. Significantly, and as would be expected from a strong, but reversible, bond between insulin and its receptor, insulin at 10^{-3}
M was effective in eluting off about 3 times more membranes
than 2% albumin as control (Table II). Consistent with the
previous observation that all of the membranes passed unretarded through the control Sepharose columns, elution with
insulin of such columns after the membranes had washed
through yielded eluates free of turbidity and hexokinase
activity. Significantly, insulin-S pretreated with AIS also
showed no binding capacity (not shown). The ability of free,
soluble insulin to reverse the binding, and the complete
inhibition of binding by AIS, all indicate a significant
degree of specificity of these insulin-Sepharose preparations
for binding to a receptor-like material on the fat cell membrane.

Effect of interposing hydrocarbon extensions between insulin and Sepharose.

On the basis of the suggestion of Cu~~trecasas and Anfinsen that extending the "arm" distance betw~~n the ligand and carrier backbone may increase the binding affinity of the ligand (19), we prepared a series of insulin-Sepharoses with progressively increasing hydrocarbon arm lengths. Two series of derivaties were prepared, one with the ε amino of the insulin β-chain lysine and the other with the N-terminal phenylalanine of insulin, each coupled to a bromoacetyl-activated hydrocarbon arm (19) linked, in turn, to cyanogen bromide-activated Sepharose (18).

In Tables III and IV it can be seen that increasing the arm lengths concomitantly increased the yields of membranes bound as determined by enzyme activity directly associated with (bound to) the column insulin-S beads and by enzyme and turbidity measurements of the collected wash fractions. There was good agreement between the turbidity of the wash fractions and the enzyme measurements of washings and beads. It is interesting that derivatives with 2-carbon-length arms were less effective in binding than those with no arm. The explanation for this is unclear. However, it suggests that, while the length is important, the components comprising the arm in themselves are not involved in the binding to the membranes. Except when designated otherwise, insulin immobilized with a 5-carbon arm *via* insulin's β-chain ε amino of lysine was selected for all further experiments.

As another means of examining the binding "capabilities" of the immobilized insulins, ^{14}C measurements were made of ^{14}C-labeled membranes derived from cells in which ^{14}C-labeled amino acids were incorporated *in vitro* into the membrane proteins (Table V). Consistent with the previous measurements, a high percentage of membranes were found to bind readily to both ins-phe-pent-S and ins-lys-pent-S. In accord with a degree of binding specificity, the ^{14}C-amino acid mixture had no affinity for these columns, and ^{14}C-membranes had no affinity for control Sepharose-4B. Because actinomycin D effectively inhibited (by 63%, not shown) the incorporation of the ^{14}C-amino acids into the membranes, the application of equal amounts of ^{14}C to each column meant that significantly more membranes from the actinomycin D-treated cells *(i.e.* with low ^{14}C specific activity*)* were applied than from the freely-incorporating, high specific activity actinomycin-untreated cells. Therefore, the lower

percentage of "actinomycin D-membranes" that were bound
(Table V, line 3) would be a reflection of the application
of an amount of low specific activity membranes that exceeded the maximum retentive capacity of the columns. Thus, although an equal "absolute" amount of membranes were likely
bound as compared to the actinomycin D-untreated cells, the
per cent bound of the total applied was significantly less.

At this point it is important to reiterate that in all
cases (see Tables I, III, IV, and V; Fig. 2) only a maximum
of about 75% of the applied total "ghost preparation" was
capable of binding to the columns. This is in accord with
the approximate per cent of ghosts present in this preparation (27).

*Effect of trypsin on insulin-sensitivity of fat cells
and on ability of membranes to bind insulin-Sepharose.*

Earlier studies by Kono revealed that trypsin at 1 mg/
ml could selectively abolish the insulin sensitivity of isolated fat cells (29). He also reported that some of this
sensitivity could be restored on reincubation of the "trypsinized" cells after inhibiting the trypsin. This loss and
restoration of sensitivity was attributed to selective effects on the insulin receptor (7,29). To test the binding
selectivity of the ins-lys-pent-S, we first repeated Kono's
findings and then tested the ability of this immobilized
insulin to bind membranes derived from such trypsin-treated
cells. In Table VI it is seen that, in agreement with Kono,
a 15 min incubation of fat cells with trypsin abolished the
sensitivity of the cells to insulin, while this treatment
had no apparent effect on the baseline utilization of ^{14}C-
glucose (i.e. in the absence of insulin). The cells remained fully hormone sensitive if, as seen in the control experiments, the action of trypsin was effectively blocked by
inclusion of soybean trypsin inhibitor (at "zero time",
Table VI). In addition, a 90 min incubation of the "trypsinized" (insulin-insensitive) cells in the presence of the
trypsin inhibitor resulted in a significant restoration of
the sensitivity. Although the trypsin pre-treatment frequently led to a reduced baseline level of ^{14}C-glucose oxidation as a result of this 1 hour incubation (e.g. from 441
to 167 cpm of ^{14}CO$_2$, Table VI), these cells exhibited a
degree of insulin sensitivity after this additional incubation comparable to the control, non-trypsin-treated re-
incubated cells. The latter cells did not exhibit a

diminished baseline rate of glucose oxidation. These experiments are in agreement with the conclusion of Kono that trypsin exerts a selective effect, possibly on the receptor, in reversibly inhibiting or destroying the insulin sensitivity of the cell. However, although a degree of selectivity of the action of trypsin is inferred by the lack of tryptic effect on the baseline rate of cellular glucose oxidation according to the assay conducted immediately after the 15 min tryptic action, a significant effect was seen if the cells were assayed *after* the stress of the additional 90 min. incubation. Thus, trypsin had, in fact, some slight but significant effect in addition to that on the cell's sensitivity to insulin.

The selectivity of the binding ability of ins-lys-pent-S as determined by comparing the binding of plasma membranes prepared from insulin-sensitive cells with those from trypsinzed cells is shown in Table VII. While 2.40 turbidity units, or 48%, of membranes prepared from cells treated with inactivated trypsin readily bound to the columns, none of the membranes from cells treated with 1 mg of trypsin/ml would bind. The lowest concentration of trypsin found to destroy most of the binding ability was about 0.25 mg/ml. The additional 90 min. incubation ("reincubation") of trypsinzed cells in the absence of added enzyme inhibitor resulted in a loss of binding capacity. However, after reincubation in the presence of the inhibitor, 1.72 or 34% of the membranes could bind as compared to 2.05 or 41% of the membranes from control cells. Thus, about 83% of the binding capacity was restored. These results coincide with the effects of trypsin on insulin sensitivity, and in that regard, are consistent with a good degree of specificity of the immobilized insulin to bind the insulin receptor on the insulin-sensitive cells. The fact that "trypsinized" cells didn't bind, in itself, shows a specific requirement of the cell membrane for binding to insulin-S.

Buoyant density demonstration of cell binding to ins-lys-pent-S.

During the course of these studies we made the interesting discovery that, in physiological media, buoyant fat cells (which float) readily associated with various insulin-S preparations (which by themselves sediment) thereby either floating the otherwise sedimentable insulin-S beads to the surface, or sinking with the beads, depending upon the ratio

of the concentration of cells to beads. The illustration
in the tube on the left of Fig. 3 shows that after mixing
Sepharose beads with viable fat cells, the beads and cells
completely separate from each other within several minutes,
leaving a distinct layer of cells at the top, a clear and
well-defined infranatant, and a distinct layer of beads at
the bottom of the tube. Microscopic examination revealed
virtually no cross contamination of beads and cells. Yet,
when this procedure was repeated under identical conditions,
except that ins-lys-pent-S was substituted for Sepharose,
all of the beads were floated to the top layer by the cells
(Fig. 3, tube on right). Conversely, it was found that an
excess of ins-lys-pent-S completely sedimented the cells,
resulting in clear and distinct supernatant and bottom phases.
By carefully decreasing the cell to bead ratio, cells associated with Sepharose were found to be dispersed throughout
the tube (not shown). It was clear that the number of cells
bound per insulin-S bead determined the buoyancy of the resultant complex. The percentage of total cells bound to the
beads was easily determined by measuring the change in volume occupied by the resultant layers of cells and beads, or
more accurately, by either ^{125}I-insulin as a radioactive
tracer to measure the insulin-S or ^{14}C-labeled cells or lipids to measure the cells.

To confirm the actual binding of isolated cells to insulin-Sepharose beads, samples were taken from the mixtures
illustrated in Fig. 3, and examined and photographed by
Nomarski interference contrast microscopy (Fig. 4). In
panel "A" of Fig. 4 is shown the random appearance of cells
with control Sepharose (derived from the mixture of cells
and Sepharose before separation). In this case most of
the Sepharose beads (seen as the larger spheres) rapidly
settled away and disappeared under cover of the pack of
smaller floating cells. In panel "B" is an identical mixture except that the sample examined consisted of the floating phase of ins-lys-pent-S:cell complexes where ins-lys-
pent-S was added in place of the control Sepharose. Clearly,
because each and every bead was surrounded by cells attract-
ed to the beads, the cells floated the beads to the surface
of the cover slide creating this organized pattern, in contrast to the random pattern seen in panel "A" of Fig. 4.

The strong binding of cells to insulin-S can also be
seen on the bottom panels of Fig. 4 as single (or double)
cell:single insulin-S complexes in more dilute solutions.

Because the free cells instantly separated away from the
plane of focus of the free beads, cells and insulin-S cannot
be seen simultaneously in focus unless they were bound to
each other, as is the case here.

In Table VIII are summarized the results of a study of
the specificity and reversibility of the bond(s) between
the intact fat cell and insulin-S, utilizing the buoyant
density procedure. As noted previously, none of the cells
were capable of binding to untreated Sepharose. Under the
conditions employed, 50% of the ins-lys-pent-S beads were
floated or suspended by binding to cells. Prior treatment
of the cells with trypsin at 1.0 mg/ml (as described in Tables VI and VII) reduced this to 25%. Higher concentrations
of trypsin more extensively abolished the receptivity of the
cells. Only 15% of the insulin-S beads without a connecting
arm were suspended or floated by binding to the cells, whereas Sepharose containing the hydrocarbon extension linked to
glycine as ligand instead of insulin, had virtually no binding affinity. Prior treatment of the cells with trypsin did
not expose any glycine-binding sites. Of considerable importance is the finding that AIS completely inhibited the
binding when added with the cells prior to the addition of
ins-lys-pent-S, and rapidly and completely *dissociated* the
complex when the AIS was added after formation of the cell:
insulin-S complex. Moreover, prior treatment of the ins-
lys-pent-S beads with AIS, followed by extensive washing of
the beads to rid excess anti-serum, completely inhibited the
beads' binding capacity. In addition, it was found that
washing the "AIS-blocked" insulin-S with 6M guanidine·HCl
completely restored the binding capacity of the beads. Thus,
AIS did not irreversibly destroy the beads or the ligand,
but acted by blocking the ligand. The finding that AIS-
coated insulin-S was incapable of binding to the cells suggests the specificity of the requirement for insulin in
preference to other proteins immobilized on Sepharose. Finally, control serum was incapable of dissociating the cell:
bead complex. These results are consistent with the interpretation that the complex is due to a strong, but reversible bond(s) between specific insulin receptor site(s) on
the cell membrane and the insulin(s) on the Sepharose. However, inasmuch as it was found that prior to treatment of
the ins-lys-pent-S beads with excess control serum also reduced the binding capacity, although to a much lesser degree
than AIS (about a 15% inhibition, not shown), some non-

specific bonds appear also to be involved.

Finally, and in accord with the insulin elution results with the membrane ghosts, free insulin at 10^{-5}M was able to inhibit the binding according to the buoyant density method (Table VIII), whereas albumin and gelatin at concentrations up to 4% had little effect. It should be pointed out that this concentration on insulin (10^{-5}M) was effective against a final concentration of 4×10^{-5}M immobilized insulin in the buoyant density procedure. Prior treatment of the insulin-S beads with excess insulin, as described for AIS above, had no effect.

Detergent-solubilized ^{125}I-*insulin-binding ghosts fractions.*

To determine the presence of ^{125}I-insulin binding fractions in solubilized plasma membranes, ghost preparations were treated with ^{125}I-insulin either before or after solublization with the non-ionic detergent Triton X-100. In Fig. 5 are shown the results of starch gel electrophoresis of fat cell ghosts that had been incubated with ^{125}I-insulin, washed to rid reversibly adsorbed ^{125}I-insulin and then solubilized (as determined by Millipore filtration) with 0.5% Triton X-100.

According to Millipore filtration of the total applied detergent-treated membrane-bound radioactivity (Fig. 5), 37% was solubilized and could be shown to be virtually 100% trichoroacetic acid insoluble, while the remainder was either not solubilized in the first place, or precipitated during the filtration step. Centrifugation at 200,000 x g in place of filtration yielded similar results. In the control experiment (Fig. 5, "Minus Triton") about 94% of the membrane-associated ^{125}I-insulin remained insoluble.

Electrophoresis of ^{125}I-insulin in the absence of membranes showed characteristic double peaks between fractions 20 and 25 with no significant peaks elsewhere (Fig. 5). However, electrophoresis of the soluble filtrate taken from the detergent-treated membrane-bound ^{125}I-insulin preparation consistently revealed the presence of two additional peaks, one at the origin and the other with a mobility coincident with fractions 8 to 12. Inasmuch as the ^{125}I-insulin-bound membranes were washed well prior to solubilization with detergent, the presence of the peaks coincident with the free ^{125}I-insulin peaks reflected the release of free ^{125}I-insulin from the membrane-associated state. Electrophoresis of detergent-solubilized membranes that had been incubated with ^{125}I-insulin *after* solubilization of the membranes, exhibited peaks qualitatively identical to those seen in Fig. 5. In other experiments not shown here, the two slow moving peaks were found to be saturable with ^{125}I-insulin and inhibited with unlabeled insulin. In view of the major radioactive peak appearing at the origin of the electrophoresis, it is possible that the soluble bound ^{125}I-insulin in the filtrate became insoluble during the electrophoresis. Consistent with this is the additional finding that electrophoresis of supernatants derived from centrifugation, or Millipore filtrates, of Triton-solubilized membrane extracts *after* incubation with ^{125}I-insulin resulted in a bound ^{125}I-insulin peak (complex) with 75% less radioactivity than those peak fractions obtained by centrifugation or filtration of the extracts *before* incubation with the labeled hormone. Thus, it would strongly appear that the binding fraction itself remains completely soluble until bound (complexed) to ^{125}I-insulin.

The electrophoretic peaks between fractions 9 and 12 (Fig. 5) and consistently seen may represent the portion of the complexed ^{125}I-insulin that remained soluble. To eliminate the possibility that fragments of degraded ^{125}I-insulin possibly could account for some of the non-^{125}I-insulin radioactivity, the extracts were precipitated with 10% trichloroacetic acid (TCA). No TCA-soluble radioactivity was observable as a consequence of the presence of membrane extracts.

The above experiments may also suggest the presence of one or more solubilized ^{125}I-insulin binding fractions. Since the major non-free ^{125}I-insulin peak did not move, its homogeneity may also be questioned. In order to compare the electrophoretic findings with those derived from a different isolation procedure, similar extracts were fractionated by gel filtration on Sephadex G-100 (Fig. 6). In addition to the major peak corresponding to free ^{125}I-insulin in fractions 18 to 27, incubation of ^{125}I-insulin with Triton-solubilized membranes ("extract") consistently yielded a larger molecular weight peak ("A" in Fig. 6) which appeared just after the void volume in fractions 5 to 12. Use of Sephadex G-200 indicated the molecular weight of this complex to be greater than 200,000. Inclusion of excess native insulin in the incubation of ^{125}I-insulin with extracts completely inhibited the appearance of the large molecular weight complex and resulted in the appearance of a free

^{125}I-insulin peak equal to the high molecular weight peak prior to competition with the native insulin. Electrophoresis of the high molecular weight complex from pooled Sephadex G-100 peak fractions yielded a major radioactive peak at the origin as well as a significant peak corresponding to free ^{125}I-insulin. Thus, the high molecular weight complex derived from Sephadex G-100 gel filtration corresponded to the previously described major bound ^{125}I-insulin peak fractions described by electrophoresis.

Using nearly identical conditions, Cuatrecasas has very recently described the presence of a similar macromolecular-bound ^{125}I-insulin complex that passes unretarded through Sephadex G-50 columns (9,10). He reported in those studies that incubation of the bound ^{125}I-insulin peak fractions with native insulin for 50 min at 37°C resulted in a *complete* displacement of the labeled with the native hormone (9). However, no control data were presented for the effect of *identical incubations* on the dissociation of the complex in the absence of added native hormone. We found that according to this important control experiment (Fig. 6), a slight but significant amount of free ^{125}I-insulin was dissociated from the complex into fractions 18 to 27. However, in repeated attempts we were unable to find that excess native insulin dissociated the complex by any more than 15% over this control (Fig. 6). Increasing the temperature, time of incubation, concentration of native insulin, or use of different buffers did not enhance the displacement by native for labeled insulin in this fraction.

Because the electrophoretic experiments suggested to us that the binding of ^{125}I-insulin to the solubilized binding fraction rendered the resultant complex relatively insoluble *(see* scheme depicted in Fig. 7), Sephadex G-100 fractionations of membranes solubilized before and after incubation with ^{125}I-insulin and subjected to Millipore filtration were compared with each other (Fig. 7). Consistent with the depicted scheme and the electrophoretic data, the Millipore step filtered out a significant amount of the ^{125}I-insulin bound macromolecular ("X") complex that was formed before treatment with detergent (*i.e.* treated with detergent and filtered *after* formation of the complex, and designated "post-solubilized X" in Fig. 7). Accordingly, the solubilized receptor-like "X" prior to incubation with ^{125}I-insulin ("pre-solubilized X" in Fig. 7) passed entirely through the Millipore thereby yielding a relatively greater amount of the large

molecular weight radioactive peak. The free ^{125}I-insulin
was likely derived from (a) the dissociation from the membranes of reversibly-adsorbed ^{125}I-insulin, (b) that bound
to the receptor-like "X" macromolecule, and (c) the excess
free ^{125}I-insulin in the "pre-solubilized"-incubation medium.

Affinity chromatographic extraction of ^{125}*I-insulin-
binding fraction.*

On the basis of the previously described evidence for
the ability of insulin-S to selectively bind plasma membrane
insulin receptor-like sites, ins-lys-pent-S was used on affinity chromatographic columns to determine if the Triton-
solubilized ^{125}I-insulin binding macromolecule ("X" fraction)
possessed properties comparable to the intact membrane sites.
A Triton-solubilized membrane extract containing the binding
fraction, as determined by Sephadex G-100 gel filtration,
was first passed through ins-lys-pent-S columns or control
Sepharose columns to compare the collected washings from
each column with each other. Measurements were made of
protein content and ability to bind ^{125}I-insulin and thereby
form the ^{125}I-insulin-"X" complex according to subsequent
Sephadex G-100 gel filtration (Fig. 8). Protein assays
showed that all of the protein applied to the Sepharose columns passed through unretarded immediately after the void
volume, while over 95% passed unretarded through the ins-lys-
pent-S column. Subsequent Sephadex fractionation of the
incubation mixtures of ^{125}I-insulin with the unretarded protein fraction from the insulin-S and Sepharose columns revealed the ability of the insulin-S column to extract a considerable proportion of the ^{125}I-insulin-binding fraction
(fractions 6 to 9, Fig. 8). As further evidence for the
validity of this interpretation, the slight increase in the
free ^{125}I-insulin peak derived from the insulin-S column
can be seen to correspond well with the loss of the large
molecular weight peak. Thus, the deficiency in binding
fraction "X" in these washings resulted in the availability,
due to decreased "trapping" by "X", of more free ^{125}I-insulin
than from the control Sepharose column.
    Clearly, the ins-lys-pent-S columns extracted the solu-
bilized insulin receptor-like binding fraction, and inasmuch
as over 95% of the protein passed unretarded through these
columns, with a good degree of selectivity. Consistent with

this, slight but significant amounts of this insulin receptor-like fraction were found in eluates from these columns
after elution with excess insulin and tracer amounts of [125]I-
insulin, and according to assay by Sephadex G-100 gel filtration.

Discussion

Several lines of evidence in the present study demonstrate the effectiveness of immobilized insulin for the study
and affinity chromatographic isolation and purification of
plasma membranes and soluble membrane fractions with insulin
receptor-like properties. Although earlier studies from
several laboratories (20,21) have shown that insulin-Sepharose
preparations were capable of exerting *in vitro* biological
activities virtually identical to those of the native hormone,
the possibility was not excluded that these activities may
have been due to the release of free, solubilized insulin
derived from the Sepharose-bound form during the period
of incubation with the cell or tissue. In the present study
a 2 hour incubation with isolated fat cells failed to release
any trichloroacetic acid-insoluble radioactivity into the
incubation medium from tracer amounts of ^{125}I-insulin coupled
to insulin-Sepharose. These and other studies with ^{125}I-insu-
lin-Sepharose, as well as those involving extensive washings
of the beads and the time-course of the action on fat cells,
all indicate that the biological activity shown in the present study was due to the hormone coupled covalently to the
Sepharose.
In contrast to the earlier studies by Cuatrecasas who
reported hormonal activities associated with insulin-lys-S
and insulin-phe-S that were quantitatively equal to that of
the soluble (free) hormone (20), we find 10% or less activity
associated with all of our preparations, including those
previously reported (20). We have noted this disparity even
at concentrations of insulin coupled to Sepharose comparable
to those reported by Cuatrecasas. The reason for these differences between laboratories is unclear. However, in view
of the present finding that only a limited and relatively
small number of cells can bind or come in contract with any
one insulin-Sepharose bead at any one time (Fig. 4), it is
unlikely that all of the insulin molecules associated with
each bead are accessible to interaction with fat cells. In

other words, there would appear to be many more hormone
molecules associated with any one bead than there are cells
accessible for interaction with the bead. In addition, it
is also likely that many insulin molecules are buried or
"masked" within the Sepharose bead and thereby also inaccessible to cells. In contrast, every free insulin molecule
should be readily accessible to fat cell receptors. Thus,
it would be expected and consistent with our present findings that less activity be associated with a large number
of hormone molecules bound to a Sepharose bead than with
an equal number of free molecules. However, other considerations such as the possible difference in binding affinities between free and immobilized hormone (see Tables III
and IV) should also have to be taken into account.

On the basis of these and the earlier findings that
insulin coupled to polysaccharide beads larger in size than
the cell retained its hormonal activity (20,21), it was
reasonably concluded that the hormone must exert its cellular actions by interacting solely with the cell membrane
(20). Nevertheless, the study of Oka and Topper (22) raised
the question of the nature of this interaction, $i.e.$ whether
an actual binding of insulin to the cell membrane is required to initiate the hormone's actions. Because they could
observe no binding of insulin-phe-Sepharose beads to mammary
epithelial cells that were sensitive to the immobilized,
but not the free, hormone, they speculated that rather than
a firm binding, the collision with, or detachment of the
hormone from, the cell may be required for the hormonal response.

Although the present studies do not definitively an
swer these questions, they do shed some light on the subject
and offer some relevant findings. Clearly, they demonstrate
that hormonally-active insulin-Sepharose beads indeed can
bind firmly to insulin-sensitive isolated adipose tissue
cells under conditions virtually identical to those in which
either native insulin or Sepharose-bound insulin stimulate
the oxidation of glucose-1-^{14}C to [14]CO$_2$ in these cells.
Thus, at $37°$ even in the presence of 4% albumin as in the
fat cell assay incubation medium of Rodbell (26), ins-lys-
pent-S beads were shown to bind readily to isolated fat
cells. The demonstrations of binding of fat cell plasma
membrane preparations to affinity columns are in accord
with this. However, these findings do not necessarily rule
out the possibility proposed by Oka and Topper (22). Thus,
because it is possible that a large number of freely-revers-

213

ible receptor:insulin bonds (complexes) may be involved at
the areas of contact between cells and beads, many of the
individual complexes may be dissociating while others could
be simultaneously reassociating. The result would be a net
effect of maintaining a sufficiently firm association of
cell to bead. It is likely that more than one insulin-receptor bond is necessary to maintain a net binding between
cell and bead. Secondly, it is possible that some non-specific as well as receptor-specific bonds may be involved in
the maintainence of the observed bond. Thirdly, the affinity
of the ins-lys-pent-S for the receptor may be much greater
than the ins-lys-Sepharose used by Oka and Topper (see Tables III and IV). Finally, and however unlikely, the recept-
or or the receptor-insulin interaction on the fat cell membrane may be different from that on the mammary epithelial
cell.

In the present study, several different lines of evidence indicate the presence of specific insulin-binding receptor-like sites on the plasma membrane of the fat cell.
These same studies also demonstrate the capability of affinity chromatography as a tool in the isolation and purification of these sites. Although all of these lines of
evidence were derived from a common cell type, the binding
fractions derived from the intact cell, membraneous ghosts
and detergent-solubilized ghosts may be different from
each other. Caution should be applied to different lines
of evidence which may be measuring different binding sites
(1-10).

However, inasmuch as all of the binding sites examined
in the present study have, in common, the relatively specific and comparable abilities to bind insulin-Sepharose and,
in particular, ins-lys-pent-S, in addition to being derived
from a common fat cell membrane source, the relevancy of
our studies to the insulin receptor appears significant.
Native insulin and anti-insulin anti-serum selectively
competed with and displaced insulin-Sepharose for binding
to intact fat cells and their ghosts, and could elute the
membranes from the affinity columns. Trypsin treatment of
fat cells, reported by Kono to destroy the receptor (7,29),
is shown in the present study to inhibit the binding capacity of the cells and "ghosts" derived from these cells.

It is interesting that despite the ability of ins-lys-
pent-S to bind 100% of the intact fat cells (implying that
all of the cells contain receptors), affinity columns with
all of the insulin-S preparations tested were found to be

incapable of binding more than about 75% of the total applied insoluble particulates from the plasma membrane "ghost preparation" of Rodbell (27). This would be in excellent agreement with the proportion of plasma membranes in this ghost preparation inasmuch as, according to Rodbell (27), this preparation consists of an appreciable percentage of free nuclei and other cell particulates not bound to the ghosts. Thus, these affinity columns appear to be capable of purifying plasma membranes from the "ghost preparation".

In addition, it is shown that insulin-Sepharose columns selectively bind a detergent-solubilized Sephadex G-100 gel-filtered membrane fraction which possessed a specific ability to bind ^{125}I-insulin. The ^{125}I-insulin receptor-like macromolecular complex could be demonstrated on starch gel electrophoresis as well as with Sephadex G-100, had an apparent molecular weight greater than 200,000, and at least to some extent, could be dissociated to yield free ^{125}I-insulin. Also to some extent, the free receptor-like binding fraction could be eluted from the insulin-Sepharose columns with excess insulin in the presence of ^{125}I-insulin as a marker. All of these findings are consistent with the insulin receptor as the membrane binding site.

It should be pointed out that, contrary to the reported findings of Cuatrecasas who is studying an apparently identical Triton X-100-solubilized insulin-binding fraction (9, 10), we could find only slight reversibility of the complex between insulin and the binding fraction. While it was claimed that virtually 100% displacement with native insulin for the ^{125}I-insulin on the complex occurred (9), we could routinely find only about 15% or less. The reason for this disparity is unclear. However, it should also be pointed out that as much as 20% or more of the ^{125}I-insulin *spontaneously* dissociated from the complex in the *absence* of added native insulin. Since Cuatrecasas did not run this important control experiment to compare the spontaneous dissociation of ^{125}I-insulin from the complex with the native insulin-induced dissociation (9), the actual reversibility in his studies is difficult to interpret. Finally, whether the inability of native insulin to displace the ^{125}I-insulin reflects a denatured complex, the physiological irreversibility of the complex, the relatively high contamination from other non-specific, irreversible binding components in the Sephadex G-100 high molecular weight fraction, or other factors, remains to be determined. Thus, further studies on the nature of the detergent-solubilized receptor-like fraction will be required in order to compare its identity with that of the "true" specific insulin-receptor.

Summary

Insulin covalently immobilized to Sepharose (S) beads directly (ins-phe-S and ins-lys-S) or indirectly through various hydrocarbon "arm" extensions of from 2 to 7 carbon lengths coupled to S (e.g. ins-lys-pent-S) were prepared and found to be biologically active on isolated adipocytes. The bioactivities were found to be due to the immobilized hormone, not to insulin released as free insulin from the immobilized state. The plasma membrane ("ghost") preparation was selectively bound to various different insulin-S affinity chromatographic columns. Increasing the "arm" length resulted in concomitant increases in amounts of membranes bound. Native insulin was found to elute the bound membranes. Membranes prepared from trypsin-treated cells lost their binding "capacities" parallel to the trypsin-induced losses of insulin sensitivity of the cells. Reincubation of trypsin-treated cells in the presence of trypsin inhibitor resulted in restorations of significant binding capacity and insulin sensitivity. The results indicated that only the plasma membrane fraction of the "ghost" preparation bound to the affinity columns not the free nuclei and other cellular particulates that contaminate this preparation. Thus, these columns may be used to purify the plasma membrane-containing fraction of the fat cell crude "ghost preparation". Utilizing a new "buoyant density" fat cell-Sepharose procedure, the firm and relatively specific binding of cells to ins-lys-pent-S beads was demonstrated. This binding (cell:bead complexes) was also demonstrated using interference contrast microscopy. Anti-insulin serum or free insulin inhibited formation of the complex, and dissociated the preformed complex. Sepharose or glycine-pent-S had no binding ability. The buoyant density results paralleled those using membranes and affinity columns.

To isolate and purify the insulin receptor, plasma membranes were solubilized with Triton X-100 and resultant extracts were subjected to starch gel electrophoresis and Sephadex gel filtration. A receptor-like fraction, capable of binding ^{125}I-insulin according to both methods, was found to have a molecular weight greater than 200,000. Contrary to a previous study elsewhere, only a relatively small per cent of the ^{125}I-insulin on the macromolecular receptor: ^{125}I-insulin complex was found to be exchangeable (*i.e.* dissociable) with native insulin, although the native hormone was fully competitive with the labeled insulin in formation of the complex. Affinity chromatography with ins-lys-pent-S successfully extracted out this receptor-like fraction selectively from the crude detergent-solubilized extract, and excess native insulin could be used to elute it off the column.

Presented by Howard M. Katzen. The authors would like to acknowledge the expert technical assistance of John Germershausen during the initial part of this study and Miss Brenda Halsey for performing many of the fat cell bioassays. We are also deeply indebted to Dr. Harry Carter of this Institute for conducting and describing to us the Nomarski interference contrast microscopic and photographic examinations.

References

1. Randle, P.J. In: G. Pincus, K.V. Thimann, and E.B. Astwood (editors), The Hormones, Vol. IV, Academic Press, Inc., N.Y. (1964), pp. 497-498.
2. Edelman, P.M. and I.L. Schwartz. Subcellular distribution of ^{131}I-insulin in striated muscle. Amer. J. Med. 40:695 (1966).
3. Garratt, C.J., R.J. Jarrett, and H. Keen. The relationship between insulin association with tissues and insulin action. Biochim. et. Biophys. Acta 121:143 (1966).
4. Wohltmann, H.J. and H.T. Narahara. Binding of insulin-^{131}I by isolated frog sartorius muscles. J. Biol. Chem. 241:4931 (1966).
5. House, P.D. and M.J. Weidemann. Characterization of an ^{125}I-insulin binding plasma membrane fraction from rat liver. Biochem. Biophys. Res. Comm.41:541 (1970).
6. Freychet, P., J. Roth, and D.M. Neville. Insulin receptors in the liver: specific binding of ^{125}-insulin to the plasma membrane and its relation to insulin bioactivity. Proc. Nat. Acad. Sci. 68: 1833 (1971).

7. Kono, T. and F.W. Barham. The relationship between the insulin-binding capacity of fat cells and the cellular response to insulin. J. Biol. Chem. 246:6210 (1971).

8. Cuatrecasas, P. Properties of the insulin receptor of isolated fat cell membranes. J. Biol. Chem. 246:7265 (1971).

9. Cuatrecasas, P. Isolation of the insulin receptor of liver and fat cell membranes. Proc. Nat. Acad. Sci. 69: 318 (1972).

10. Cuatrecasas, P. Properties of the insulin receptor isolated from liver and fat cell membranes. J. Biol. Chem. 247:1980 (1972).

11. Silman, I. and E. Katchalski. Water-insoluble derivatives of enzymes, antigens, and antibodies. Ann. Rev. Biochem. 35:873 (1966).

12. McCormick, D.B. Specific purification of avidin by column chromatography on biotin-cellulose. Anal. Biochem. 13:194 (1965).

13. Bar-Ell, A. and E. Katchalski. Preparation and properties of water-insoluble derivatives of trypsin. J. Biol. Chem. 238:1690 (1963).

14. Axen, R., J. Porath and S. Ernback. Chemical coupling of peptides and proteins to polysaccharides by means of cyanogen halides. Nature 214:1302 (1967).

15. Porath, J., R. Axen and S. Ernback. Chemical coupling of proteins to agarose. Nature 215:1491 (1967).

16. Cuatrecasas, P., M. Wilchek and C. Anfinsen. Selective enzyme purification by affinity chromatography. Proc. Nat. Acad. Sci. 61:636 (1968).

17. Wilchek, M. Enzyme purification by affinity chromatography. Israel J. Chem. 7:124p (1969).

18. Axen, R. and S. Ernback. Chemical fixation of enzymes to cyanogen halide activated polysaccharide carriers. Eur. J. Biochem. 18:351 (1971).

19. Cuatrecasas, P. and C. Anfinsen. In: W. B. Jakoby (editor), Methods in Enzymology, Vol. XXII, Academic Press, Inc., N.Y. (1971), pp. 345-378.

20. Cuatrecasas, P. Interaction of insulin with the cell membrane: the primary action of insulin. Proc. Nat. Acad. Sci. 63:450 (1969).

21. Blatt, L.M. and K-H Kim. Regulation of hepatic glycogen synthetase: stimulation of glycogen synthetase in an *in vitro* liver system by insulin bound to Sepharose. J. Biol. Chem. 246:4895 (1971).

22. Oka, T. and Y.J. Topper. Insulin-Sepharoses and the dynamics of insulin action. Proc. Nat. Acad. Sci. 68: 2066 (1971).

23. Soderman, D.D., J. Germershausen and H.M. Katzen. Specific binding of insulin-Sepharose to isolated fat cells and affinity chromatography of receptor-containing membranes. Fed. Proceedings. 31:486 (1972).

24. Greenwood, F.C., W.M. Hunter and J.S. Glover. The preparation of ^{131}I-labelled human growth hormone of high specific radioactivity. Biochem. J. 89:114 (1963).

25. Gavin, J.R., J. Roth, P. Jen and P. Freychet. Insulin receptors in human circulating cells and fibroblasts. Proc. Nat. Acad. Sci. 69:747 (1972).

26. Rodbell, M. Metabolism of isolated fat cells. I. Effects of hormones on glucose metabolism and lipolysis. J. Biol. Chem. 239:375 (1964).

27. Rodbell, M. Metabolism of isolated fat cells. V. Preparation of "ghosts" and their properties; adenyl cyclase and other enzyme J. Biol. Chem. 242:5744 (1967).

28. Lowry, O.H., N.J. Rosebrough, A.L. Farr and R.J. Randall. Protein measurement with the folin-phenol reagent. J. Biol. Chem. 193:265 (1951).

29. Kono, T. Destruction and restoration of the insulin effector system of isolated fat cells. J. Biol. Chem. 244:5777 (1969).

30. Katzen, H.M. In: G. Weber (editor), Advances in Enzyme Regulation, Vol. 5, Pergamon Press, N.Y. (1967), p. 335.

31. Katzen, H.M., D.D. Soderman and C. Wiley. Multiple forms of hexokinase: Activities associated with sub-cellular particulate and soluble fractions of normal and streptozotocin diabetic rat tissues. J. Biol. Chem. 245:4081 (1970).

32. Unpublished observations.

33. Rodbell, M. Metabolism of isolated fat cells. VI. The effect of insulin, lipolytic hormones, and theophylline on glucose transport and metabolism in ghosts. J. Biol. Chem. 242:5751 (1967).

TABLE I

RETENTION OF FAT CELL GHOSTS ON
INS-LYS-SEPHAROSE COLUMNS

*Total beads on each column were stained after final washings;
low and high insulin-S refer to 1.52 and 2.64 mg of insulin
coupled/ml of settled Sepharose, respectively. Ghosts derived from 2.6 g of adipose tissue were divided into three
0.5 ml aliquots with a net O.D. at 280 nm of 7.58 per aliquot,
one aliquot applied per column. Other details are as in
Fig. 2 and are given in Methods.*

Turbidimetric assays of pooled collected washings

Column	O.D. at 280 nm
Sepharose 4B	7.52
Ins-S (1.52 mg /ml)	5.78
Ins-S (2.64 mg /ml)	5.24

Hexokinase staining intensities of collected wash
fractions and of washed column beads

Fraction No. or Beads	Sepharose	Low Ins-S	High Ins-S
1	0	0	0
2	10+	4+	4+
3	4+	2+	1+
4	1+	1+	1+
5	1+	1+	1+
6	0	0	0
7	0	0	0
Beads	0	8+	10+

TABLE II

ELUTION OF GHOSTS BOUND TO INS-LYS-S COLUMNS

Ghosts were first applied to each column resulting in the equivalent of 15.4 turbidity (0.D. at 450 nm) units bound to the ins-S column and none that was observable bound Sepharose column. Columns were then thoroughly washed, as described in Table I, prior to elution with 5 ml of buffer, 5 mM insulin, or 2.0% albumin, as designated. The turbidity represents net 0.D. at 450 nm of the total pooled eluates collected off of each column. Other details are in Table I.

Assay	Total eluate from:				
	Ins-lys-S			Sepharose	
	buffer + insulin + albumin			buffer + insulin	
Hexokinase	0	+3	+1	0	0
Turbidity	0	1.201	0.476	0	0

TABLE III

BINDING OF GHOSTS TO COLUMNS OF INS-LYS-S DERIVATIVES
WITH INCREASING HYDROCARBON ARM LENGTHS

*A total equivalent of 12.90 turbidity units (O.D. at 280 nm)
of membrane preparation was applied to each column. After
fraction 4 (final washing), resultant washed "beads", each
collected wash fraction, and total pooled washings were
estimated for hexokinase activities, and turbidities were
measured as designated. All ins-Sepharoses were prepareed
with insulin added during the preparation at a concentration
of 8 mg/ml of settled Sepharose. Further details are given
in Table I and Methods.*

Column	Beads	Washings	Wash fractions				
			0	1	2	3	4
	Hexokinase	Turbidity	Hexokinase				
Sepharose	0	12.79	0	8	5	2	1
Ins-lys-S	2+	10.15	0	5	3	2	1
Ins-lys-ethyl-S	1+	11.64	0	5	3	2	1
Ins-lys-propyl-S	2+	9.97	0	3	2	2	1
Ins-lys-butyl-S	4+	8.64	0	3	2	1	1
Ins-lys-pentyl-S	8+	6.24	0	2	1	1	0
Ins-lys-heptyl-S	7+	4.33	0	2	1	1	0

TABLE IV

BINDING OF GHOSTS TO COLUMNS OF INS-PHE-S DERIVATIVES
WITH INCREASING HYDROCARBON ARM LENGTHS

*A total equivalent of 9.05 O.D. turbidity units of membrane
preparation was added to each column. Other details are as
in Table III.*

Column	Pooled washings	Washed beads
	turbidity at 280 nm	hexokinase - NBT
Sepharose	8.99	0
ins-phe-S	6.57	1+
ins-phe-ethyl-S	8.97	0
ins-phe-propyl-S	5.23	3+
ins-phe-pentyl-S	1.90	6+

TABLE V

AFFINITY COLUMN BINDING DETERMINED
BY USING ^{14}C-LABELED GHOSTS

*Percentages are based upon comparison of cpm of ^{14}C applied
to each column compared to ^{14}C washed through ("pooled washings"), as well as to the ^{14}C directly bound to the beads
after final washing ("washed beads"). ^{14}C-ghosts were prepared from fat cells treated with a mixture of ^{14}C-amino
acids to incorporate ^{14}C-amino acids into membrane protein.
"Act-D" refers to cells treated with actinomycin-D to block
incorporation. Further description and details are given
in Methods and Results.*

Column	Applied	Pooled Washings	Beads
		% bound	
ins-lys-pent-S	^{14}C-ghosts	75	70
ins-lys-pent-S	^{14}C-amino acids	0	0
ins-lys-pent-S	^{14}C-ghosts (Act.D.)	26	30
ins-phe-pent-S	^{14}C-ghosts	65	58
Sepharose	^{14}C-ghosts	8	6

TABLE VI

EFFECT OF TRYPSIN ON INSULIN-SENSITIVITY OF FAT CELLS,
AND REGENERATION OF SENSITIVITY

*Insulin sensitivity was determined by measurement of oxida-
tion of glucose-1-^{14}C to $^{14}CO_2$ during a 1 hour incubation
in the presence and absence of insulin in fat cell bioassay.
The effect of trypsin was determined (29) by incubating cells
for 15 min at 37°C in K-R-bicarbonate buffer (pH 7.4), in
the presence and absence of trypsin (1 mg/ml); soybean trypsin inhibitor (29) was incubated separately with the trypsin
for 5 min prior to 15 min incubation with cells (designated
"zero time"), or immediately after the incubation (designated
"15 min"). Cells were assayed "immediately", as designated,
or after a 90 min additional incubation (designated "after
reincubation") in the presence of 1 mM glucose and inhibitor.
Further description is given in Results.*

| | | | Assay | |
| | Trypsin | | | after |
Trypsin	Inhibitor	± insulin	immediately	reincubation
			$(cpm\ ^{14}CO_2)$	
−	−	−	527	441
−	−	+	1359	1265
+	15 min	−	461	167
+	15 min	+	497	460
+	zero time	−	423	600
+	zero time	+	1330	1308
+	zero time	−	449	−
+	zero time	+	4009	−
+	15 min	−	505	−
+	15 min	+	650	−

TABLE VII

TRYPSIN-INDUCED LOSS AND RESTORATION OF BINDING OF GHOSTS
TO INSULIN-PENT-LYS-S COLUMNS

*Cells were incubated with trypsin (1 mg/ml or as designated)
for 15 min, as described in Table VI, in the presence and
absence of soybean trypsin inhibitor, and ghosts were prepared from an aliquot of treated cells after the addition
of inhibitor. The resultant ghosts ("after trypsin treatment") were subsequently tested for their ability to bind
to insulin-S, as designated. The remaining aliquot of trypsin-treated cells was subjected to an additional incubation
(designated "reincubation") for 90 min at 37°C in the absence (line designated "A") and presence (as designated) of
inhibitor, after which inhibitor was added as necessary and
ghosts were prepared to test their binding capacity. Binding capacities were determined by turbidity measurements as
described in Fig. 2. "ΔO.D." refers to membranes bound as
determined by difference between turbidities (at 450 nm)
applied and washed off of columns. Other details are as in
Table VI and are described in Methods.*

	Ghosts Bound After:			
Cell treatment	Trypsin-treatment		Reincubation	
	$\Delta O.D.$	%	$\Delta O.D.$	%
inhibitor + trypsin	2.40	48	2.05	41
trypsin (4 mg/ml)	0.00	0	–	–
trypsin (1 mg/ml)	0.00	0	–	–
trypsin (0.25 mg/ml) ("A")	0.85	17	0.00	0.00
"A" reincubated with				
inhibitor	0.85	17	1.72	34

TABLE VIII

DETERMINATION OF FAT CELL BINDING TO INSULIN-S BEADS
BY BUOYANT DENSITY PROCEDURE

*Ins-lys-pent-S at 750 µg insulin coupled/ml of settled Seph-
arose and ins-lys-S at 450 µg/ml were used. Glycine-pent-S
was prepared using a concentration of glycine identical to
that of the insulin used for ins-lys-pent-S. The ratio of
cells to ins-lys-pent-S was adjusted arbitrarily so as to
obtain half of the ins-S beads in the suspended (buoyant)
phase, the remaining half in the sedimentable phase. A similar ratio was used for the other Sepharose preparations.
"Percent Suspended" refers to percent of beads suspended as
determined by volume and radioactivity measurements of resultant floating and sedimented phases of unlabeled and ^{125}I-
insulin-labeled insulin-S beads, and cells. AIS and other
designated supplements at 0.02 ml were added to the cell
suspension immediately before addition of the beads. Serum
at the same protein concentration as the AIS, insulin at
$10^{-5}M$ and albumin at 1% were used. Cells were treated with
trypsin (as designated) at 1 mg/ml prior to buoyant density
assay. Other details are given in Methods and in Results.*

Components mixed with cells	Trypsin-treated cells	% Suspended (Buoyancy)
Sepharose	±	0
ins-lys-pent-S	−	50
ins-lys-pent-S	+	25
ins-lys-S	−	15
glycine-pent-S	±	3
ins-lys-pent-S + AIS	−	0
ins-lys-pent-S + Serum	−	55
ins-lys-pent-S + insulin	−	5
ins-lys-pent-S + albumin	−	53

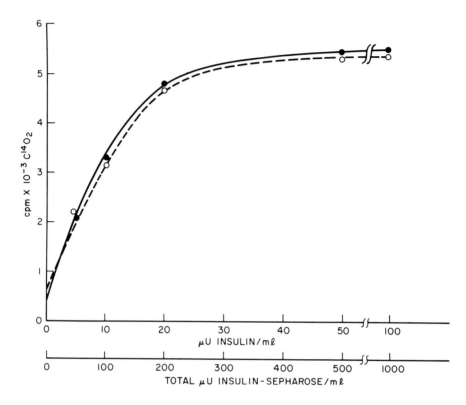

Fig. 1. *Biological activity of insulin-Sepharose preparations.*
Native insulin (-•-•-) and ins-lys-pent-S (--o--o--) were assayed by the isolated fat cell method of Rodbell (26). According to amino acid analysis 450 µg of insulin were coupled per ml of settled Sepharose.

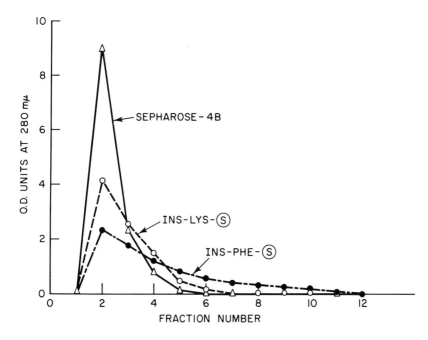

Fig. 2. *Affinity chromatography profiles of turbidity measurements at 280 nm of collected wash-fractions.* Ins-lys-S and Ins-phe-S were coupled at 1.52 and 2.15 mg of insulin per ml of settled Sepharose, respectively. Ghosts suspended in Krebs-Ringer bicarbonate buffer (pH 7.4), were derived from 4.1 g of adipose tissue and were divided equally into three 0.5 ml aliquots, and 0.5 ml were applied to each column containing 1 ml of settled Sepharose per column. Columns were washed with buffer, and 1.5 ml per fraction were collected. "(S)" refers to Sepharose. Other details are given in Methods.

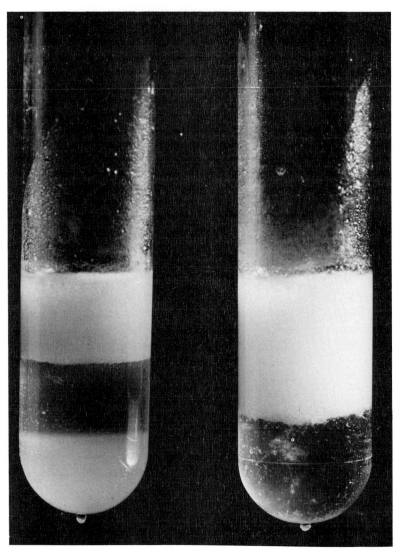

Fig. 3. *Spontaneous buoyant density distribution of fat cells, Sepharose beads and ins-lys-pent-S.* The distributions were at 30°, 5 minutes after thorough mixing of cells and beads in K-R-bicarbonate buffer containing 0.2 per cent albumin. To each tube were added diluted aliquots of beads equivalent to 0.50 ml of either settled Sepharose (tube on left) or ins-lys-pent-S (2.6 mg insulin coupled per ml settled Sepharose, tube on right), and 0.5 ml of packed floating fat cells (packed by 450 x *g* centrifugation) and buffer to a final volume of 1.5 ml. Other details are given in Results and Methods.

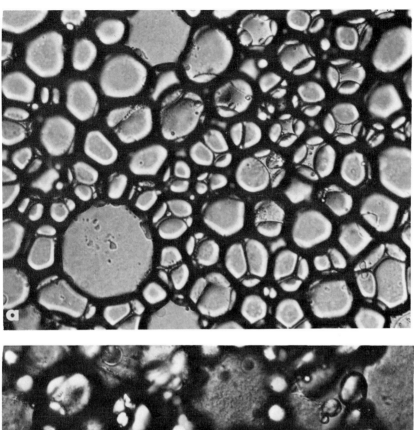

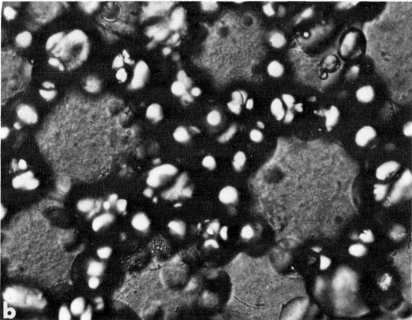

Fig. 4. *Nomarski interference contrast microscopy (500 x magnification) of mixtures of fat cells and Sepharose beads (panel "A"), and cells and ins-lys-pent-S beads ("B"), and diluted mixture of cells and ins-lys-pent-S ("C" and "D"). Larger spheres are beads and smaller ones cells.* Other details are as in Fig. 3. See page 232 for c and d

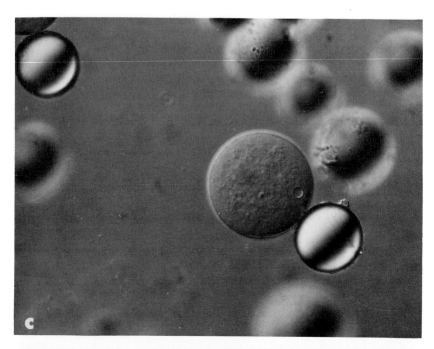

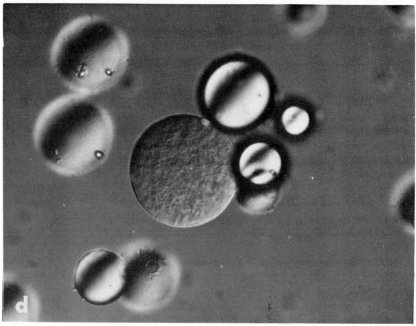

FILTRATION	cpm ^{125}I	PERCENT
PLUS TRITON		
TOTAL APPLIED	5422	—
INSOLUBLE	3236	60
FILTRATE	2001	37
MINUS TRITON		
INSOLUBLE	5026	94
FILTRATE	280	5

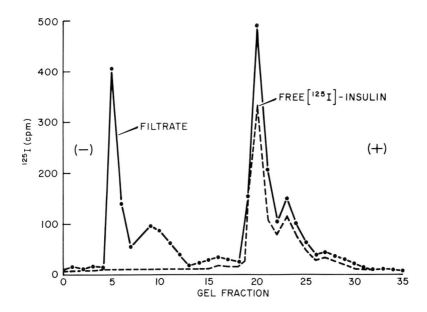

Fig. 5. *Starch gel electrophoresis of Triton-Solubilized, membrane-bound ^{125}I-insulin.* After 30 min incubation in K-R phosphate buffer (pH 7.4) of fat cell ghosts from 3 g of adipose tissue with 0.5 μCi ^{125}I-insulin, ghosts were washed twice with buffer, solubilized with 0.5% Triton X-100, filtered through 0.45 μ HAWP Millipore filter paper, and the resultant filtrate applied to gel origin. ^{125}I-insulin, in the absence of ghosts, was added as a marker to a separate origin on the gel. Each gel fraction was counted as a 0.5 cm slice. Other details are given in Methods.

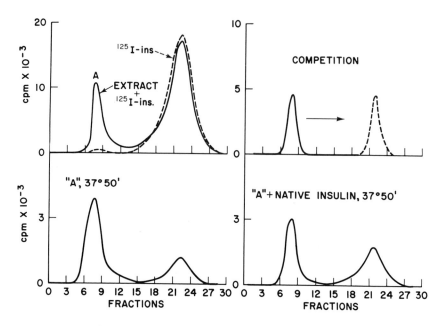

Fig. 6. *Sephadex G-100 gel filtration profiles of Triton-solublized ghosts ("Extract") incubated with* ^{125}I-*insulin.*
On upper left, 10 ng of ^{125}I-insulin (---) in the absence
of ghosts was used as a marker. In "Competition" experiment,
2 ng of ^{125}I-insulin was incubated with solubilized ghosts
from 2.5 g of adipose tissue in the absence (——) and in the
presence (----) of 20 μg of native insulin in final volume
of 0.5 ml of K-R-phosphate buffer containing 0.1% bovine
plasma albumin. Arrow designates displacement of peak on
left with peak on the right due to presence of native insulin. On the bottom 2 panels, pooled peak fractions from
peak "A" were incubated in the absence and presence of 1 mg/
ml of native insulin. Fractions of 1 ml each were collected.
Columns were equilibrated with buffer containing 0.5 per cent
Triton. Other details are as in Fig. 5.

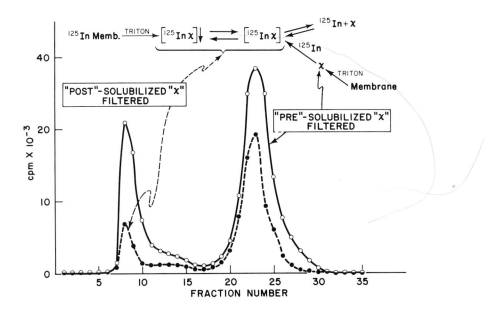

Fig. 7. *Sephadex G-100 gel filtration profiles of fat cell ghosts ("Memb.") solubilized with Triton and then Millipore filtered ("Filtered") before incubation ("Pre") of solubilized ghosts and after ("Post") incubation of intact ghosts with 5 μl of* ^{125}I-*insulin (*^{125}In*).* Other details are described in Text and in Figs. 5 and 6.

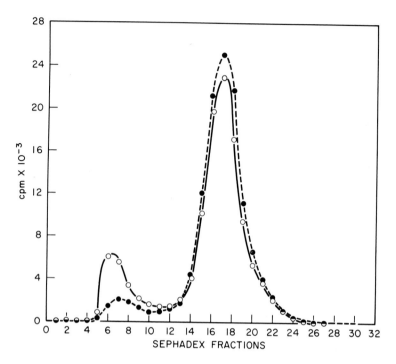

Fig. 8. *Sephadex G-100 gel filtration profiles of Triton-solubilized ghosts that were incubated with* [125]*I-insulin after prior passage of the solubilized ghosts through affinity chromatographic columns of ins-lys-pent-S (●) and control Sepharose (o).* All columns were equilibrated with buffer containing 0.5 per cent Triton. Further description of procedure is given in Results and Methods, and details of Sephadex gel filtration are as in Fig. 6.

THE INTERACTION OF INSULIN WITH FAT CELLS:
ITS PHYSIOLOGICAL SIGNIFICANCE

Tetsuro Kono and Oscar B. Crofford

Introduction

As one of the many fascinating functions of cell membranes, it has long been hypothesized that the plasma membranes of certain cell types are equipped with specific
hormone receptors that have a capacity to interact with
specific hormones and thereby generate and transmit the intracellular hormonal signals to the metabolic processes.
One such hormone receptor is that for insulin. In this
presentation, I wish to describe how the concept of the insulin receptor, which was originally introduced as a purely
operational term, has been substantiated empirically during
the course of the past 20 years.

In 1952 and 1953, Stadie *et al.* (1,2) reported that
certain insulin derivatives labeled with either ^{131}I or ^{35}S
tightly bound to rat diaphragm *in vitro* and showed the expected biological activity. However, as in the cases of
other pioneer work, their observations were challenged by
others. First,it was noted by Kono and Colowick (3) that
the binding of iodoinsulin to rat diaphragm was reversible
and, therefore, it was difficult to make a clear cut distinction between the bound insulin and the interstitial
free hormone. This technical difficulty was subsequently
overcome by the work of Wohltmann and Narahara (4), who
found that the binding of iodoinsulin to frog sartorius
muscle was practically irreversible at $0°$, although it was
reversible at $19°$. This observation was later confirmed
with fat cells (5), fat cell membranes (6), and liver cell
membrane preparations (7). Second,several investigators
noted that certain iodoinsulin preparations had little or
no biological activities [*cf.*(8,9)]. This problem was
later solved by Garratt (8) and Izzo *et al.* (9), who showed
that iodoinsulin preparations that contained only one, or

less than one, iodine atom per insulin molecule retained
almost the full biological activity. Although it was possible that a "monoiodo"-insulin preparation was a mixture of
native insulin and polyiodoinsulin, it was recently noted
that the binding characteristics of $[^{125}I]$-iodoinsulin to
fat cells were similar to those of native insulin (5). In
this connection, it was noted by Antoniades and Gershoff
(10) and Crofford (11) that diaphragm, adipose tissue, or
isolated fat cells could take up not only labeled iodoinsulin but also unlabeled native insulin. Third, a number of
investigators noted that the binding of either native or
iodinated insulin to muscle or fat cell preparations was
not saturated at the hormone concentration where the typical biological effect of insulin was saturated (4,5,11,12,
13,14,15,16). For example, Kono and Barham noted that
glucose utilization in fat cells was stimulated to the half-
maximal when the insulin concentration $[K_e'$;e for effector]
was approximately 50 pM (4,17) but the binding of the hormone to the cells reached the half-maximal point only when
the hormone concentration (K_e) was 5 (18) to 7 nM (5). Incidentally, the normal insulin concentration in rat blood
is less than 1 nM [$e.g.$ (19)]. Consequently, it was previously suggested that either there was little correlation
between the binding and physiological effects of insulin
(12,13) or there might be specific (or active or physiological) and non-specific (or inactive or non-physiological)
insulin bindings in cells or tissues (4,14). However,
recent studies by Kono and Barham on the characteristics
of trypsin-treated fat cells (5) indicated that there can be
be a new interpretation, as discussed below in detail.

Results and Discussion

*Proteolytic modification of the insulin receptor in
fat cells.*

When adipose tissue or isolated fat cells of rats were
exposed to trypsin (1 mg/ml) for 15 min (in the presence of
crude serum albumin) the cells were rendered unresponsive
to insulin even at high hormone concentrations (17,20,21).
Under the same conditions, trypsin also rendered fat cells
either totally or partially unresponsive to glucagon (100%),

ACTH[1] (20-50%), or epinephrine (0-20%) (17,20,21,22). However, the enzyme did not significantly alter the other cellular parameters such as the glucose-transport capacity, the contents of ATP or fat, or the adenylate cyclase-phosphodiesterase activity (20,21). These observations, which were first noted by Kono (20,21,22) and later confirmed by others (23,24,25), are consistent with the view that trypsin modifies certain hormone receptors, which are presumably located in the cell surface, without affecting the other components in the cell (5,23).

When trypsin-treated fat cells were subsequently incubated with buffer alone for 1 to 2 hours after trypsin was inactivated with soybean trypsin inhibitor, the cells regained their responsiveness to insulin (21). However, it should be emphasized at this point that the cells *recovered* from trypsin treatment were less sensitive to insulin as compared to the untreated control, although their maximal metabolic response to the hormone (at high concentrations) was almost comparable to the control (17,22). It may appear, therefore, that *recovered* cells are equipped with modified insulin receptors that have a low affinity for the hormone. However, according to the data of Kono and Barham (5) the affinity of insulin with *recovered* cells was almost the same with that of the untreated control, while the maximal insulin binding capacity of *recovered* cells was considerably smaller than the control; thus, the observed K_e value (dissociation constant) of the insulin-fat cell complex was approximately 7 nM (5); whereas, the B_{max} values (the maximal insulin binding capacity) of untreated and *recovered* cells were 4.1 and 0.27 pmoles, respectively, per g of fat cells (5). Incidentally, the former figure indicates that untreated fat cells are equipped with approximately 21 receptors per μm^2 of their cell surface if the receptors are evenly distributed (5).

Relationship between the binding and physiological effects of insulin.

In order to explain the puzzling characteristics of

---

[1]*The abbreviations used in this article are: ACTH, adrenocorticotropic hormone; cyclic AMP, adenosine 3',5'-monophosphate.*

recovered cells described in the previous section, Kono
and Barham (5) proposed a hypothesis, which is schematically
presented in Fig. 1. It is assumed in this figure (a) that
the action of insulin in fat cells is mediated by an unknown hormonal signal and (b) that the maximal insulin
binding capacities (B_{max}) of untreated and *recovered* cells
are A and B. As it was noted earlier, the K_e' (for glucose
utilization) and K_e (for binding) of insulin in fat cells
are 50 pM and 7 nM, respectively. As it may be seen in the
figure, when the B_{max} value is reduced from A to B (without changing the K_e value), the system cannot maintain
the maximal metabolic response unless the hormone concentration is increased from a to b. Although no particular
line is provided in the figure, it may be apparent that
when the B_{max} value is reduced to less than a certain
critical point, the system cannot maintain the maximal
metabolic response even in the presence of insulin in high
concentrations. It appears, therefore, that this model
system is consistent, at least qualitatively, with the
above mentioned experimental data that trypsin-treated
fat cells which had a minimum number of insulin receptors
were unresponsive to insulin even at high hormone concentrations and that *recovered* cells equipped with a certain
small number of newly formed receptors can respond to the
hormone in full if the hormone concentration was sufficiently high.

The quantitative aspect of the above hypothesis was
tested by the experiment summarized in Table I. As it may
be seen, the observed data were in good agreement with the
theoretical values that were estimated from the B_{max} and
K_e values by the law of mass action. In this connection,
it was shown in a separate experiment that glucose utilization in various types of fat cell preparations(*i.e.*,
those that were untreated or *recovered* from different
lengths of trypsin treatment) were stimulated almost maximally when the binding of insulin to fat cells was 0.1pMole
per g (5). This suggests that fat cells can generate a
hormonal signal which is strong enough to stimulate glucose
utilization maximally when the cells are interacted with
0.1 pMole insulin per g (5), or approximately 4,000 insulin
molecules per single cell (5). It is of interest to note
that the last figure is very close to the value estimated
by Crofford and Minemura [3,000; *cf*. (30)] by a different
method.

According to the hypothesis in Fig. 1, there is no reason why the K_e value for binding should be equal to K_e' value for a certain metabolic process. In fact, it is possible to postulate that a number of metabolic processes with different K_e' values are regulated by a common insulin signal transmitted from a single type of receptor, since individual metabolic processes may be stimulated half-maximally at certain levels of the common insulin signal (18). This idea is consistent with the experimental data that a number of metabolic processes in fat cells are regulated half-maximally at different insulin concentrations (11,18), while only one K_e value (for binding) was noted by Kono and Barham (5). Naturally, the above discussion does not imply that all the insulin sensitive metabolic processes are regulated by the same mechanism. The mechanisms involved between the individual metabolic processes and the common insulin signal mentioned above may be very complex and different.

Conclusion

It may be concluded from the considerations described above that (a) fat cells, and presumably other insulin-sensitive cells as well, are equipped with the specific insulin receptor which possesses essential peptide elements and is distinct from the glucose-transport or the adenylatecyclase-phosphodiesterase system in the cell (20,21),and (b) at least in the case of fat cells, most (if not all) of the observed binding of insulin are those of the specific, or physiologically active, type (5). Although only a fraction of the total available receptors may be occupied by insulin under the physiological conditions, the presence of receptors that are unoccupied by insulin does not necessarily indicate that there are nonspecific, or spare, receptors (5). Instead, it is suggested that the presence of a large number of unoccupied (but fully active) receptors has a great physiological significance since the apparent metabolic sensitivity of cells to the hormone can be dependent on the B_{max} value (Fig. 1). It may be added in this connection that the model system presented in Fig. 1 is applicable not only to the insulin system in fat cells but also the glucagon system in rat liver, as discussed elsewhere (18). Incidentally, the presence of a low-K_e receptor

in fat cells was reported by Cuatrecasas (26). The relationship between this low-K_e receptor and the high-K_e receptor
observed by others (5,11,15) is not clear.

As it is suggested by the observation that the insulin
receptor is readily modifiable with trypsin, the receptor
is probably located on the cell membrane. This view was
substantiated by the work of Crofford and Okayama (27),
who showed that the plasma membranes prepared from untreated
fat cells had a capacity to take up insulin but those from
trypsin-treated cells did not. This observation was recently confirmed by Cuatrecasas (28) and Soderman et $al.$ (29),
who, furthermore, were successful in solubilizing an insulin-
binding protein from the plasma membranes of liver and fat
cells (28,29). The regeneration of the insulin receptor
after the initial trypsin treatment is tentatively considered
to be a result of the turnover of the cell membrane; the
rate of regeneration of the receptor was a few per cent of
the untreated control per hour (5). In this connection, it
was shown previously that the recovery of physiological response was inhibited by puromycin or cycloheximide (21).
Although it was noted earlier that the binding of insulin
to the receptor was reversible (3,5,6), it was recently
suggested by Crofford, Rogers, and Russell (30) that the
dissociation of insulin, hence the termination of the hormonal action, is facilitated by the insulin-decomposing
activity of the cell membrane.

As for the physiological effects of insulin, it has
been well documented that the hormone (a) stimulates protein
synthesis and glucose transport across the cell membrane in
muscle and fat cells [$cf.$ (31)], and (b) inhibits lipolysis
and glucose release in rat cells [$cf.$ (31)] and liver (32),
respectively. Some of these effects of the hormone are
probably related to its ability to lower the cellular levels
of cyclic AMP [$cf.$(31)]. However, it is still obscure at
the present time how the interaction of insulin with the
specific cellular receptor induces these regulatory effects
in the cell.

---

*Presented by Tetsuro Kono. The preparation of this article
was supported by United States Public Health Service Grants
RO1 AM06725 and 07462-AMP.*

References

1. Stadie, W.C., N. Haugaard, and M. Vaughan. Studies of insulin binding with isotopically labeled insulin. J. Biol. Chem. 199:729-739 (1952).

2. Stadie, W.C., N. Haugaard, and M. Vaughan. The quantitative relation between insulin and its biological activity. J. Biol. Chem. 200:745-751 (1953).

3. Kono, T. and S.P. Colowick. Isolation of skeletal muscle cell membrane and some of its properties. Arch. Biochem. Biophys. 93:520-533 (1961).

4. Wohltmann, H. and H.T. Narahara. Binding of insulin-^{131}I by isolated frog sartorius muscle. J. Biol. Chem. 241:4931-4939 (1966).

5. Kono, T. and F.W. Barham. The relationship between the insulin-binding capacity of fat cells and the cellular response to insulin. J. Biol. Chem. 246:6210-6216 (1971).

6. Cuatrecasas, P. Properties of insulin receptor of isolated fat cell membranes. J. Biol. Chem. 246:7265-7274 (1971).

7. Cuatrecasas, P., B. Desbuquois, and F. Krug. Insulin-receptor interactions in liver cell membranes. Biochem. Biophys. Res. Commun. 44:333-339 (1971).

8. Garratt, C.J. Effect of iodoinsulin on the biological activity of insulin. Nature 201:1324-1325 (1964).

9. Izzo, J.L., A. Roncone, M.J. Izzo, and W.F. Bale. Relationship between degree of iodination of insulin and its biological, electrophoretic, and immunochemical properties. J. Biol. Chem. 239:3749-3754 (1964).

10. Antoniades, H.N., S.N. Gershoff. Inhibitory effects of bound insulin on insulin uptake by isolated tissues. Diabetes 15:655-662 (1966).

11. Crofford, O.B. The uptake and inactivation of native insulin by isolated fat cells. J. Biol. Chem. 243:362-369 (1968).

12. Malaisse, W. and J.R.M. Franckson. Application des radioisotopes a l'etude de la consommation de glucose par le diaphragme de rat normal. Arch. int. Pharmacodyn. 155:484-494 (1965).

13. Bewsher, P.D. Effects of nethalide on insulin activity and binding by rat muscle and adipose tissue. Mor. Pharmacol. 2:227-236 (1966).

14. Garratt, C.J., J.S. Cameron, and G.Menzinger. The association of ^{131}I-iodoinsulin with rat diaphragm

muscle and its effect on glucose uptake. Biochim. Biophys. Acta 115:176–186 (1966).

15. Garratt, C.J., R.J. Jarrett, and H. Keen. The relationship between insulin association with tissues and insulin action. Biochim. Biophys. Acta 121:143–150 (1966).

16. Balázsi, I. Insulin uptake by isolated rat fat cells. Acta Physiol. Acad. Sci. Hungaricae 38:351–356 (1970).

17. Kono, T. and F.W. Barham. Insulin-like effects of trypsin on fat cells. J. Biol. Chem. 246:6204–6209 (1971).

18. Kono, T. The insulin receptor of fat cells. In: The Proceeding of Symp. on Insulin Action. I. B. Fritz (Editor). Academic Press, New York (1972) pp. 171–203.

19. Morgan, C.R. and A. Lazarow. Immunoassay of insulin. Diabetes. 12:115–126 (1963).

20. Kono, T. Destruction of insulin effector system of adipose tissue cells by proteolytic enzymes. J. Biol. Chem. 244:1772–1778 (1969).

21. Kono, T. Destruction and restoration of the insulin effector system of isolated fat cells. J. Biol. Chem. 244:5777–5784 (1969).

22. Kono, T. Insulin effector system of fat cells. In: Adipose Tissue. B. Jeanrenaud and D. Hepp (Editors). Georg Thieme Verlag, Stuttgart, and Academic Press, New York, pp. 108–111 (1970).

23. Fain, J.N. and S.C. Loken. Response of trypsin treated brown and white fat cells to hormones. J. Biol. Chem. 244:3500–3506 (1969).

24. Czech, M.P. and J.N. Fain. Insulin protection against fat cell receptor inactivation by trypsin. Endocrinology 87:191–194 (1970).

25. Rodbell, M., L. Birnbaumer, and S.L. Pohl. Adenyl cyclase in fat cells. (III). J. Biol. Chem. 245:718–722 (1970).

26. Cuatrecasas, P. Insulin-receptor interaction in adipose tissue cells. Proc. Natl. Acad. Sci. U.S.A. 68:1264 (1971).

27. Crofford, O.B. and T. Okayama. Insulin-receptor interaction in isolated fat cells. Diabetes. 19:369 (1970).

28. Cuatrecasas, P. Properties of the insulin receptor isolated from liver and fat cell membranes. J. Biol. Chem. 247:1980–1991 (1972).

29. Soderman, D.D., J. Germershausen, and H.M. Katzen. Specific binding of insulin-sepharoses to isolated fat cells and affinity chromatography of receptor-containing membranes. Fed. Proc. 31:486 (1972).

30. Crofford, O.B., N.L. Rogers, and W.G. Russell. The effect of insulin on fat cells. Diabetes (in press).

31. Crofford, O.B., T. Minemura, and T. Kono. Insulin-receptor interaction in isolated fat cells. Advances in Enzyme Regulation 8:219-238 (1970).

32. Exton, J.H. and S.C. Harper. Role of cyclic AMP and glucocorticoid in the action of hepatic gluconeogenesis by diabetes. Fed. Proc. 31:243 (1972).

TABLE I

EFFECTS OF THE B_{MAX} VALUE ON THE BINDING
OF INSULIN TO FAT CELLS

This table shows the insulin concentrations when the binding of the hormone to fat cells was 0.1 pmole per g. The binding of insulin was estimated using [^{125}I]-iodoinsulin as the tracer. The theoretical values were calculated from the given B_{max} and K_e values by the law of mass action. [The figures were calculated from the data of Kono and Barham (5)].

Cell Preparations	B_{max} [a]	Insulin concentrations when binding is 0.1 pMole/g	
		Observed	Calculated
	pMole/g	*pM*	
Untreated	4.1	173	166
Recovered from 15 sec[b]	0.60	1133	1333
Recovered from 15 min[b]	0.27	4533	4000

[a]K_e = 6.7 nM, in all cases.

[b]*Time for treatment of cells with trypsin (1mg/ml).*

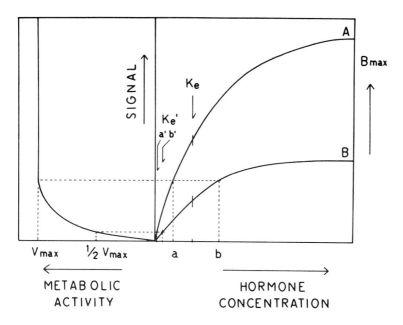

Fig. 1. *A schematic presentation of a hypothetical action of a hormone to a metabolic process.* The figure indicates that when the action of a hormone is mediated by an intracellular signal, the K_e value (for binding) and K_e' value (for metabolic effect) of the hormone are not necessarily the same. The figure also shows that when the B_{max} value (maximal hormone binding capacity) of the cells is reduced from A to B without changing the K_e value, one has to increase the hormone concentration from a to b in order to maintain the original maximal metabolic activity. (Kono: unpublished drawing).

THE ROLE OF PHOSPHOLIPIDS IN THE ACTIVATION OF MYOCARDIAL ADENYLATE CYCLASE BY GLUCAGON, HISTAMINE, AND THE CATECHOLAMINES

Gerald S. Levey

Introduction

The actions of many hormones appear to be related to their capacity to increase the activity of the membrane-bound enzyme adenylate cyclase, which catalyzes the conversion of ATP to adenosine 3',5'-cyclic monophosphate (cyclic AMP). Important in this scheme of hormone action is the receptor which serves as the binding site for the hormone on the external cell surface. Current evidence suggests that hormone receptors consist of proteins and phospholipids (1, 2). In this regard, we have reported the preparation of a solubilized myocardial adenylate cyclase utilizing a nonionic detergent, Lubrol-PX (3, 4). The solubilized myocardial adenylate cyclase in the presence or absence of detergent is unresponsive to the hormones which activate the particulate enzyme, norepinephrine, glucagon, histamine, and thyroxine (3). We have studied the role of phospholipids as they relate to the hormone-responsiveness of solubilized myocardial adenylate cyclase using a preparation freed of detergent by DEAE-cellulose chromatography. The data show that phosphatidylserine restores hormone activation of the adenylate cyclase by glucagon and histamine and that phosphatidylinositol restores the norepinephrine-activation.

Methods

Preparation of detergent-free, solublized adenylate cyclase

Normal cats were anesthetized with pentobarbital, 25-

35 mg per kg intraperitoneally, and the heart was quickly excised. The left ventricle was dissected free of endocardium and epicardium and about 300 mg of muscle was homogenized in 4.5 ml of a cold solution containing in final concentration sucrose, 0.25 M; Tris HCl, 10 mM, pH 7.7; Lubrol-PX, 20 mM; and EDTA-magnesium chloride, 1 mM. The homogenate was centrifuged at 12,000 x g for 10 minutes at 4°C. Approximately 1.3 ml of the 12,000 g supernatant containing the solubilized myocardial adenylate cyclase and having a protein concentration of 4 mg/ml was applied to a 1.0 x 12.0 cm DEAE-cellulose column equilibrated at 4°C in Tris-HCl, 10 mM, pH 7.7. The flow rate was approximately 0.20 ml/min. The column containing the enzyme was washed with 15-20 volumes of Tris-HCl, 10 mM, pH 7.7. Adenylate cyclase was eluted with Tris HCl, 1 M, pH 7.7. The fraction containing adenylate cyclase activity has been shown to be totally free of detergent using Lubrol-PX labeled with ^{14}C in the ethylene oxide moiety (4).

Adenylate cyclase assay

Adenylate cyclase was assayed by the method of Krishna, Weiss, and Brodie (5). The fractions for assay containing 0.025 to 0.05 mg protein in a total volume of 0.06 ml were incubated at 37°C for five minutes with ATP, 1.6 mM α-^{32}P-ATP, 2.5-3.5 x 10^6 cpm; theophylline 8 mM; Mg Cl$_2$, 2 mM; Tris-HCl, 21 mM, pH 7.7; and human serum albumin, 0.8 mg/ml. Phosphatidylserine dispersed in Tris-HCl, 10 mM, pH 7.7, and histamine were added to the enzyme at 1°C, to the other components which were at 23°C. After five minutes the incubations were stopped and the ^{32}P-cyclic 3',5'-AMP accumulated was determined as previously described (6).

Preparation of phospholipids

Phosphatidylserine (25 mg/ml) and phosphatidylinositol (10 mg/ml) were obtained as solutions in CHCl$_3$. The required amount was placed in a 10 x 75 mm glass test tube and the CHCl$_3$ was removed by evaporation with a stream of nitrogen. One milliliter of Tris-HCl, 10 mM, pH 7.7, was added to the residue and the lipid was dispersed by sonication with a Sonifier Cell Disrupter, Model W185, Branson

Sonic Power Company, until there was no apparent change in clarity of the solution, generally one half to one minute. Both phospholipids yielded one spot with thin-layer chromatography in either of two separate solvent systems; either $CHCl_3:CH_3OH:CH_3COOH:H_2O$ (100:60:16:8), or $CHCl_3:CH_3OH:H_2O$ (65:25:4).

Materials

Chromatographically pure phosphatidylinositol was prepared from bovine brain by Dr. S. Ramachandran, Applied Science Laboratories, State College, Pennsylvania. Histamine phosphate and crystalline glucagon were gifts from Eli Lilly and Co., Indianapolis, Indiana; diphenhydramine hydrochloride (Benadryl) was from Parke, Davis and Co., Detroit, Michigan. L-norepinephrine bitartrate was from Sigma Chemical Co., St. Louis, Missouri. D,L-propranolol was from Ayerst Laboratories, New York. Lubrol-PX was a gift from ICI America Inc., Stanford, Connecticut. Alpha labeled ^{32}P-ATP was from International Chemical and Nuclear Corp., Irvine, California.

Results

Effect of phosphatidylserine on hormone-responsiveness of solubilized myocardial adenylate cyclase

Figure 1A shows that the solubilized myocardial adenylate cyclase freed of detergent by DEAE-cellulose chromatography is unresponsive to stimulation by concentrations of glucagon ($1 \times 10^{-5}M$), histamine ($8 \times 10^{-5}M$), and norepinephrine ($5 \times 10^{-5}M$), which maximally activate the particulate myocardial adenylate cyclase (7-10). The addition of phosphatidylserine (8 µg/incubation, 128 µg/ml) restores the responsiveness to glucagon and histamine but not to norepinephrine (Fig. 1B).

Concentration-response curves for glucagon and histamine in the presence of phosphatidylserine

Glucagon (Fig. 2A) and histamine (Fig. 2B) activated the solubilized myocardial adenylate cyclase in the pres-

ence of phosphatidylserine over similar concentration
ranges reported for these hormones with the particulate
enzyme (7, 9). Half maximal activation occurred at 5 x
10^{-7}M for glucagon and 2 x 10^{-5}M for histamine.

*Effect of diphenhydramine on the glucagon and hista-
mine-mediated activation of adenylate cyclase*

The activation of the particulate myocardial adenylate
cyclase by histamine is abolished by the antihistamine
diphenhydramine (9). In an attempt to ascertain whether
the phosphatidylserine-reconstituted system for glucagon
and histamine activation conformed to the receptor-specifi-
city observed in particulate preparations we examined the
effect of diphenhydramine on the glucagon and histamine-
mediated activation of the solubilized adenylate cyclase.
Table I shows that diphenhydramine, 8 x 10^{-5}M, abolished
the accumulation of cyclic AMP produced by histamine, 8
x 10^{-5}M, but not that produced by glucagon, 1 x 10^{-5}M.

Effective concentrations of phosphatidylserine

The concentration of phosphatidylserine half-maximally
effective in restoring the activation produced by glucagon
and histamine, was 2 µg/incubation or 32 µg/ml. Concentrations less than 1 µg/incubation (16 µg/ml) were without
effect and concentrations greater than 4 µg/incubation (64
µg/ml) were maximally effective.

*Restoration of catecholamine-responsiveness by
phosphatidylinositol*

Another acidic phospholipid, phosphatidylinositol,
restored responsiveness of adenylate cyclase to norepinephrine, but did not restore responsiveness to glucagon
and histamine. As shown in Fig. 3, norepinephrine activated the solubilized adenylate cyclase in the presence of
phosphatidylinositol over the concentration range 5 x 10^{-8}M
to 1 x 10^{-5}M, half-maximal activation occurring at a concentration of norepinephrine of 8 x 10^{-8}M. The sensitivity of adenylate cyclase to norepinephrine in this system

as judged by threshold and concentration producing half-maximal activation is approximately 100 times greater than that observed in particulate preparations (6, 10).

Effect of D,L-propranolol on the norepinephrine-mediated activation of adenylate cyclase

Table II shows that D,L-propranolol, 1 x 10^{-6}M, abolished the activation of adenylate cyclase produced by 2 x 10^{-6}M norepinephrine. Similar findings have been reported for the particulate enzyme (7).

Effective concentrations of phosphatidylinositol

Phosphatidylinositol, 0.05 μg/incubation (0.8 μg/ml), was half-maximally effective in restoring norepinephrine responsiveness. Concentrations of phosphatidylinositol less than 0.025 μg/incubation (0.4 μg/ml) were ineffective and greater than 0.25 μg/incubation (4 μg/ml) maximally effective.

Discussion

A number of investigations have served to emphasize the importance of phospholipids in hormone sensitive adenylate cyclase systems. Solubilized preparations of adenylate cyclase from brain (11), heart (11), skeletal muscle (11), and liver (11, 12) are unresponsive to the hormones which activate the membrane-bound enzyme. In addition, certain phospholipases decrease the effects of hormones on their target tissues (12-14) and decrease the binding of glucagon to isolated liver membranes (15). Direct evidence for the importance of phospholipids was provided by Pohl and coworkers who demonstrated that addition of pure phosphatidylserine partially restored glucagon responsiveness of adenylate cyclase in phospholipase A-treated liver membranes and the binding of glucagon to these membranes (15).

The data in this report demonstrate that two acidic phospholipids have the capacity to selectively restore

253

responsiveness of the solubilized myocardial adenylate cyclase to three of the hormones which activate the particulate enzyme. Phosphatidylserine restored responsiveness to glucagon and histamine and phosphatidylinositol to norepinephrine. Concentration response curves to glucagon and histamine were virtually identical to those found in particulate preparations. Interestingly, a marked increase in sensitivity was noted for norepinephrine in the presence of phosphatidylinositol as compared to concentration response curves noted with the particulate enzyme and norepinephrine (6). The degree of sensitivity in the reconstituted system approaches that found in intact physiologic preparations (16). The reason for this striking increase in sensitivity is obscure, but suggests that the process of homogenization alone alters the lipid-enzyme relationship resulting in decreased sensitivity of the enzyme to hormonal stimulation in particulate preparations.

It is of great interest that the phospholipids not only restored hormone-responsiveness of solubilized adenylate cyclase, but hormone receptor specificity was retained as well. This was clearly shown by the results with diphenhydramine and propranolol. Diphenhydramine abolished the activation of solubilized adenylate cyclase by histamine in the presence of phosphatidylserine, but not that by glucagon. D,L-propranolol, a specific beta adrenergic blocking agent, abolished the activation of adenylate cyclase by norepinephrine in the presence of phosphatidylinositol. These data concerning receptor specificity would appear to add greater significance to this *in vitro* system in terms of its usefulness in understanding the molecular components which compose these cardiac hormone receptors *in vivo*. It should also be noted that the enzyme fraction is impure and therefore other factors may be present and necessary to provide a functional hormone receptor.

The precise site and mechanism of action of the phospholipid is unclear. These phospholipids may induce a specific conformational change in the enzyme molecule necessary for binding of the hormone and subsequent activation of the enzyme. Clearly the catalytic subunit of the adenylate cyclase does not require phospholipid since the solubilized enzyme retains fluoride responsiveness (3,4, 12). Phospholipid would seem to be required either at the receptor site or at an intermediate coupling site between receptor and catalytic site. On the basis of their studies,

Rodbell and coworkers have postulated the phospholipid to act on the coupling site (17).

Summary

Several investigations have demonstrated that phospholipids play an important role in hormone sensitive adenylate cyclase systems. Particulate preparations of myocardial adenylate cyclase are activated by glucagon, histamine, and norepinephrine whereas solubilized preparations are not. The addition of certain phospholipids restore the hormone responsiveness of the solubilized cat myocardial adenylate cyclase. Phosphatidylserine restored the activation produced by glucagon and histamine but not norepinephrine. Concentration response curves to glucagon and histamine were almost identical to those obtained in particulate preparations. Receptor specificity was demonstrated since the antihistamine, diphenhydramine, abolished the histamine-activation but not that due to glucagon. Phosphatidylinositol restored responsiveness to norepinephrine but not to glucagon or histamine. Sensitivity of the solubilized adenylate cyclase to norepinephrine in the presence of phosphatidylinositol was increased almost 100-fold compared to particulate preparations. The beta adernergic blocking agent D,L-propranolol abolished the norepinephrine-activation. The site and mechanism of action of these lipids is unclear. They may act on the coupling site between the receptor and catalytic sites producing the necessary molecular configuration of the enzyme for specific hormone activation.

Presented by Gerald S. Levey. The experimental work reported in this paper was supported in part by United States Public Health Service Grant 1 RO1 HE13715-01 and Florida Heart Association Grant 20 AG 71. Dr. Levey is an investigator of the Howard Hughes Medical Institute.

255

References

1. Waud, D.R. Pharmacological receptors. Pharmacol. Rev. 20:49-88 (1968).
2. Ehrenpreis, S., J.H. Fleish, and T.W. Mittag. Approaches to the molecular nature of pharmacological receptors. Pharmacol. Rev. 21:131-181 (1969).
3. Levey, G.S. Solubilization of myocardial adenyl cyclase. Biochem. Biophys. Res. Commun. 38:86-92 (1970).
4. Levey, G.S. Solubilization of myocardial adenyl cyclase: Loss of hormone-responsiveness and activation by phospholipids. Ann. N.Y. Acad. Sci. 185:449-457 (1971).
5. Krishna, G., B. Weiss, and B.B. Brodie. A simple, sensitive method for the assay of adenyl cyclase. J. Pharmacol. Exp. Ther. 163:379-385 (1968).
6. Levey, G.S., C.L. Skelton, and S.E. Epstein. Decreased myocardial adenyl cyclase activity in hypothyroidism. J. Clin. Invest. 48:2244-2250 (1969).
7. Levey, G.S. and S.E. Epstein. Activation of adenyl cyclase by glucagon in cat and human heart. Circ. Res. 24:151-156 (1969).
8. Murad, F. and M. Vaughan. Effect of glucagon on rat heart adenyl cyclase. Biochem. Pharmacol. 18:1053-1059 (1969).
9. Klein, I. and G.S. Levey. Activation of myocardial adenyl cyclase by histamine in guinea pig, cat and human heart. J. Clin. Invest. 50:1012-1015 (1971).
10. Murad, F., Y.-M. Chi, T.W. Rall, and E.W. Sutherland. Adenyl cyclase III. The effect of catecholamines and choline esters on the formation of adenosine 3',5'-phosphate by preparations from cardiac muscle and liver. J. Biol. Chem. 237:1233-1238 (1962).
11. Sutherland, E.W., T.W. Rall, and T. Menon. Adenyl cyclase I. Distribution, preparation, and properties. J. Biol. Chem. 237:1220-1227 (1962).
12. Birnbaumer, L., S.L. Pohl, and M. Rodbell. The glucagon-sensitive adenyl cyclase system in plasma membranes of rat liver II. Comparison between glucagon- and fluoride-stimulated activities. J. Biol. Chem. 246:1857-1860 (1971).
13. Rodbell, M., H.M.J. Krans, S.L. Pohl, and L. Birnbaumer. The glucagon-sensitive adenyl cyclase system in plasma membranes of rat liver III. Binding of glucagon: Method of assay and specificity. J. Biol. Chem. 246:1861-1871 (1971).

14. Macchia, V. and I. Pastan. Action of phospholipase C on the thyroid. Abolition of the response to thryoid-stimulating hormone. J. Biol. Chem. 242:1864-1869 (1967).
15. Pohl, S.L., H.M.J. Krans, V. Kozyreff, L. Birnbaumer, and M. Rodbell. The glucagon sensitive adenyl cyclase system in plasma membranes of rat liver. VI. Evidence for a role of membrane lipids. J. Biol. Chem. 246: 4447-4454 (1971).
16. Buccino, R.A., J.F. Spann, Jr., P.E. Pool, E.H. Sonnenblick, and E. Braunwald. Influence of the thyroid state on the intrinsic contractile properties and energy stores of the myocardium. J. Clin. Invest. 45:1669-1682 (1967).
17. Rodbell, M., L. Birnbaumer, and S.L. Pohl. Hormones, receptors, and adenyl cyclase activity in mammalian cells. In: T.W. Rall, M. Rodbell, and P.G. Condliffe (Editors), The Role of Adenyl Cyclase and Cyclic 3',5'-AMP in Biological Systems, Government Printing Office, Washington, D.C. (1971), pp. 59-76.

TABLE I

EFFECT OF DIPHENHYDRAMINE ON THE GLUCAGON AND HISTAMINE
ACTIVATION OF ADENYLATE CYCLASE

	Diphenhydramine $(8 \times 10^{-5}M)$	
	Absent	Present
Cyclic 3',5'-AMP Accumulated/5 min/mg protein		
Control[a]	510 ± 90	680 ± 100
Glucagon $(1 \times 10^{-5}M)$	780 ± 100	990 ± 90
Histamine $(8 \times 10^{-5}M)$	1000 ± 80	660 ± 40

[a]*Each value represents the mean ± S.E. of 6-8 samples.*
Phosphatidylserine present at 8 μg per incubation.

TABLE II

EFFECT OF PROPRANOLOL ON THE NOREPINEPHRINE ACTIVATION
OF ADENYLATE CYCLASE

| | D,L-Propranolol $(1 \times 10^{-6}M)$ | |
	Absent	Present
Cyclic 3',5'-AMP Accumulated/5 min/mg protein		
Control[a]	840 ± 60	680 ± 200
Norepinephrine $(2 \times 10^{-6}M)$	1020 ± 120	2400 ± 200

[a]*Each value represents the mean ± S.E. of 4 samples.
Phosphatidylinositol present at 5 µg per incubation.*

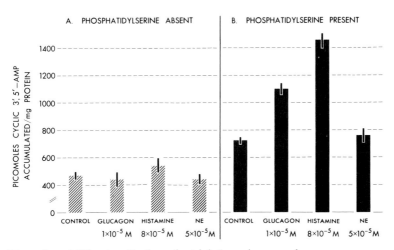

Fig. 1. *Effect of phosphatidylserine on hormone-responsiveness of sulubilized myocardial adenylate cyclase.*
Each value represents the mean ± S.E. of 6-15 samples.

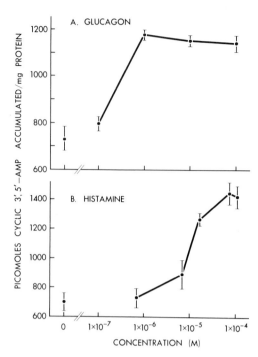

Fig. 2. *Concentration response curves for glucagon and histamine.* Each value represents the mean ± S.E. of 6-13 samples. Phosphatidylserine present at 8 μg per incubation.

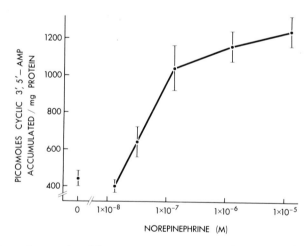

Fig. 3. *Concentration response curve for norepinephrine.* Each value represents the mean ± S.E. of 10-23 samples. Phosphatidylinositol present at 5 μg per incubation.

CHARACTERIZATION AND PURIFICATION OF THE CARDIAC β-ADRENERGIC RECEPTOR

Robert J. Lefkowitz

Introduction

Sutherland and co-workers (1) first described the stimulation of hepatic adenyl cyclase by epinephrine. Since that time the action of a host of hormones has been shown to be mediated via stimulation of this enzyme activity in the plasma membranes of various target tissues (2). Despite its ubiquitous distribution in virtually all mammalian tissues, the range of hormones which will stimulate the cyclase in any given tissue is quite narrow. Thus ACTH stimulates the adrenal cyclase, TSH the thyroid cyclase, epinephrine the cardiac cyclase, *etc*. This remarkable "tissue specificity" is felt to be due to structures called "receptors," which in some way recognize or discriminate which hormone structure will bind to and activate the cyclase in any given tissue.

Although studies of adenyl cyclase have been actively pursued over the past 10 years, it is only quite recently that attempts to study directly the interaction of labelled hormones with their receptors in cell membranes have been successful (3-7).

Recently we have been able to demonstrate *in vitro* binding of [^{3}H]-norepinephrine to a membrane fraction of ventricular myocardium (8). The characteristics and specificity of this binding were as one would expect for the physiologic cardiac β-adrenergic receptor. Catecholamines compete for binding to these sites, activating a cyclase with an identical potency series which parallels the *in vitro* potency of catecholamines in stimulating myocardial contractility (9,10).

The receptor has been solubilized using a variety of detergents and the solublized receptors have been extensively purified by affinity chromatography. The specificity of these highly purified receptors is identical to that of the membrane bound receptors though the kinetic characteristics are some-

261

what altered (11).

Methods

Preparation of ventricular microsomal particles has been described in detail elsewhere (8). The fraction sedimenting after 78,000 x g for one hour was generally used. For solubilization of receptors, membrane fractions were homogenized in buffered solutions of Lubrol PX (ICI America) or sodium deoxycholate, generally in a concentration of 0.25%. The material was then centrifuged for 1 hour at 100,000 x g and supernatant used as a source of soluble receptors (11).

Receptor binding activity was assayed by incubating 1 ml aliquots of membrane preparations (100-200 μg/ml of membrane protein) or soluble preparations ($\sim$ 500 μg/ml) with [^{3}H]-norepinephrine (10^{-9} to 10^{-8} M; $\sim$ 10Ci/mM, New England Nuclear) for 1 to 2 hours. After the incubation the receptor bound [^{3}H]-norepinephrine was separated from free [^{3}H]-norepinephrine and quantitated by liquid scintillation counting. For the receptors in membrane or particulate form receptor bound norepinephrine was isolated by millipore filtration on filters of 0.45μ pore size. For the soluble material, receptor bound [^{3}H]-norepinephrine was separated from free [^{3}H]-norepinephrine on small columns of G-25 fine sephadex (8,11).

Norepinephrine-agarose conjugates for use as adsorbents for affinity chromatography purification of soluble β-receptors were prepared by coupling norepinephrine via a 30 Å side chain to insoluble agarose beads. Detailed methods have been published elsewhere (11,12). The side chain consists of alternating dipropylamino and succinate units (Fig. 1). The preparations generally contained about 7.0 μmoles of norepinephrine per ml of agarose. When soluble preparations of the receptors were passed over columns of this material, 80 to 100 % of the receptors were absorbed to the agarose-norepinephrine. The receptors could then be quantitatively eluted with concentrated solutions of epinephrine at low pH (11).

Results

Membrane Bound β-Adrenergic Binding Sites

When ventricular microsomal particles are incubated with [^{3}H]-norepinephrine, rapid binding of the catecholamine to sites in the particles occurs (8,9) (Fig. 2). The binding is temperature dependent. Particles concentrated [^{3}H]-norepinephrine 500-1000x in 2 hours at 37°C. The specificity of the binding was similar to that of the cardiac β-adrenergic receptor as determined from *in vivo* studies. β-active drugs displaced [^{3}H]-norepinephrine from the *in vitro* binding sites in a potency series parallel to that for their *in vivo* effects on cardiac contractility. Figure 3 indicates that, on a molar basis, isoproterenol was most potent in competing for the binding site, followed by epinephrine, norepinephrine, dopamine, and DOPA. α-active and indirectly active amines were much less potent as indicated in Fig. 4. Metabolites such as normetanephrine and vanillylmandelic acid (VMA) were inert in all concentrations up to 10^{-4}M. The parent compound β-phenethylamine, lacking both ring hydroxyl groups as well as the side chain hydroxyl, was inert at 10^{-2}M.

From data such as this, the structural requirements for binding to the *in vitro* receptor can be deduced. Figure 5 tabulates these and compares them with the structure-activity relationships of the β-receptor as determined from physiological studies and with those for binding of [^{3}H]-norepinephrine to other known uptake mechanisms. It is apparent that the 2 ring hydroxyl groups are essential for binding to the β-receptor *in vivo* and *in vitro*. The side chain OH group, though not required, enhances binding. Finally, substitution on the amino N increases binding, thus isoproterenol is more potent than norepinephrine. Binding of [^{3}H]-norepinephrine to isolated nerve storage granules or to neuronal uptake sites has a totally different specificity (13,14,15).

Figures 6 and 7 indicate that β-adrenergic blockers such as propranolol and dichlorisoproterenol inhibit [^{3}H]-norepinephrine binding whereas α-blockers such as phentolamine do not.

Binding of [^{3}H]-norepinephrine to the *in vitro* receptors is reversible. Figure 8 indicates that after addition of excess unlabelled norepinephrine, there is an initial, rapid dissociation of receptor bound [^{3}H]-norepinephrine followed by very little further dissociation during the time period studied. Nonetheless, at any time up to 2 hours virtually all of the receptor bound [^{3}H]-norepinephrine could be dissociated by addition of 1M HCl. The dissociated [^{3}H]-norepinephrine was biologically active (*i.e.* could bind to fresh receptors) and was chromatographically identical to native norepinephrine (ascending paper chromatography; butanol: acetic acid: water, 4:1:5) (9,16).

Table I indicates that a variety of reagents and treatments also dissociated the norepinephrine-receptor complex.

In as much as *in vitro* binding of [^{3}H]-norepinephrine to nerve storage granules has previously been demonstrated (13,14), it seemed important to distinguish the current binding phenomenon to receptors from that to components of the sympathetic nervous system. Reserpine which potently blocks binding to nerve storage vesicles at 10^{-7}M and ATP which stimulates nerve storage vesicle binding at 10^{-3}M (17) were both without effect on this system at concentrations of 10^{-5} and 10^{-3}M respectively (9).

To further exclude the possibility of binding to nerve storage vesicles, a series of animals was sympathectomized using the drug 6-hydroxydopamine. This compound accumulates in sympathetic nerve terminals throughout the body and causes them to degenerate (18) thus producing an effective "chemical sympathectomy." Our treated animals showed a decline of more than 90% in measurable myocardial norepinephrine levels. Nonetheless, ventricular microsomal particles prepared from these animals bound [^{3}H]-norepinephrine to essentially the same extent as untreated animals (9) (Table II).

Since the effects of catecholamines on myocardial contractility are thought to be mediated via stimulation of adenyl cyclase (19), it seemed of interest to study the relationship of binding to cyclase activation in the microsomal particles. Adenyl cyclase activity was present in the particles and could be stimulated by catecholamines (9). Figures 9a and b compare the relative efficacy of β-adrenergic agents in blocking binding of [^{3}H]-norepinephrine to the receptors and stimulating the cyclase. The potency series are seen to be parallel and essentially identical to that for stimulation of myocardial contractility *in vivo* (20).

When Scatchard plots (21) of binding data for the interaction of [^{3}H]-norepinephrine with the particulate receptor were constructed (Fig. 10), two orders of binding sites were identified. One possessed an association constant of 1.04×10^7/M, the other 1.33×10^6/M. The free energy changes, ΔF, for combination of [^{3}H]-norepinephrine with receptors of each type were -9.96 and -8.70 Kcals/mole, respectively (10).

Figure 11 shows a pH curve for the binding reaction. Maximum binding occurred at physiological pH 7.4-7.5 with rapid fall in binding below pH 7.4. The marked inhibition of binding even at pH values achieved during severe clinical acidosis (7.0-7.1) may provide a partial explanation for the known clinical ineffectiveness of catecholamines in acidotic patients, *i.e.* an inability to bind to physiologic receptor sites.

When membrane preparations were exposed to a variety of enzymes prior to [³H]-norepinephrine, only the proteolytic enzymes trypsin and subtilisin adversely affected the binding (Fig. 12).

The sulfhydryl reagent parachloromercuribenzoate (PMB) inhibited binding which could be in part reversed by subsequent exposure to cysteine (Fig. 13).

Taken together these findings suggest that the receptor is at least in part a protein with free-SH groups crucial for activity.

Solubilized Receptors

To gain further insight into the structure and function of the isolated β-adrenergic receptors, attempts were made to solubilize the norepinephrine binding activity with a variety of detergents (11). As noted in Table III, effective solubilization could be achieved with the non ionic detergent Lubrol-PX or the ionic detergent sodium deoxycholate. Triton was less satisfactory.

The receptors could then be purified by the technique of affinity chromatography (12). This widely applicable method can be used to purify macromolecules which have as one of their properties reversible binding to another known compound. In this case, one utilizes norepinephrine to purify the β-adrenergic receptor binding site. The adsorbents were prepared [*see* Methods; *also* (11)] by covalently binding norepinephrine to agarose via a 30 Å side chain. A schematic representation of the affinity chromatography purification sequence is shown in Fig. 14. When soluble preparations were passed over columns of the absorbent, the adrenergic receptors were adsorbed. Other proteins and receptors pass through unretarded. After washing the column extensively with buffer, the adsorbed receptors could be successfully eluted with 0.1M epinephrine (pH 3.8). The receptor-bound epinephrine was then removed by extensive dialysis. In experiments of this type (11), virtually all the protein added to the column is recovered in the column run-through and buffer wash. The epinephrine eluate, generally containing 110-120% of the original binding activity, contained too little protein to accurately measure by Lowry technique (22). In other experiments, using 1^{125} radioiodinated receptors, we have found the purification of receptors achieved by a single passage over the affinity column to be approximately 300 fold.

The binding characteristics of the purified soluble receptors were very similar to those of the original particulate receptors. Thus, binding was quite rapid, reaching equilibrium within 10 minutes at $37^{\circ}C$ (Fig. 15). The binding was also reversible. The specificity of the binding was also identical to that of the particulate receptors. When β-active catecholamines were tested for their ability to inhibit binding of [^{3}H]-norepinephrine to the purified receptors (Fig. 16), the order of potency was isoproterenol > norepinephrine or epinephrine > dopamine > DOPA. Figure 17 shows data for α-active and indirectly active amines, which were much less potent. Figure 18 indicates that the α-blocker phentolamine and the metabalite VMA did not inhibit binding at $10^{-4}M$, whereas the β-blocker propranolol did.

It is of note that although the specificity of binding to the purified receptor is essentially identical to that of the particulate receptor, somewhat higher concentrations of drugs are required for inhibition of binding. This indicates that the association constant for interaction with the purified receptor is somewhat lower. The Scatchard plot shown in Fig. 19 indicates that only a single order of sites was present in the purified preparations and the association constant for this site was approximately equal to 2×10^5 L/M.

An indication of the molecular weight of the receptors was obtained by chromatographing aliquots of [^{3}H]-norepinephrine bound to soluble receptors on columns of sepharose 4B (Fig. 20). Two peaks of "bound" norepinephrine were identified. By comparison with the elution profiles of substances of known molecular weight on the same column, these 2 peaks were found to correspond to approximate molecular weights of 40,000 and 160,000. These two fractions can also be separated by DEAE cellulose chromatography. Only the larger fraction is associated with adenyl cyclase activity (23).

Discussion

The data presented indicate that it is possible to prepare

a membrane fraction from canine ventricular tissue which
contains a binding site with many of the properties to be
expected of the physiological cardiac β-adrenergic receptor.
The site can be readily distinguished from other catecholamine binding sites derived from various components of the
sympathetic nervous system. It binds norepinephrine rapidly
and reversibly without altering the biological activity of
the bound amine. The binding specificity of the particulate
receptor parallels that of adenyl cyclase present in the
same preparations, as well as that of the β-receptor as
determined from physiological studies, *i.e.* isoproterenol >
epinephrine or norepinephrine > dopamine > DOPA, with α-
active amines and metabolites much less active or inert.
The significance of the 2 orders of sites is not yet entirely
clear, but has been found to be characteristic of similar
binding phenomena in a number of other systems (4, 24). This
may provide for a more even response over a wider range of
hormone concentrations (4). The respone to β but not α-
blocking agents is also typical of a "β-receptor." In this
regard it should be noted that the concentrations of blocking
agents required to achieve effects were considerably higher
than those required for effects in *in vivo* preparations.
The reason for this discrepancy is not clear, though similar
observations have been made in *in vitro* studies of catecholamine binding to liver and erythrocyte membrane receptors
(25,26). β-adrenergic blockade may be more complex than
simple competition for receptor sites (10,26).

The receptors, which appear to be sulfhydryl proteins,
could be solubilized and extensively purified by affinity
chromatography. The purified receptors retained many of the
properties of the particulate binding sites, including the
same specificity. The lower association constant may be
due to disruption of the membrane structure required for
optimal functioning of the receptors. The presence of only
one order of binding site in the purified preparations presumably is a reflection of the purification. The presence
of receptor binding activity in two molecular weight forms,
40,000 and 160,000, only the latter of which is associated
with adenyl cyclase activity, is consistent with a subunit
structure for the β-receptor-cyclase unit. Such a structure
is, however, in no way proven in the current studies.

Recent investigations in collaboration with Dr. G. Levey
have provided new insights into the coupling between norepinephrine-receptor interaction and adenyl cyclase activation

(27). Solubilized preparations of cat myocardium were found
to contain both the β-adrenergic binding site and the adenyl
cyclase. Nonetheless, activation of the cyclase by norepinephrine required further addition of phosphatidyl inositol.
The phospholipid was not required for and did not affect the
binding reaction. These results suggest that:
    1) β-receptor binding and adenyl cyclase activation
are discrete processes and
    2) The coupling of the two phenomena appears to involve
membrane phospholipids such as phosphatidyl inositol.
    Current studies are directed toward achieving complete
purification and characterization of the cardiac β-adrenergic
receptor and a further understanding of the mechanism of
its interaction with adenyl cyclase.

*Presented by Robert J. Lefkowitz. Supported by USPHS Grant
#HE-5196, NASA #9-10891 and SCOR #HE-14150. Original invest-
igations reported here were done in collaboration with
Drs. G. Sharp, D. O'Hara and E. Haber and have been previously
reported (8-11).*

References

1. Sutherland, E. W. and T. W. Rall. The relation of adeno-
sine-3'5' phosphate and phosphorylase to the actions of
catecholamines and other hormones. Pharmacol. Rev. 12:
265 (1960).
2. Pastan, I. and R. Pearlman. Cyclic AMP in metabolism.
Nature New Biology, 229: 5 (1971).
3. Lefkowitz, R. J., J. Roth, W. Pricer and I. Pastan.
ACTH receptors in the adrenal: Specific binding of
ACTH-^{125}I and its relation to adenyl cyclase. Proc.
Nat. Acad. Sci. 65: 745 (1970).
4. Lefkowitz, R. J., J. Roth and I. Pastan. ACTH-receptor
interaction in the adrenal: A model for the initial
step in the action of hormones that stimulate adenyl
cyclase. Ann. N. Y. Acad. Sci. 185: 195 (1971).
5. Rodbell, M., H. M. J. Krans, S. L. Pohl and L. Birnbaumer
The glucagon sensitive adenyl cyclase system in plasma
membranes of rat liver III: Binding of glucagon: Method
of assay and specificity. J. Biol. Chem 246: 1861 (1971).
6. Rodbell, M., H. M. J. Krans, S. Pohl and L. Birnbaumer.
The glucagon sensitive adenyl cyclase system in plasma
membranes of rat liver IV: Effects of guanyl nucleotides on binding of ^{125}I-glucagon. J. Biol. Chem. 246:

L872 (1971).
7. Tomasi, V. S., T. K. Ray, J. K. Dunnick and G. V. Marinetti. Hormone action at the membrane level II. The binding of epinephrine and glucagon to the rat liver plasma membrane. Biochim. Biophys. Acta 211: 31 (1970).
8. Lefkowitz, R. J. and E. Haber. A fraction of the ventricular myocardium that has the specificity of the cardiac beta adrenergic receptor. Proc. Nat. Acad. Sci. 68: 1773 (1971).
9. Lefkowitz, R. J., G. W. G. Sharp and E. Haber. Studies on the identification of the cardiac beta adrenergic receptor II: Relation to nerve storage vesicles, adenyl cyclase and thyroid hormones. Submitted for publication.
10. Lefkowitz, R. J. and E. Haber. Studies on the identification of the cardiac beta adrenergic receptor III. Interaction with [^{3}H]-norepinephrine. Submitted for publication.
11. Lefkowitz, R. J., E. Haber and D. O'Hara. Studies on the identification of the cardiac beta adrenergic receptor IV: Solubilization and purification by affinity chromatography. Submitted for publication.
12. Cuatrecasas, P. Protein purification by affinity chromatography. J. Biol. Chem. 245: 3059 (1970).
13. Von Euler, U. S. and F. Lishajko. Effect of directly and indirectly acting sympathomimetic amines on adrenergic transmitter granules. Acta Physiol. Scand. 73: 78 (1968).
14. Kirshner, N. Uptake of catecholamines by a particulate fraction of the adrenal medulla. J. Biol. Chem. 237: 2311 (1962).
15. Burgen, A. S. V. and L. L. Iversen. The inhibition of noradrenaline uptake by sympathomimetic amines in the rat isolated heart. Brit. J. Pharmacol. 25: 34 (1965).
16. Shepherd, D. M. and G. B. West. Detection of some precursors of adrenaline by paper chromatography. Nature 171: 1160 (1953).
17. Potter L. and J. Axelrod. Properties of norepinephrine storage particles of the rat heart. J. Pharmacol. Exp. Ther. 142: 299 (1963).
18. Tranzer, N. P. and H. Thoenen. An electron microscopic study of selective, acute degeneration of sympathetic nerve terminals after administration of 6-hydroxydopamine. Experientia 15: 2 (1968).
19. Epstein, S. E., G. S. Levey and C. L. Skelton. Adenyl cyclase and cyclic AMP biochemical links in the regulation

of myocardial contractility. Circulation 43: 437 (1971).

20. Ahlquist, R. P. A study of the adrenotropic receptors. Amer. J. Physiol. 153: 586 (1948).

21. Scatchard, G. The attractions of proteins for small molecules and ions. Ann. N. Y. Acad. Sci. 51:660 (1949).

22. Lowry, O. H., N. J. Rosebrough, A. L. Farr and R. J. Randall. Protein measurement with the folin phenol reagent. J. Biol. Chem. 193:265 (1951).

23. Lefkowitz, R. J., G. W. G. Sharp and D. O'Hara. Unpublished Data.

24. Schlatz, L. and G. V. Marinetti. Hormone-calcium interactions with the plasma membrane of rat liver cells. Science 176: 175 (1972).

25. Dunnick, J. K. and G. V. Marinetti. Hormone action at the membrane level III. Epinephrine interaction with the rat liver plasma membrane. Biochim. Biophys. Acta 249: 122 (1971).

26. Schramm, M., H. Feinstein, E. Naim, M. Lang and M. Lasser. Epinephrine binding to the catecholamine receptor and activation of the adenylate cyclase in erythrocyte membranes. Proc. Nat. Acad. Sci. 69: 523 (1972).

27. Lefkowitz, R. J. and G. S. Levey. Norepinephrine: Dissociation of β-receptor binding from adenylate cyclase activation in solubilized myocardium. Submitted for publication.

28. Krishna, G., B. Weiss and B. B. Brodie. Adenyl cyclase. J. Pharm. Exp. Therap. 163: 379 (1968).

TABLE I

STABILITY OF NOREPINEPHRINE-ADRENERGIC RECEPTOR COMPLEX

The effectiveness of each of the compounds or treatments on dissociating receptor bound [^3H]-norepinephrine was tested. Value shown is the amount dissociated in 30 minutes. Each value is mean of four samples ± SD.

Compound Added or Treatment	[^3H]-Norepinephrine Dissociated
	%
None	None
Urea (2M, final concentration)	20%±5
(4M)	26%±1
(5M)	46%±1
(6M)	52%±1
PMB (0.001M)	65%±2
Boiling water (10 min)	78%±2

TABLE II

EFFECT OF CHEMICAL SYMPATHECTOMY ON MICROSOMAL
β ADRENERGIC BINDING OF [^{3}H]-NOREPINEPHRINE

"Post treatment" dogs had been treated with serial intravenous injections of 6-hydroxydopamine (9) to achieve a "chemical sympathectomy."

Experimental Conditions	Mean Control Heart Rate	Mean Peak Heart Rate After Atropine	Binding of [^{3}H]-Norepinephrine
			pmoles/mg Microsomes[a]
Pretreatment Dogs (7)	114±7	183±20	6.8±1.5
Post-treatment Dogs (4)	102±4	104±5	6.04±1.7
P	<0.05	<0.001	NS

[a]*mean of 12 animals*

TABLE III

SOLUBILIZATION OF RECEPTORS WITH DETERGENTS

Membrane fractions were homogenized with detergents at the concentrations shown. Each value is the mean of duplicates.

Material		[^{3}H]-Norepinephrine Bound
		pmoles/mg protein
Original microsomal particles		17.0
Particles after treatment with 0.25% deoxycholate		2.1
105,000 xg supernatant		
Deoxycholate	0.5%	10.6
	0.25%	11.6
	0.15%	7.4
Lubrol-PX	0.5%	9.3
	0.25%	9.1
Triton X-100	0.5%	2.5
	0.25%	1.5
	0.15%	1.4

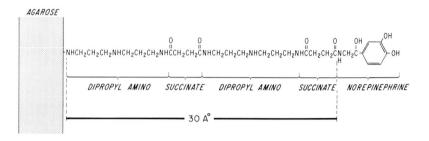

Fig. 1. *Structure of the agarose-norepinephrine affinity chromatography adsorbent.*

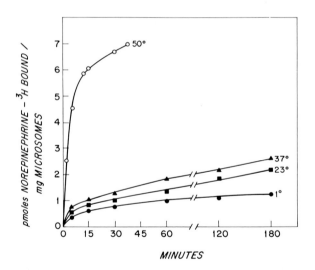

Fig. 2. *Time course of binding of [³H]-norepinephrine.*

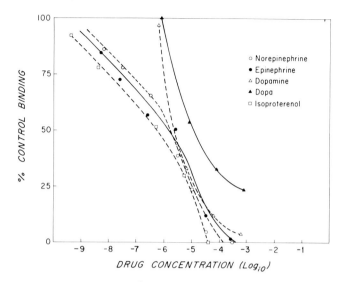

Fig. 3. *Inhibition of [³H]-norepinephrine binding to membrane receptors by β-adrenergic agents.* □ , isoproterenol; •, epinephrine; o, norepinephrine; Δ, Dopamine; ▲, DOPA.

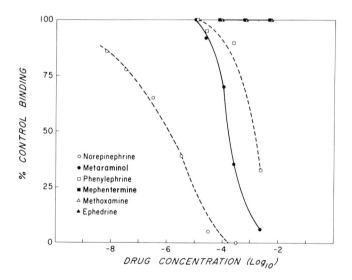

Fig. 4. *Inhibition of [³H]-norepinephrine binding to membrane receptors by α-adrenergic agents and indirectly-active β-adrenergic agents.*

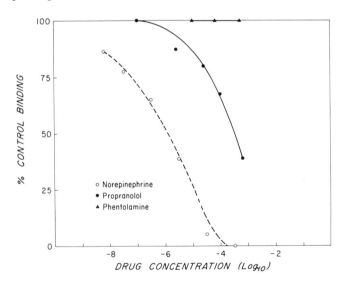

		Inhibition of ^{3}H-Norepinephrine		
Substituents	β-Adrenergic Inotropy and Chronotropy	Binding to Cardiac Microsomes	Uptake by Neural Vesicles	Uptake by whole heart
Required for activity	3 - OH 4 - OH	3 - OH 4 - OH	None	None
Not required but enhanced activity	β - OH R=CH$_3$,CH(CH$_3$)$_2$	β - OH R=CH$_3$,CH(CH$_3$)$_2$	β - OH	3 - OH 4 - OH
Decrease activity			R=CH$_3$CH(CH$_3$)$_2$	β - OH R=CH(CH$_3$)$_2$

Fig. 5. *Structure-activity relationships for inhibition of* [^3H]-*norepinephrine binding to membrane receptors by adrenergic agents.*

Fig. 6. *Inhibition of* [^3H]-*norepinephrine binding to membrane receptors by adrenergic blocking agents.*

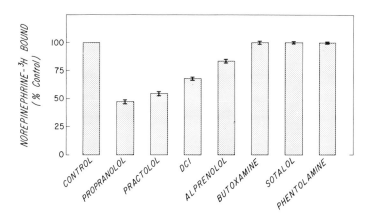

Fig. 7. *Effect of adrenergic blocking agents on* [^3H]-*norepinephrine binding.* Drugs were added at a final concentration of 1 x 10^{-4}M. Control binding was 7.0 pmoles [^3H]-norepinephrine bound/mg microsomal particles. Bars indicate ± SD for 4 determinations.

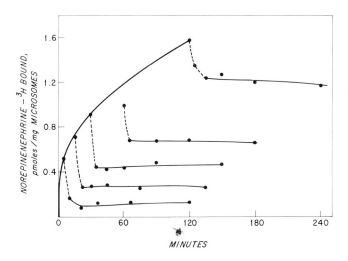

Fig. 8. *Dissociation of Receptor Bound* [^3H]-*norepinephrine.* At each of the time points indicated, 10^{-4}M norepinephrine was added and the dissociation of receptor bound [^3H]-norepinephrine measured serially.

277

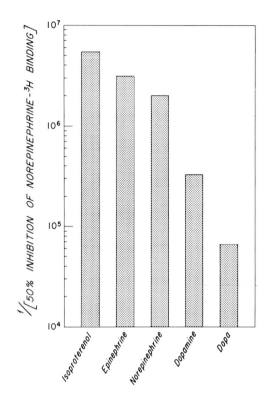

Fig. 9a. *Affinity of β-adrenergic drugs for in vitro cardiac receptors.* Association constants have been approximated by computing the reciprocals of concentrations of each drug required to 50% inhibit the binding of [^{3}H]-norepinephrine. Each value differs significantly ($p < 0.05$) from all other values except for the difference between epinephrine and norepinephrine.

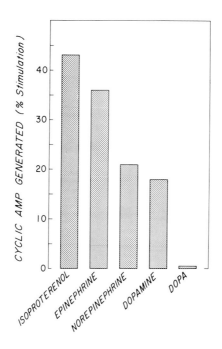

Fig. 9b. *Stimulation of cardiac microsomal adenyl cyclase by β-adrenergic drugs.* Cyclic AMP generated in a 20 minute incubation was determined by the method of Krishna (28). Detailed methods are presented elsewhere (9). Catecholamines were added at a final concentration of 1 x 10^{-5}M. Each value is the mean of 8 to 10 values from 4 or 5 experiments. The following differences were significant at the 0.05 level: isoproterenol > norepinephrine, dopamine, and DOPA; epinephrine > dopamine and DOPA; norepinephrine > DOPA; dopamine > DOPA. In the absence of added drugs an average of 317 pmoles of cyclic AMP was generated.

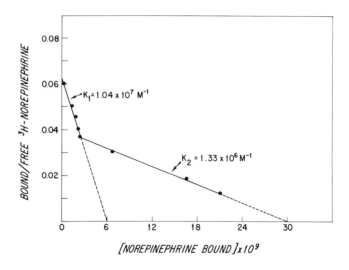

Fig. 10. *Scatchard plot for [³H]-norepinephrine binding to particulate β-adrenergic binding sites.*

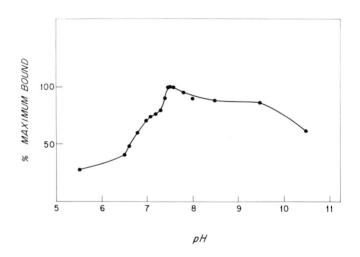

Fig. 11. *Effects of pH on norepinephrine binding.*

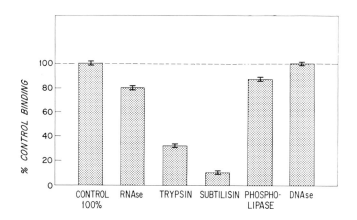

Fig. 12. *Effects of enzymes on norepinephrine binding.*
Enzymes (4 μg of enzyme protein) were incubated with microsomes for 30 minutes at 37° prior to incubation with [³H]-
norepinephrine. Bars indicate ± SD of triplicates.

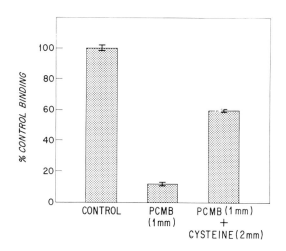

Fig. 13. *Effect of sulfhydryl reagents on binding of [³H]-
norepinephrine.* Bars indicate ± SD of 4 determinations.

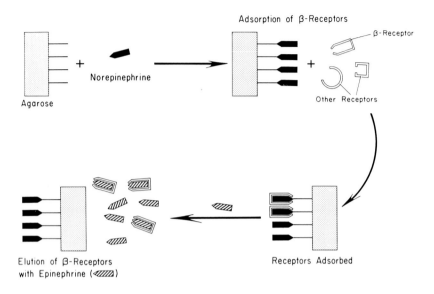

Fig. 14. *Affinity chromatography of soluble β-adrenergic binding sites.* See text for details.

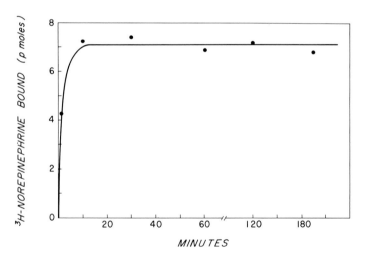

Fig. 15. *Time course of binding of* [³H]-*norepinephrine to soluble β-adrenergic binding sites.*

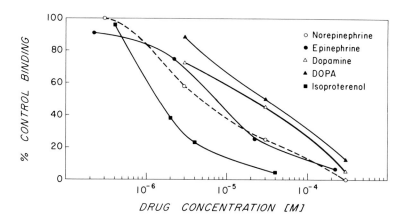

Fig. 16. *Inhibition of* [³H]-*norepinephrine binding to soluble binding sites by β-adrenergic agents.*

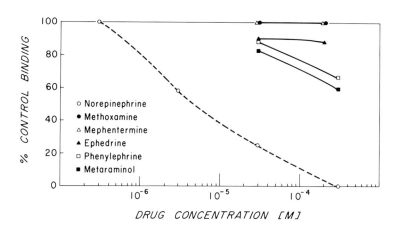

Fig. 17. *Inhibition of* [³H]-*norepinephrine binding to soluble binding sites by α-adrenergic and indirectly active agents.*

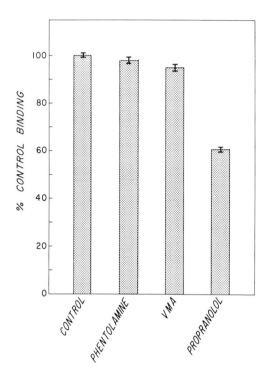

Fig. 18. *Effects of adrenergic blocking agents and Vanillyl-mandelic acid on binding of* [^3H]*-norepinephrine to soluble β-adrenergic binding sites.*

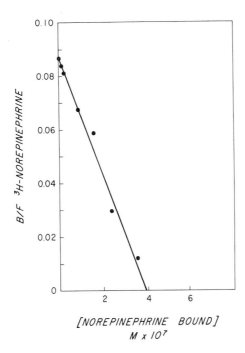

Fig. 19. *Scatchard plot for [³H]-norepinephrine binding to soluble β-adrenergic binding sites.*

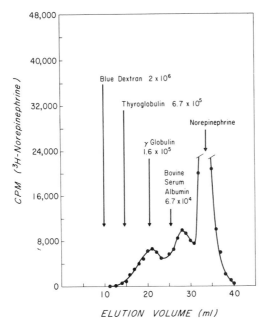

Fig. 20. *Sepharose chromatography of [³H] norepinephrine bound to soluble β-adrenergic binding sites.*

INTERACTION BETWEEN Na$^+$-DEPENDENT TRANSPORT SYSTEMS:
POSSIBLE MECHANISTIC SIGNIFICANCE

*George Kimmich, Anne Marie Tucker, Eugene Barrett and
Joan Randles*

Introduction

The nature of energy transduction events associated
with biological membranes represents one of the great un-
solved problem areas of modern biochemistry. Whether one
considers the mechanism of oxidative phosphorylation in
mitochondrial membranes, of photophosphorylation in chloroplasts, or of active transport of ions and organic molecules
across plasma membranes it is readily apparent that our
understanding of the means by which membrane-bound systems
convert energy from one form to another is shallow indeed.
    In the case of active transport processes, chemical
energy is expended and partially conserved in the new form
of an electrochemical gradient for a specific biologically
important molecule. Most animal cells have this type of
capability for supporting the accumulation of amino acids (1).
In addition, certain cells, such as those lining the lumen
of the proximal kidney tubule or the small intestine, have
the capability for active uptake of both amino acids and
certain monosaccharide sugars (1). It is the nature of the
energy input events related to these transport systems which
I would like to consider here.
    One striking aspect of the active accumulation systems
for sugars and amino acids in animal cells is that they
exhibit a set of rather characteristic features regardless
of the tissue of origin or the species. These features can
be summarized as follows:

    1) sensitivity to metabolic inhibitors (although
        transport may not necessarily be directly energized
        by ATP).
    2) an absolute dependence on Na$^+$ for accumulation of
        metabolite against a concentration gradient.

3) inhibition by elevated K^+ concentrations.
4) sensitivity to ouabain and other inhibitors of Na^+ transport.
5) a general correlation between the magnitude of the trans-membrane Na^+ gradient and the ability for cells to accumulate substrate.
6) a mutually inhibitory interaction between sugar and amino acid transport in those tissues where both systems occur.

A number of these characteristics (particularly #s 2-5 above) suggest that a rather close relationship exists between cellular Na^+ transport and the Na^+-dependent transport of substrates. In light of this suspected relationship, Christensen and his colleagues (2) first suggested a possible explanation, which was later developed more explicitly by Crane (3-5). The fundamental premises of the Crane hypothesis have become rather widely accepted and are worth considering briefly before proceeding further.

The Crane model suggests that any assymetry in substrate distribution able to be generated across the cell membrane is dependent upon, and a consequence of, an opposite assymetry in sodium ion distribution. Mobile membrane carriers are envisioned which have binding sites not only for a substrate molecule but also for Na^+. Kinetic evidence indicates that the carriers have higher affinity for substrate when Na^+ is bound than when in the Na^+-free state (6). Consequently, in the relatively Na^+-rich environment characteristic of extra-cellular fluids, a Na^+-substrate-carrier ternary complex with high substrate affinity forms readily, simply by mass action considerations. When the complex reaches the relatively Na^+-poor environment at the inner membrane surface, dissociation occurs, and consequently the carrier exists primarily in a form with low affinity for its substrate. Extrusion of Na^+ by the sodium pump maintains the system poised for further substrate entry. Accumulation should continue until the degree of saturation of the carrier with substrate is equivalent at the two membrane surfaces. Before this occurs, a higher cellular substrate concentration is required, due to the difference in carrier affinity at the two sides, which in turn is dependent on the inwardly directed Na^+ gradient.

Two ideas are implicit in the ion gradient model. First, no input of ATP is required directly at the locus of the substrate carrier. ATP is expended only at the sodium pump and may occur at a completely independent cellular site. Second, the system should exhibit symmetry: if the normal sodium gradient is imposed in the opposite sense, then the cell should actively extrude substrate. Only when the Na^+ concentration is equal at each surface would one expect equal steady-state substrate concentrations on each side of the membrane.

Methods

All of the work discussed below was performed using suspensions of intestinal epithelial cells prepared from chick intestine by methods discribed previously (7). Accumulation of 3-OMG, galactose, and valine was evaluated by monitoring the uptake of the appropriate radioactive substrate by the cells with the use of millipore filtration techniques for rapid separation of cells from the suspending medium. A detailed account of this procedure has also appeared in an earlier publication (8). The usual incubation medium contained 80 mM Na Cl, 80mM mannitol, 20 mM Tris-Cl (pH 7.4), 3 mM K_2 HPO_4, 1 mM Mg Cl_2, 1 mM Ca Cl_2, and 1 mg/ml BSA in addition to substrate (1mM-10mM). Variations from the standard medium are noted in the text. Changes in Na^+ or K^+ concentration were made by concomitantly adjusting the mannitol concentration in order to maintain a total tonicity of 280 m osmolar. Isotopes were added to provide a final activity of 0.15 μc/ml.

Results and Discussion

Our earlier work has focused primarily on the prediction stated above with regard to the symmetry which a Na^+-dependent carrier should exhibit. Working with isolated intestinal epithelial cells prepared from chicken we attempted to reverse the cellular sodium gradient from normal and study the effects on sugar fluxes (8). A representative experiment is illustrated in Fig. 1. The cells were pre-loaded with Na^+ and galactose at 0° in media containing the appropriate isotopic tracers. At time 0 the pre-loaded cells were introduced to Na^+-free medium containing ^{14}C-galactose at the same concentration and specific activity as during the pre-incubation. The dilution decreased extra-cellular $[Na^+]$ from

289

80 mM to 20 mM. Loss of cellular $^{22}Na^+$ even in the presence
of 200 μM DNP indicates the cells had indeed been loaded
with Na^+ to a concentration greater than 20 mM. The steady
state cellular content of $^{22}Na^+$ which is approached in the
presence of DNP should be an indication of the point at
which cellular Na^+ activity matches that in the medium (7,8).
Note that the non-inhibited cells require approximately 1.5
minutes to reduce their $^{22}Na^+$ content to this level; and
can be expected to have a Na^+ gradient reversed from normal
until that interval is elapsed. In spite of the unfavorable
Na^+ gradient imposed during the early part of the experiment,
the cells were able to actively accumulate ^{14}C-galactose as
the up-sweeping curve in Fig. 1 indicates. Furthermore, the
accumulation rate is as rapid during the first minute as at
any subsequent 1 minute interval. The ion gradient hypothesis would predict *extrusion* of ^{14}C-galactose until a
normally directed Na^+ gradient begins to be re-established
(*i.e.* at least 1.5 min.). Whereas, no gradient of galactose
is expected for 1.5 minutes if the premises of the Crane
model are correct; a 2 fold gradient is in fact established
during this time. Lack of a ^{14}C-sugar flux in the presence
of 200 μM DNP, indicates that the cell water had equilibrated
with galactose in the medium during the pre-incubation
period, as expected. Using the same basic approach, we
have generated a good deal of evidence which is difficult to
reconcile with the idea that the primary energy input for
sugar accumulation is derived from the trans-membrane sodium
gradient. For a more detailed account the reader is referred
to our earlier publications (7-9).

   More recently we have evaluated the possibility that
cellular K^+ gradients might provide an energy input, but
again have been unable to observe sugar fluxes consistent
with that idea (9,10). We recognize that such data is
difficult to reconcile with reports of substrate gradients
(amino acids) generated by ion gradients experimentally
imposed on metabolically inhibited cell populations (11-13).
On the other hand, a number of other situations have been
described in which reversed ion gradients imposed on normally
energized cell populations did not prevent continued active
amino acid accumulation (14-16). These latter observations
are consistent with those shown in Fig. 1. Apparently the
energy status of the cell plays an essential role in energy
transduction events associated with the cell membrane as
one might predict.

   All of the work cited above suffers from at least one

serious limitation. In every case it is assumed that measured cell Na^+ is uniformly distributed in the cell water. Sodium concentrations are calculated making use of that assumption for lack of more definitive information regarding actual intracellular distribution. At the same time, it is logical to expect that the concentration within cellular organelles, such as nuclei, may be much higher than that in the extra-nuclear regions. Average cellular $[Na^+]$ calculated as described might be a serious under-estimate for nuclear $[Na^+]$ and an equally serious over-estimate for cytoplasmic compart-ments. In addition, localized cellular environments relatively depleted of Na^+ might be expected to occur near sites of active sodium extrusion in normally energized cells. These cellular micro-environments would tend to be created near the inner surface of the plasma membrane in particular. It is possible that a normally directed Na^+ gradient still exists in such membrane micro-environments even in situations where average cellular $[Na^+]$ exceeds extra-cellular $[Na^+]$.

At first consideration, the possibility of ruling out the participation of localized cellular Na^+ gradients in supporting substrate accumulation, seems remote. However, certain aspects of recently proposed explanations for the interaction between Na^+ dependent transport systems suggest a realistic approach to the problem. As we have already mentioned, an interaction between the Na^+-dependent trans-port system for sugars and amino acids in intact intestinal tissue is well known (17-21). It has been suggested that a partial dissipation of the trans-membrane Na^+ gradient occurs when one substrate is transported due to co-transport of Na^+, leaving less energy inherent in that gradient to support transport of a second substrate (1,20). If this concept is accurate, there should be a high degree of correlation between the rate of transport of a particular substrate species and its' ability to act as an inhibitor. The faster a substrate enters, the more rapidly Na^+ should enter in co-transport, and consequently the greater the degree of discharge of the Na^+ gradient. The activity of any other transport system dependent on the Na^+ gradient should of course reflect the degree to which that gradient dissipates.

Rate of substrate transport and interaction between transport systems are two easily evaluated parameters. As shown in Fig. 2, a marked interaction between valine and 3-OMG entry systems can be demonstrated using the isolated intestinal cell preparation. Ten millimolar 3-OMG inhibits

291

the uptake of 1 mM valine by 60%. Considering only the active valine uptake (DNP sensitive) the sugar is 70% effective as an inhibitor. Higher 3-OMG concentrations caused only slightly more inhibition than that shown for 10 mM. The converse experiment is shown in Fig. 3. Valine at a concentration of 10 mM inhibits only 20% of the total and 25% of the active transport of 1 mM 3-OMG. Valine concentrations higher than 10 mM cause no further degree of inhibition. Thus, for the conditions used, 3-OMG is almost 3 times more effective than valine as an inhibitor. Considering the concepts presented earlier, one would therefore predict that the rate of transport of 3-OMG would be approximately three fold faster than valine if rates are measured at a substrate concentration of 10 mM.

Figure 4 shows the uptake of 10 mM valine by the isolated cells. Transport was monitored only for a short interval in an attempt to obtain influx rates uncomplicated by backflux. The observed deviation from linearity for uptake over the first three minutes indicates this objective was not completely achieved. Nevertheless a near linear rate of influx was maintained for 1 minute and this interval was used to estimate unidirectional influx rates. The slope of the initial portion of the curve shown in Fig. 4 indicates an uptake rate of about 19 n moles/min/mg protein. It is important to recognize, however, that this value represents the total rate of valine entry, and includes both carrier mediated and diffusional events. A correction for diffusional entry must be considered, as valine fluxes occuring by diffusion will not contribute to discharge of the cellular sodium gradient. One method for evaluating diffusional entry is to monitor uptake of valine in the presence of a high concentration of another amino acid which can effectively compete for the valine carrier. Leucine appears to satisfy this requirement as illustrated by the lower line in Fig. 4. In the presence of 25 mM leucine, the rate of uptake of 1 mM valine by the cells is constant over the entire 3 minute interval monitored. We have also shown that the uptake of valine at low concentrations (<1 mM) is a linear function of valine concentration, under these conditions, as expected if only diffusional, or low-affinity carrier-mediated fluxes can occur. Valine concentrations above 1 mM were avoided in this experiment in order to be certain that leucine was completely effective in competitively blocking active accumulation of valine via the Na^+-dependent carrier. Under these conditions, 1 mM valine enters at the rate of 0.4

n moles/min/mg protein (11). If this value can be taken to vary linearly with valine concentration at valine concentrations greater than 1 mM, then the diffusional entry rate at a concentration of 10 mM must be approximately 4 n moles/min/ mg protein. The dashed line in Fig. 4 represents this calculated passive entry rate. Carrier-mediated valine entry is therefore about 15 n moles/min/mg protein.

A similar approach can be used to calculate carrier-mediated entry rates for 3-OMG accumulation. In this case, diffusional entry rates are determined in the presence of phlorizin which specifically inhibits sodium dependent sugar accumulation. The difference between total and diffusional entry rates is approximately 9 n moles/min/mg protein as shown in Fig. 5.

The predicted correlation between substrate entry rates and intensity of interaction with another Na^+ dependent transport system does not appear to be valid. Valine is transported nearly twice as rapidly as 3-OMG, yet is less than half as effective as an inhibitor. Of course a difference in the stoichiometry of entry between Na^+ and substrate might account for the observed discrepancy. However, data obtained with rabbit ileum indicates a nearly identical stoichiometry for Na^+ entry with 3-OMG (1:1) (22), as compared to Na^+ entry with valine (0.8:1) (23), when extracellular Na^+ is 80 mM. While data of this type for chick intestine is not available, the characteristics of Na^+ dependent transport systems from a wide variety of species are fundamentally similar. Even if the stoichiometry of Na^+ co-transport with valine is 80% that obtained with 3-OMG, one would expect valine to be more effective than 3-OMG as an inhibitor; as shown in Table I. There is nearly a 4 fold discrepancy between the predicted ratio for Na^+ entry with the two substrates and their relative effectiveness as inhibitors.

Considering the facts presented above, we feel it is unlikely that the interaction between Na^+-dependent transport systems reflects a partial collapse of the transmembrane sodium gradient. Furthermore, the approach used here is valid in dealing with the possibility that microenvironments near membrane surfaces might determine substrate carrier characteristics. In order to have Na^+ which is delivered on one carrier affect the activity of a second carrier the two carriers must be sensing a common intracellular compartment. This compartment may be either a membrane microenvironment or involve the cytoplasmic compartment as a whole. If Na$^+$ delivered to this compartment on the sugar carrier can inhibit 70% of the active entry of valine, it is difficult to envision how a greater rate of sodium delivery on the valine carrier can be less effective as an inhibitor of sugar transport. If the two carriers differ in their sensitivity to cellular sodium one would expect agents which inhibit active sodium extrusion, such as ouabain to differentially inhibit the two transport systems, with valine transport exhibiting greater sensitivity. Instead, nearly the same degree of inhibition is obtained with low concentrations of ouabain as shown in Fig. 6. In fact, 3-OMG entry may be slightly more sensitive than valine entry.

If the observed interaction between transport systems cannot be related to discharge of the Na$^+$-gradient, what is the explanation? Alvarado has suggested the possibility that interaction is a reflection of competition for sterically interacting sites on a common multi-functional carrier (19,24). We feel this alternative is unlikely for the following reasons. If the substrate binding sites interact sterically, then agents which bind to the sugar carrier, such as phlorizin, would be expected to partially inhibit amino acid transport. In fact, phlorizin is able to completely overcome sugar induced inhibition of valine uptake (Fig. 7), in spite of a molecular size which is significantly larger than that for monosaccharides. Also, it has thus far been impossible to detect counter-transport phenomena between the two substrate groups (25,26). Finally, the inhibitory interaction disappears in cells de-energized by treatment with DNP (Fig. 8) in contrast to what would be expected for interaction produced by steric interference between substrates binding to closely positioned membrane carriers (27).

What mechanism can be envisioned to account for an interaction between transport systems which is dependent on the energy status of the cell? In order to answer this question it is important to recall that the characteristics of Na$^+$-dependent transport systems suggest that a close relationship exists between active transport systems for sodium and those for certain organic molecules. The relationship may be much more direct than that envisioned by the ion gradient hypothesis. For instance, it is tempting to speculate that a single set of basic energy transduction events might serve in support of a variety of energy-dependent transport systems. In this regard, the membrane bound phosphorylated intermediates which have been described for $[Na^+ + K^+]$ activated ATPase (28,29) may have broader significance than commonly recognized. The inter-mediates are thought to represent energized forms of the enzyme which are important in conserving a portion of the free energy of hydrolysis of ATP. The energized inter-mediates apparently can be expended and the energy released be partially conserved and used to impel ions across the membrane boundary against an electrochemical gradient. It seems possible that membrane components which have classic-ally been associated with separate transport systems might have the capability for tapping energy from the same set of intermediates. This possibility is illustrated in scheme 1. Reactions 1, 2, and 3 are those partial reactions which have been described for $[Na^+ + K^+]$ activated ATPase. X, Y, and Z are envisioned as closely associated membrane com-ponents (carriers?) which are substrate specific for sugars, amino acids, and K^+ respectively, and which can tap energy inherent in $E_2{\sim}P$ to support active transport. In this sense, K^+ transport is regarded as simply another form of Na^+-dependent transport.

These concepts provide us with a model which can ex-plain all of the basic characteristics of Na^+-dependent transport events, but which does not demand an energy input derived from the trans-membrane Na^+ gradient.

1. The transport systems are Na^+-dependent because in the absence of Na^+ the proper energized inter-mediates are not generated.

2. A general correlation between sodium transport and metabolite transport is expected because each system derives energy from a common energy transduction event.

3. Oligomycin and ouabain are expected to inhibit both ion and metabolite transport because each agent interacts with components common to both transport systems.

4. All transport systems are dependent on a supply of ATP and hence should be susceptible to metabolic inhibitors.

5. Elevated K^+ concentrations would be expected to be inhibitory to substrate transport by diverting energy from $E_2{\sim}P$ toward components responsible for K^+ transport; at the same partially depriving

substrate transport components of their normal
supply of $E_2{\sim}P$.

6. An interaction between sugar and amino acid transport is also expected because each system competes
for the $E_2{\sim}P$ energized intermediate.

In addition, active substrate transport would still
occur in normally energized cells even when the Na^+ gradient
is reversed from normal, as we have observed (8,9,14,16). On
the other hand, in deenergized cells, an imposed ion gradient
would generate $E_2{\sim}P$ which in turn could support substrate
uptake as has also been reported (11,13). This possibility
simply depends on the reversibility of $[Na^+ + K^+]$ activated
ATPase, a fact which has been demonstrated (30). It in no
way implies that the ion gradient normally energizes substrate transport any more than the fact that discharge of
mitochondrial K^+ gradients with net production of ATP (31)
implies a role for the K^+ gradient in the mechanism of oxidative phosphorylation. We have previously (8) emphasized the
analogy between the model described above, and the so called
chemical model for oxidative phosphorylation. In each case,
a membrane bound energized intermediate is regarded as
providing energy for a variety of energy dependent events.
A more formal analogy can be drawn from the recent work of
Roseman and his collaborators on the PEP energized monosaccharide transport systems of certain bacteria (32,33).
In this situation, PEP phosphorylates a cytoplasmic protein
(HPr), which in some species (e.g. *E. coli*) can then phosphorylate a sugar non-specific protein in the cell membrane.
The phosphorylated membrane protein apparently represents
an energized intermediate which can be tapped by a number of
sugar-specific transport systems (33). Energy transfer in
this situation occurs in part by a phosphorylation of the
sugar molecule as it traverses the cell membrane. Each
sugar entry system is separately inducible indicating a set
of different membrane components exists, each of which may
tap the membrane bound energized intermediate. Mutually
inhibitory interactions between transport systems have
been observed (32), and would be expected for reasons entirely analogous to those postulated here as a basis for interactions between the transport of sugars and amino acids in
mammalian cells.

Several predictions can be derived from our model which
can be easily evaluated experimentally. One of the most

important concerns the role which K^+ plays as an inhibitor. If our model is accurate, the inhibitory effect of K^+ should disappear in cells depleted of their energy reserves by pre-incubation with DNP. K^+ is envisioned as an inhibitor only indirectly by virtue of its ability to compete for an energized intermediate. In contrast, in terms consistent with the ion gradient hypothesis it has been suggested that K^+ acts directly on the substrate carrier by competing for the Na^+ site and forming a complex which has poor substrate affinity (6). A mode of action of this sort should not depend on the energy status of the cell.

Figures 9 and 10 show that the inhibitory effect of K^+ is entirely dependent on an energized cell population. As little as 36 mM K^+ will inhibit more than 40% of the active accumulation of ^{14}C-3-OMG in untreated cells. On the other hand, the same K^+ concentration has no significant effect in cells pre-incubated with 200 μM DNP for 10 minutes. The de-energized cells do exhibit a dependency on Na^+ for sugar uptake, however. It is for this reason that a role for extra-cellular Na^+ at the substrate carrier has been included in our model. This carrier requirement for Na^+ is considered as secondary to the role Na^+ plays in generating the appropriate energized intermediate. However, an effect directly at the sugar carrier might contribute to sugar accumulation by de-energized cell populations in high $[Na^+]$ environments.

Finally, if our model is valid, it may be possible to find agents which interact rather specifically with membrane components responsible for one transport system with consequent adjustments in the activity of others dependent on the same energy source. For instance if such agents could prevent carrier energization and preserve energy in the form of $E_2 \sim P$ it might be possible to demonstrate a decreased accumulation of one substrate group and stimulation of another. We have already indicated that phlorizin is a rather specific inhibitor of Na^+-dependent sugar transport (34), and it was therefore of interest to determine its' effects on amino acid uptake. As shown in Fig. 11, a significant stimulation of valine transport occurs when phlorizin is present. In order to determine whether the transport systems exhibit these characteristics with other inhibitors of sugar transport we also examined phloretin, a potent inhibitor of carrier-mediated passive sugar transport in red blood cells (35). To our surprise, exactly the converse results were obtained (Figs. 11 and 12). Phloretin acts as a modest inhibitor of valine accumulation, but

markedly stimulates 3-OMG uptake. While it is too early to
recognize the full meaning of these interesting relationships,
it is tempting to speculate that they imply a direct relationship between energy transduction events occuring in the
membrane in support of sugar and amino acid transport. In
this regard, it is interesting to note that phlorizin and
phloretin inhibit a variety of enzymatic reactions, many of
which involve phosphorylated intermediates (36-39). Perhaps
the fact that these agents modify Na^+-dependent substrate
accumulation is in itself an indication that phosphorylated
intermediates play a role in the mechanism of transport.

Summary

A number of observations reported here and elsewhere
seem difficult to reconcile with premises implicit in the
ion gradient hypothesis.

1. Normally energized intestinal cell populations
   actively accumulate sugars and amino acids even
   when a reversed Na^+ gradient is imposed. Similar
   results have been obtained with ascites cells (14,
   16).
2. In ascites cells, Na^+ dependent transport systems
   seem more responsive to the ATP content of the
   cell, than to the magnitude or direction of the
   ion gradients (16).
3. Reversed gradients of both Na^+ and K^+ are also not
   effective in preventing Na^+-dependent substrate
   uptake, if metabolic activity is not inhibited
   (9,10); although elevated K^+ concentrations do
   decrease transport rates.
4. The inhibitory effects of K^+ disappear completely
   in cells de-energized by pre-incubation with DNP.
5. There is no correlation between rate of transport
   of a given substrate and its ability to inhibit
   transport of a second substrate which enters by
   another Na^+ dependent system.

We propose that there may be fundamental energy transduction events associated with the plasma membrane which
are common to a variety of energy dependent transport systems. An attractive possibility for Na^+-dependent transport systems envisions the participation of energized

intermediates already described for energy transfer events associated with [Na^+ + K^+] activated ATPase. This idea can explain many of the rather unique characteristics observed for Na^+-dependent transport, including the general correlation between cellular Na^+ gradients and activity of the substrate transport systems. At the same time, a strict dependence of substrate transport on the Na^+ gradient is non-essential.

An important ramification of our hypothesis is the recognition that interacting transport systems need not necessarily imply competition for common membrane carriers as has frequently been assumed. Even closely related molecules such as two different monosaccharides might use different carriers, but compete for energy generated at limited rates by basic transduction events common to both carriers. We have drawn an analogy between this concept for mammalian cells, and the better documented PEP-energized sugar transport systems of certain bacteria (33). Expansion of transport capability to include new substrates might be regarded simply as an elaboration of membrane components which can tap a common energy transducing unit, rather than development of new carriers each with different requirements for energy transfer. While these concepts must be treated as speculative, it is well worth noting that nature frequently solves apparently diverse problems with mechanisms of remarkably similar fundamental design.

From the Department of Radiation Biology and Biophysics, University of Rochester School of Medicine and Dentistry, Rochester, New York 14642. Supported in part by a grant from the Public Health Service #1 RO1 AM 15365-01 Division of Arthritis and Metabolic Diseases, and in part by U. S. Atomic Energy Commission Contract No. AT(11-1)3490, and assigned as Report No. UR-3490-118.

References

1. Schultz, S. G. and P. F. Curran. Coupled transport of sodium and organic solutes. Physiol. Rev. 50:637 (1970).
2. Riggs, T. R., L. M. Walhen and H. N. Christensen. Potassium migration and amino acid transport. J. Biol. Chem. 233: 1479 (1958).
3. Crane, R. K., D. Miller and I. Bihler. The restrictions

on possible mechanisms of intestinal active transport of sugars. In: A. Kleinzeller and A. Kotyk (Editors), Membrane transport and functions, Academic Press, Inc., New York (1960), p. 439.

4. Crane, R. K. Hypothesis of mechanism of intestinal active transport of sugars. Fed. Proc. 21:891 (1962).

5. Crane, R. K. Absorption of sugars. Aliment. Canal 3: 1323 (1968).

6. Crane, R. K., G. Forstner and A. Eicholz. Studies on the mechanism of the intestinal absorption of sugars. X. An effect of Na$^+$ concentration on the apparent Michaelis constant for intestinal sugar transport, *in vitro*. Biochim. Biophys. Acta. 109: 467 (1965).

7. Kimmich, G. A. Preparation and properties of mucosal epithelial cells isolated from small intestine of the chicken. Biochemistry 9: 3559 (1970).

8. Kimmich, G. A. Active sugar accumulation by isolated intestinal epithelial cells. A new model for sodium-dependent metabolite transport. Biochemistry 9: 3669 (1970).

9. Kimmich, G. A. Sodium-dependent accumulation of sugars by isolated intestinal cells. Evidence for a mechanism not dependent on the sodium gradient. (In press, 1972).

10. Kimmich, G. A. and J. P. Randles (Manuscript in preparation).

11. Vidaver, G. A. Glycine transport by hemoloyzed and restored pigeon red cells. Biochemistry 3: 795 (1964).

12. Eddy, A. A., M. F. Mulcahy and P. J. Thompson. The effects of sodium ions and potassium ions on glycine uptake by mouse-tumor cells in the presence and absence of selected metabolic inhibitors. Biochem. J. 103: 863 (1967).

13. Eddy, A. The effects of varying the cellular and the extra-cellular concentrations of sodium and potassium ions on the uptake of glycine by mouse ascites-tumor cells in the presence and absence of sodium cyanide. Biochem. J. 108: 489 (1968).

14. Schafer, J. A. and J. A. Jacquez. Evidence against the sodium gradient hypothesis for amino acid transport in the Ehrlich ascites cell. Federation Proc. 27: 516 (1968).

15. Jacquez, J. A. and J. A. Schafer Sodium and potassium electrochemical potential gradients and the transport of AIB in Ehrlich ascites tumor cells. Biochim. Biophys. Acta. 193: 368 (1969).

16. Potashner, S. J. and R. M. Johnstone. Cation gradients, ATP and amino acid accumulation in Ehrlich ascites cells. Biochim. Biophys. Acta 233: 91 (1971).
17. Newey, H. and D. H. Smyth. Effects of sugars on intestinal transfer of amino acids. Nature 202: 400 (1964).
18. Hindmarsh, J. T., D. Kilby and G. Wiseman. Effect of amino acids on sugar absorption. J. Physiol. 186: 1966 (1966).
19. Alvarado, F. Transport of sugars and amino acids in the intestine: evidence for a common carrier. Science 151: 1010 (1966).
20. Read, C. P. Studies on membrane transport. I. A common transport system for sugars and amino acids. Biol. Bull. 133: 630 (1967).
21. Chez, R. A., S. G. Schultz and P. F. Curran. Effects of sugars on transport of alanine in intestine. Science 153: 1012 (1966).
22. Goldner, A. M. S. G. Schultz and P. F. Curran. Sodium and sugar fluxes across the mucosal border of rabbit ileum. J. Gen. Physiol. 53: 362 (1969).
23. Curran, P. F., S. G. Schultz, R. A. Chez and R. E. Fuisz. Kinetic relations of the Na-amino acid interaction at the mucosal border of intestine. J. Gen. Physiol. 50: 1261 (1967).
24. Alvarado, F. Amino acid transport in hamster small intestine: Site of inhibition by D-galactose. Nature 289: 276 (1968).
25. Munck, B. G. Amino acid transport by the small intestine of the rat. Evidence against interactions between sugars and amino acids at the carrier level. Biochim. Biophys. Acta 156: 192 (1968).
26. Kimmich, G. A. Interaction between sugar and amino acid transport in isolated intestinal epithelial cells. Proc. Int. Union Physiol. Sci 9: 303 (1971).
27. Frizzell, R. A. and S. G. Schultz. Distinction between galactose and phenylalanine effects on alanine transport in rabbit ileum. Biochim. Biophys. Acta 233: 485 (1971).
28. Fahn, S., G. J. Koval and R. W. Albers. Sodium-potassium activated adenosine triphosphatase of *Electrophorous* electric organ. I. An associated sodium-activated transphosphorylation. J. Biol. Chem. 241: 1882 (1966).

29. Sen, A. K., T. Tobin and R. L. Post. A cycle for ouabain inhibition of sodium-and potassium-dependent adenosine triphosphatase. J. Biol. Chem. 244: 6596 (1969).
30. Garrahan, P. J. and J. M. Glynn. The incorporation of inorganic phosphate into adenosine triphosphate by reversal of the sodium pump. J. Physiol. 192: 237 (1967).
31. Cockrell, R. S., E. J. Harris and B. C. Pressman. Synthesis of ATP driven by a potassium gradient. Nature 215: 1487 (1967).
32. Roseman, S. The transport of carbohydrates by a bacterial phosphotransferase system. J. Gen. Physiol. 54: 138S (1969).
33. Kundig, W. and S. Roseman. Sugar Transport II. Characterization of constitutive membrane-bound enzymes II of the *Escherischia coli* phosphotransferase system. J. Biol. Chem. 246: 1407 (1971).
34. Caspary, W. F., N. R. Stevenson and R. K. Crane. Evidence for an intermediate step in carrier mediated sugar translocation across the brush border membrane of hamster small intestine. Biochim. Biophys. Acta. 193: 168 (1969).
35. LeFevre, P. G. and J. K. Marshall. Attachment of phloretin and analogues to human erythrocytes in connection with inhibition of sugar transport. J. Biol. Chem. 234: 3022 (1959).
36. Lygre, D. G. and R. C. Nordlie. Rabbit intestinal glucose-6-phosphate phosphohydrolase and inorganic pyrophosphate-glucose phosphotransferase inhibition by phlorizin. Biochim. Biophys. Acta. 185: 360 (1969).
37. Robinson, J. L. Effects of phlorizin on membrane cation-dependent adenosine triphosphatase and p-nitrophenyl phosphatase activities. Mol. Pharmacol. 5: 584 (1969).
38. Uribe, E. G. Phloretin: an inhibitor of phosphate transfer and electron flow in spinach chloroplasts. Biochemistry 19: 2100 (1970).
39. Izawa, S., G. D. Winget and N. E. Good. Phlorizin, a specific inhibitor of photophosphorylation and phosphorylation-coupled electron transport in chloroplasts. Biochem. Biophys. Res. Commun. 22: 223 (1966).

Table I

COMPARISON OF RATES OF ENTRY FOR 10 mM VALINE AND 10 mM 3-OMG AND EXPECTED RELATIVE EFFECTIVENESS AS INHIBITORS

Substrate	Total	Passive	Carrier Mediated	Na^+ Coupling Coefficient	Expected Na^+ Entry	$\frac{Na^+ Entry_{val}}{Na^+ Entry_{3-OMG}}$	$\frac{\%I_{val}}{\%I_{3-OMG}}$
				n moles/min/mg protein			
Valine	19.0	4.0	15.0	0.8[a]	12.0[b]		
						1.33	0.36
3-OMG	12.5	3.5	9.0	1.0	9.0		

[a]Values reported for rabbit ileum at 80 mM Na^+ (22, 23).

[b]Carrier mediated substrate entry x Na^+ coupling coefficient

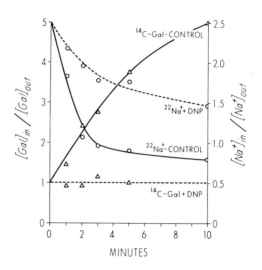

Fig. 1. *Fluxes of* $^{22}Na^+$ *and* ^{14}C-galactose following reversal of the Na^+-gradient in isolated intestinal epithelial cells. Cells were pre-loaded at 0° in media with 80 mM $^{22}Na^+$ and 1.25 mM ^{14}C-galactose. Incubation at 37° and 20 mM Na^+. Details are given in the text. The cell protein concentration was 3.0 mg/ml. The sample size was 200 μl. (Reprinted by permission from Biochemistry 9: 3669)

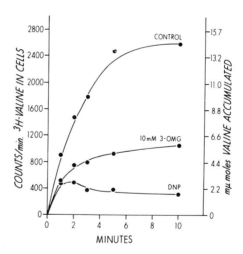

Fig. 2. *Effect of 10 mM 3-OMG on accumulation of 1 mM valine by isolated intestinal cells.* Three and three-tenths milligram cell protein per milliliter were used.

304

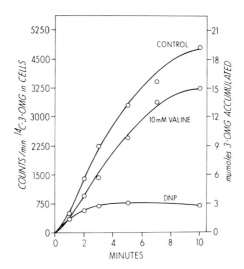

Fig. 3. *Effect of 10 mM valine on accumulation of 1mM 3-OMG by isolated intestinal cells.* Three and five-tenths milligram cell protein per milliliter were used.

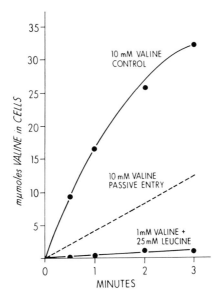

Fig. 4. *Influx of valine into isolated intestinal epithelial cells.* Passive entry of 1 mM valine was monitored in the presence of 25 mM leucine which competes for the same entry system. Passive entry for 10 mM valine is taken simply as 10 x that illustrated for 1 mM. The cell protein concentration was 5.0 mg/ml. The sample size was 200 µl.

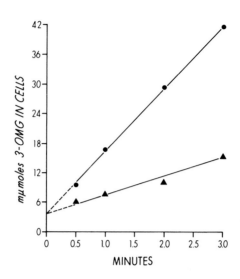

Fig. 5. *Influx of 10 mM 3-OMG in the presence and absence of phlorizin.* The cell protein concentration was 5.0 mg/ml and the sample size was 200 µl; •, control; Δ, control plus 200 µM phlorizin.

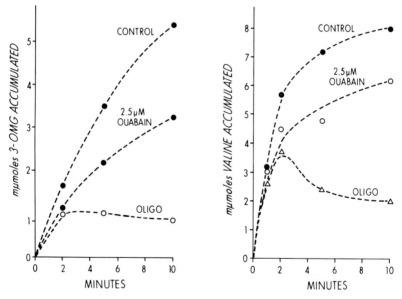

Fig. 6. *Effect of sub-optimal concentrations of ouabain on the accumulation of 3-OMG and valine by isolated intestinal epithelial cells.* Oligomycin was used at a concentration of 5 µg/ml. Cell protein concentration was 2 mg/ml.

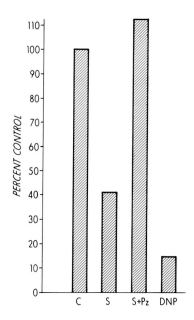

Fig. 7. *Release of 3-OMG induced inhibition of 1 mM valine accumulation by phlorizin.* C, control; S, 10 mM 3-OMG added; DNP, 200 μM; S + Pz, 10 mM 3-OMG plus 200 μM phlorizin.

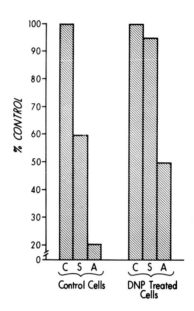

Fig. 8. *Loss of 3-OMG induced inhibition of valine uptake in DNP treated cells.* Valine concentration was 1 mM. Treated cells were pre-incubated for 10 min at 37° with 200 µM DNP. C, control; S, 10 mM 3-OMG added; A, 5 mM alanine added.

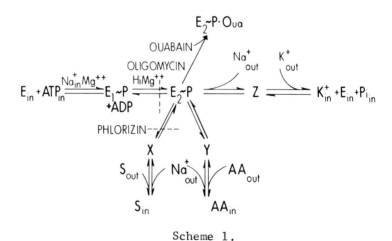

Scheme 1.

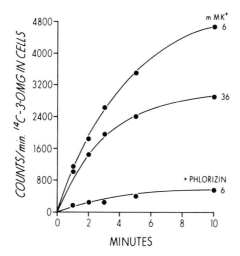

Fig. 9. *Effect of elevated K⁺ concentration on the accumulation of 3-OMG by isolated intestinal epithelial cells.* Potassium ion was increased by replacing a portion of the mannitol in the medium with an osmotically equivalent amount of KCl.

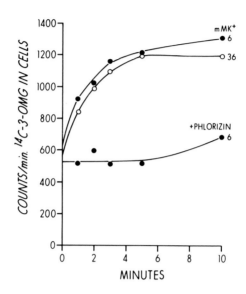

Fig. 10. *Effect of elevated K^+ concentration on the uptake of 3-OMG in DNP treated intestinal cells.* The cells were pre-incubated for 10 minutes at 37° with 200 μM DNP in Na^+-free medium. Incubation was at 60 mM Na^+ so that a normally directed Na^+ gradient was initially imposed. One millimolar ^{14}C-3-OMG (0.1 μc/ml) was included in both the pre-incubation and experimental phase.

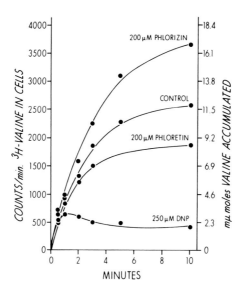

Fig. 11. *Effect of phlorizin, phloretin and DNP on uptake of 1 mM valine by isolated intestinal epithelial cells.*

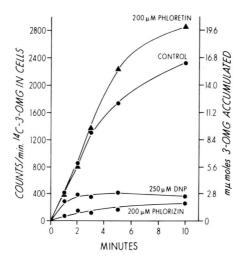

Fig. 12. *Effect of phloretin, phlorizin, and DNP on uptake of 1 mM 3-OMG by isolated intestinal epithelial cells.*

THE STIMULATION OF CORTICOSTEROIDOGENESIS IN ISOLATED RAT ADRENAL CELLS BY AGAROSE-ACTH

Morton Civen

Introduction

The chemical linkage of protein and peptide hormones to inert support materials such as cellulose (1), agarose (2-5), polyacrylamide (6) and dextran (7,8) has been effected with retention of some, if not all, of the bioactive character- istics of the unbound hormones. These macroscopic polymer bound hormones have proven useful as instruments to explore interactions between protein and peptide hormones and cell surfaces (2-6, 9-12) and to isolate cell membrane macro- molecules involved in the hormone protein-membrane inter- action (10,13-15).

Our work is mainly concerned with the demonstration that adrenocorticotropin (ACTH) can be covalently linked to agarose with retention of biological activity, and with the nature of the interaction between agarose-ACTH and isolated adrenal cells.

Methods

Porcine β^{1-39} Corticotropin (Armour & Co., 20 iu/mg), synthetic α^{1-24} corticotropin (Cortrosyn, Organon, Inc.), synthetic β^{1-24} corticotropin (Synacthen, Ciba-Geigy, Inc.) and synthetic D-Ser^{1}NLe^4- (Val-NH$_2$)^{25}-β^{1-25} corticotropin (DW-75, Sandox, Ltd.) were diazotized to 3 - [3'-(4 amino- benzamido)-propylamino]-propylamine agarose by a method re- ported by Selinger and Civen (4) and Cuatrecasas (16).

*Preparation of 3-(3'-4-aminobenzamido)-propylaminoaga-
rose from 3-(3'-aminopropylamino)-propylamine agarose.*

Fifteen milliliters of 3-(3'-aminopropylamino)-propyl-
amine agarose (AF 102; 8-9 µM amine/ml; Biorad Corp., Rich-
mond, California) is measured into a siliconized graduated
cylinder and transferred to a fritted glass filter of coarse
porosity. The gel is washed 2 times with 200 ml of 0.5 M
sodium borate (pH 9.5). The gel is transferred into a teflon beaker with 40 ml of 0.5 M sodium borate (pH 9.5). With
stirring at 4°, 40 ml of 100% redistilled N,N-dimethyl for-
mamide (DMF) is added slowly. Ten milliliters of 0.2 M p-
nitrobenzoylazide (Eastman) in 100% DMF is added and the
reaction mixture permitted to stand at room temperature for
4 hours. The gel beads gave no color reaction with sodium
picrylsulfonate (Pierce Chemical Co.) as described by
Cuatrecasas (16).

The gel is transferred to a sintered glass filter and
washed over a period of 6 to 8 hours with 3 **liters of 50%**
DMF, followed by a wash with 200 ml of 0.5 M $NaHCO_3$ (pH 8.5).
The gel is suspended as a slurry in 45 ml of 0.5 M $NaHCO_3$
(pH 8.5) in a teflon beaker. At this point, the gel is
stable.

Solid sodium dithionite is added to a final concentration of 0.1 M. The reaction mixture is held at 40° in the
water bath for 90 minutes, is then transferred to a fritted
glass filter and washed with 500 ml of 0.1 M sodium bicarbonate. The color test with sodium picrylsulfonate is red-
orange. The gel is washed finally with 200 ml of 0.5 N HCl.

*Diazotization of α^{1-24} corticotropin (Cortrosyn) to 3-
(3'-4-aminobenzamido)-propylaminoagarose.*

Five milliliters of gel (settled volume) is suspended
in a teflon beaker in 10 ml of 0.5 N HCl and 0.5 ml of a
freshly prepared 0.1 M sodium nitrite solution is added.
This is permitted to react for 7 minutes at 4°, then is
transferred rapidly to a fritted glass filter and washed
with 30 ml of ice cold distilled water. The gel is transferred with 12 ml of cold 0.25 M sodium borate buffer (pH 9.5)
into a teflon beaker and 2 mg[1] (3.6 nmoles/µmole of agarose
bound amine) of α^{1-24} corticotropin (Cortrosyn) is added
rapidly. The gel diazo derivative and the ACTH are permitted

314

to react for 2 hours at room temperature. The final pH of the reaction mixture was 9.2.

α^{1-24} corticotropin also was reacted with agarose diazo derivative in 0.2 M sodium phosphate (pH 7.0).

The diazoagarose derivatives of porcine corticotropin, β^{1-24} corticotropin and D-Ser^{1}NLe^4-(Val-NH$_2$)^{25} β^{1-25} corticotropin also were prepared using the above procedure.

In order to remove any physically adsorbed ACTH, the gel preparations were washed with the following solutions: 1) 1700 ml of 0.2 M sodium phosphate (pH 7.0); 2) 650 ml of 1 N HCl; 3) 200 ml of 5 M guanidine HCl (pH 5.0); 4) 750 ml of 8 M urea; 5) 500 ml of 0.2 M ammonium acetate (pH 6.7); 6) 500 ml of 0.1 N HCl; and 7) 1000 ml 4% (w/v) Fraction V bovine serum albumin (Pentex) in 0.2 M sodium phosphate (pH 7.0). Complete removal of non-covalently linked ACTH was ascertained by adding 500,000-1,000,000 cpm of ACTH-^{125}I during the diazotization, and then carrying out the above mentioned washes until radioactivity in the washes reaches background levels.

Preparation of free adrenal cells for ACTH stimulation of corticosterone formation.

Eight to forty male rats (Charles River Breeding Laboratories), 350 to 500 gms, were sacrificed by decapitation and were exsanguinated. The adrenals were removed, placed in iced 0.9% NaCl, and trimmed of extraneous tissue. Quartered adrenals were then reduced by either the trypsin digestion procedure of Sayers *et al.* (17) or the bacterial collagenase digestion procedure of Haning *et al.* (18). To increase the sensitivity of the latter method, a further modification of the collagenase[2] disruption procedure was made.

---

[1]*The following amounts of α^{1-24} corticotropin were also diazotized: 387.2 nmoles and 1720 nmoles/µmole of agarose bound amine. In all cases corticosteroidogenic activity was proportional to the amount of α^{1-24} corticotropin linked.*

[2]*It is essential to test several batches of collagenase (Worthington) and Fraction V albumin (Pentex) to obtain cells which are optimally stimulated by ACTH.*

Cells prepared by the collagenase digestion method were suspended in Krebs-Ringer bicarbonate glucose (KRBG) containing 100 mg of crystalline trypsin (Worthington)/ml at a concentration of 1 to 1.5×10^6 cells/ml. The cell suspension was then incubated 3 minutes at 37° under 95% O_2-5% CO_2. The cells were centrifuged at 100 x g for 10 min at 22° and were resuspended in 1.5 ml of KRBG containing 0.5% Fraction V bovine serum albumin (Pentex) and 7.65 mM $CaCl_2$ (KRBGA, high Ca^{++}). Lima bean trypsin inhibitor (Worthington) was added in 0.5 ml of the same buffer, in an amount to exactly inhibit the trypsin added. The cells were centrifuged at 100 x g for 10 min and resuspended in KRBGA-high Ca^{++} to a concentration of 2.5×10^5 Cells/ml for hormonal stimulations. The adrenal (0.9 ml, 2.5×10^5 cells/ml) cells were incubated in a total volume of 1 ml in teflon beakers. The incubations were carried out at 37°, 90 revolutions/minute under 95% O_2-5% CO_2 in a Dubnoff type incubator for 2 hours.

Standard solutions of porcine ACTH or other corticotropin peptides were dissolved in 0.9% NaCl, 0.5% bovine serum albumin, and 0.1 N HCl (ACTH vehicle).

Agarose-ACTH preparations were also suspended in ACTH vehicle. In order to obtain uniform suspensions of agarose-ACTH, the gel beads were stirred with a magnetic stirrer during the addition of agarose-ACTH beads to the incubation mixture.

The adrenal cell assay manifests a limitation in that consecutive cell harvests do not exhibit identical steroidogenic potentials: fixed numbers of cells do not generate reproducibly the same quantity of corticosterone on different days (19). However, within a single harvest of trypsinized cells, individual aliquots have identical baseline and inducible levels of corticosterone production.

The corticosterone content of incubates is determined fluorimetrically. ACTH-agarose itself is not fluorogenic and did not interfere with the determination of corticosterone (4).

Cyclic adenosine 3,5 monophosphate (cAMP) in the cell incubates was extracted and purified according to the method of Manganello et al. (20). Cyclic AMP levels were measured using the competitive binding method of Gilman (21).

Results and Discussion

Both the free and covalently linked β^{1-24} corticotropin

induce the production of corticosterone by free adrenal cells
(Fig. 1). The steroid output elicited by the gel varies
regularly with the weight of gel used (sigmoid on a semi-log
scale). Uniform responses are obtained with gel weights as
low as 0.0001 g; however, below this weight β^{1-24} corti-
cotropin-agarose exhibited stochastic variations in its induction potential, which are due, presumably, to the non-un-
iform distribution of ACTH molecules among the gel particles.
Gel bound ACTH generally induced a higher maximal steroidogenic response than the free hormone (Fig. 1).

Four different ACTH derivatives have been linked to
agarose; porcine β^{1-39} corticotropin, synthetic α^{1-24} and
β^{1-24} corticotropin, and D-Ser^1 NLe^4-(Val-NH$_2$)^{25} β^{1-25} corticotropin. All show steroidogenic activity in relation to
their known biological potencies and show similar dose response relationships to that observed in Fig. 1.

Different quantities of α^{1-24} corticotropin (see foot-
note 1) have been linked to agarose and the steroidogenic
activity was found to be proportional to the amount of
hormone reacted.

Agarose α^{1-24} corticotropin stimulated steroidogenesis
(22) in cells from monolayer cultures of murine adrenal
cortex tumors (23). These cells, which are extremely insensitive to free ACTH compared to trypsinized rat adrenal
cells, required greater than 200 times the amount of agarose-
α^{1-24} corticotropin derivative (1.72 μmoles of α^{1-24} corti-
cotropin/μmole agarose bound amine) needed to stimulate maximally rat adrenal cells.

Figure 3 shows that agarose α^{1-24} corticotropin also
stimulated increases in cAMP levels in a manner similar to
free ACTH (24). The particular α^{1-24} corticotropin derivative was prepared using a ratio of 1.72 μmoles of α^{1-24} cor-
ticotropin/μmole of agarose bound amine. It can be seen
from Fig. 3 that greater than 10 mg of agarose-α^{1-24} corticotropin was required to produce maximal increases in cAMP
levels. In contrast to this, only 50 to 100 μg of this
agarose derivative was required to stimulate corticosteroidogenesis maximally. This large difference between the amount
of ACTH needed to stimulate maximally these two parameters
has also been observed with free ACTH (25).

Reduction of the diazo bond between the agarose "arm"
and the tyrosyl and histidyl groups of the ACTH moiety should
release ACTH from the agarose support if it is covalently
linked to it. Agarose-ACTH (porcine) was reduced with 0.2 M

sodium dithionite in 0.5 M NaHCO$_3$ (3 hours, 40°) and rinsed
with 200 ml of 1 M NaCl. The dithionite reduction changed
the color of the agarose–ACTH gel from orange (due to the
diazo group) to colorless. However, Fig. 2a shows that in
spite of dithionite reduction the ACTH activity is strongly
retained by the gel. Since peptides have a tendency to be
strongly adsorbed by agarose, an attempt was made to elute
the adsorbed ACTH by several washes with 6 M guanidine HCl
(pH 5) and other peptide eluting solvents (see gel washing
procedures in Methods). If the agarose–ACTH washed extensively with such solvents, it can be seen that the adsorbed ACTH is almost completely removed (Fig. 2b).

Stimulation of steroidogenesis by both agarose–ACTH and
free ACTH was strongly depressed when Ca^{++} ion was omitted
from the incubation medium. Detailed comparisons between
the free and agarose bound ACTH with respect to dependency
of steroidogenesis on Ca^{++} ion concentration were not made.
Thus it remains to be determined whether or not linking of
ACTH to agarose affects this parameter in the same way as
does free ACTH.

The various diazoagarose–ACTH derivatives are highly
stable, and when stored at 2° in 0.1 N HCl, retain their
activity with little change for at least several months.

It is of interest that the trypsin digested agarose
derivative inhibits the endogenous secretion of corticoster-
oids by the free rat adrenal cells (Table I). Assuming
diazotization of both the tyrosines and histidine of ACTH,
tryptic degradation of porcine ACTH would leave residual
peptides from the N-terminal serine to arginine^{-8} and from
valine^{-22} to C-terminal phenylalanine. It is possible that
either one or both of these peptides is an inhibitor of
corticosterone secretion.

Agarose–β$^{1-24}$ corticotropin was preincubated with adrenal cells to determine whether or not a specific inactivating
interaction related to hormonal induction occurred. Such an
inactivation could involve scission of corticotropin from
the gel matrix, breaking of peptide bonds, or binding of an
inhibitor. Agarose–β$^{1-24}$ corticotropin was preincubated
with trypsinized adrenal cells for 15 min, 60 min and 120
min; washed twice with 0.1 M phosphate buffer (pH 7.6);
washed twice with ACTH vehicle; and stored in the latter reagent at 4° for 24 hours. The samples were assayed for
steroidogenic potential versus untreated gel (Fig. 4).
Through the first hour of preincubation with cells only a

very slight decrease in steroidogenic capacity of the gel-
ACTH occurred. However, after the second hour of preincubation there was significant reduction in the agarose bound
ACTH activity. Similar results were obtained when adrenal
cells were preincubated with agarose-β^{1-39} corticotropin
(4). Since trypsinized adrenal cells have been found to
lyse easily (24), it is possible that lytic principles are
released during the incubation which bring about the observed hormonal inactivation. However, it is clear that at
least during the first hour when linear corticosteroidogenesis is proceeding (Fig. 5), little destruction of agarose-
ACTH occurs.

Equilibration of anti-human ACTH antibody (at 1:25,000
ilution, bound/free = 1) with agarose-β^{1-39} corticotropin
(porcine) for 3 days at 4° resulted in a total loss of
steroid stimulating activity by the agarose-ACTH.

The agarose-ACTH can be sequestered during cellular
incubation by the use of nylon screens (nylon microfilament
cloth, 37 μ mesh opening) which gives the cells access to
the agarose-ACTH beads, but allows removal of the agarose-
ACTH from the incubate at a given time. The beaded gel has
a minimum diameter approximately three times that of the
free adrenal cells. Figure 5 shows an experiment in which
the cells and agarose-ACTH were removed together, or the
agarose-ACTH beads were removed at 2 min, 15 min, and 30
min, and the cellular incubation then allowed to proceed
for the remainder of the 120 min. Removal of the cells and
beads together at different times shows similar kinetics
of stimulation of corticosteroid formation to that of free
ACTH (25). There is an initial 15 minute lag followed by
essentially linear corticosteroidogenesis for the remaining
105 minutes. Removal of the beads alone at 2, 15 and 30
minutes resulted in markedly reduced steroidogenesis, indicating that the continued contact of the cells with agarose-
ACTH is necessary for maximal stimulation of steroidogenesis.
However, it is also clear that a small but significant amount
of corticosteroid formation takes place after the beads are
removed at 2, 15 and 30 minutes. The same amount of corticosteroid was produced when the beads were removed during
the lag phase as when they were removed during the linear
phase. Although the agarose-ACTH beads were washed extensively with reagents which seemed to remove completely any
adsorbed ACTH it is conceivable that a very small amount of
extremely tightly adsorbed ACTH is removed by binding to the
ACTH receptor sites on the cell membrane.

The removal of tightly bound ACTH from the agarose beads is deemed unlikely, since it was shown (Fig. 4) that if agarose beads are shaken with cells for up to sixty minutes no significant ACTH activity is lost from the beads. Thus it is conceivable that the short exposure of the cells to agarose-ACTH can produce lasting stimulatory effects. More detailed studies on the kinetics of the residual corticosteroid formation after short exposures of adrenal cells to agarose-ACTH are being carried out.

When a soluble ACTH-^{125}I binding extract was prepared from rabbit adrenal tissue by the method of Lefkowitz et $al.$ (27) and passed through a short column (1/2 x 5 cm) of agarose-β^{1-39} corticotropin, the ACTH-^{125}I binding molecules were completely removed. Passage through an unmodified agarose column allowed full recovery of ACTH-^{125}I binding activity in the column filtrate. These results indicate that agarose-ACTH derivatives will be useful in the purification of the ACTH receptor protein from both adrenal and fat cells.

Conclusions

ACTH linked to an agarose support exhibits characteristics identical with those of the free molecule. It induces steroidogenesis and increases in cyclic AMP levels in free adrenal cells; its activity is calcium dependent; and it is susceptible to tryptic digestion.

Microscopic observation of incubates of the agarose-ACTH and adrenal cells suggest that there is no specific adherence between the two particles. The minimum gel-ACTH size is 3 times that of the adrenal cells, therefore induction occurs at the cell surface without passage of the corticotropin into the cell. If adrenal cells are exposed to agarose-ACTH for 30 min or less, and the incubation allowed to continue for 2 hours, the corticosteroid formed is only a small fraction of that produced when the agarose-ACTH beads are continually present. This indicates that continuous contact of agarose-ACTH with the cell surface is necessary to maintain steroidogenesis. The agarose-ACTH does not lose significant activity after incubation with adrenal cells for 1 hour, suggesting that destruction of the corticotropin does not accompany the induction process.

ACTH-^{125}I binding activity is quantitatively removed by agarose-ACTH from adrenal tissue extracts suggesting that agarose-corticotropin derivatives will be useful tools in the purification of ACTH binding substances.

Summary

Corticotropin and its synthetic analogues coupled by an azo linkage to an agarose support induces steroidogenesis in free adrenal cells in the same manner as does free ACTH. Observation of incubates of adrenal cells and agarose-ACTH indicates that 1) agarose-ACTH is not adherent to the cell surface, 2) entrance of ACTH into the cell may not be a prerequisite to the initiation of steroidogenesis, 3) the continuous presence of ACTH is necessary to maintain maximal steroid production in cellular incubates, 4) induction does not alter significantly the functional integrity of the bound corticotropin, and 5) ACTH-^{125}I binding macromolecules are trapped on columns of agarose-ACTH.

Presented by Morton Civen.

References

1. Schimmer, B.P., K. Veda, and G.H. Sato. Site of action of adrenocorticotropic hormone (ACTH) in adrenal cell cultures. Biochem. Biophys. Res. Comm. 32:806-810 (1968).
2. Cuatrecasas, P. Interaction of insulin with the cell membrane: the primary action of insulin. Proc. Natl. Acad. Sci. 63:450-457 (1969).
3. Turkington, R.W. Stimulation of RNA synthesis in isolated mammary cells by insulin and prolactin bound to sepharose. Biochem. Biophys. Res. Comm. 41:1362-1367 (1970).
4. Selinger, R.C.L. and M. Civen. ACTH diazotized to agarose: effects on isolated adrenal cells. Biochem. Biophys. Res. Comm. 43:793-799 (1971).
5. Johnson, C.B., M. Blecher and N.A. Giorgio, Jr. Hormone receptors I. Activation of rat liver plasma membrane adenyl cyclase and fat cell lipolysis by agarose-glucagon. Biochem. Biophys. Res. Comm. 46:1035-1041 (1972).
6. Richardson, M.C. and D. Schulster. β^{1-24} Adrenocorticotrophin diazotized to polyacrylamide: effects on isolated adrenal cells. Biochem. J. 120:60 p (1971).

7. Kågedahl, L. and Å. Kerström. Covalent binding of proteins to polysaccharides by cyanogen bromide and organic cyanates. I Preparation of soluble glycine-, insulin- and ampicillin-dextran. Acta Chem. Scand. 25: 1855-1859 (1971).

8. Armstrong, K.J., M.W. Noall, and J.E. Stouffer. Dextran-linked insulin: a soluble high molecular weight derivative with biological activity *in vivo* and *in vitro*. Biochem. Biophys. Res. Comm. 47:354-360 (1972).

9. Soderman, D.D., J. Germerhausen, and H.M. Katzen. Specific binding of insulin-sepharoses to isolated fat cells and affinity chromatography of receptor-containing membranes. Fed. Proc. 31:486 (1972).

10. Katzen, H.M. Affinity chromatography, solubilization and isolation of fat cell membrane insulin receptor. Chapter 9, this volume.

11. Topper, Y.J. On the development of the mammary epithelial cell *in vitro*. Chapter 16, this volume.

12. Venter, J.C., J.E. Dixon, P.R. Maroko, and N.O. Kaplan. Biologically active catecholamines bound to glass beads. Proc. Natl. Acad. Sci. 69:1141-1145 (1972).

13. Lefkowitz, R.J. Hormone receptors and the adenyl cyclase system: *in vitro* studies of isolated cardiac beta adrenergic receptors. Chapter 12, this volume.

14. Blecher, M. Detection and isolation by affinity chromatography of glucagon-binding proteins from solubilized rat liver plasma membranes. Chapter 18, this volume.

15. Cuatrecasas, P. Affinity chromatography and purification of the insulin receptor of liver cell membranes. Proc. Nat. Acad. Sci. 69:1277-1281 (1972).

16. Cuatrecasas, P. Protein purification by affinity chromatography. J. Biol. Chem. 245:3059-3065 (1970).

17. Sayers, G., R.L. Swallow and N.D. Giordano. An improved technique for the preparation of isolated rat adrenal cells: a sensitive, accurate and specific method for the assay of ACTH. Endocrinology 88:1063-1068 (1971).

18. Haning, R, S.A.S. Tait, and J.F. Tait. *In vitro* effects of ACTH, angiotensins, serotonin and potassium on steroid output and conversion of corticosterone to aldosterone by isolated adrenal cells. Endocrinology 87:1147-1167 (1970).

19. Vernikos-Danellis, J., E. Anderson, and L. Trigg. Changes in adrenal corticosterone concentration in rats: method of bioassay for ACTH. Endocrinology 79:624-630 (1966).

20. Manganiello, V., W.H. Evans, T.P. Stossel, R.J. Mason and M. Vaughan. The effect of polystyrene beads on cyclic 3',5'-adenosine monophosphate concentrations in leukocytes. J. Clin. Invest. 50:2741-2744 (1971).
21. Gilman, A.G. Protein binding assay for adenosine 3'-5'-cyclic monophosphate. Proc. Natl. Acad. Sci. 67:305-312 (1970).
22. Civen, M. and R. Wishnow. Unpublished results.
23. Buonassisi, V., G. Sato and A.I. Cohen. I. Hormone-producing cultures of adrenal and pituitary origin. Proc. Natl. Acad. Sci. 48:1184-1190 (1962).
24. Civen, M. and C.B. Brown. Unpublished observations.
25. Sayers, G., R.J. Beall and S. Seelig. Isolated adrenal cells: ACTH, calcium, steroidogenesis and cyclic adenosine monophosphate. Sci. 175:1131-1132 (1972).
26. Beall, R.J. and G. Sayers. Isolated adrenal cells: Steroidogenesis and cyclic AMP accumulation in response to ACTH. Arch. Biochem. Biophys. 148:70-76 (1972).
27. Lefkowitz, R.J., J. Roth, W. Pricer and I. Pastan. ACTH receptors in the adrenal: specific binding of ACTH-^{125}I and its relation to adenyl cyclase. Proc. Natl. Acad. Sci. 65:745-752 (1970).

Table I

AGAROSE–ACTH ACTIVITY AFTER TRYPSIN DIGESTION

Ten milligrams of agarose-ACTH were incubated 2 hours at 37°
in 0.1 M sodium phosphate (pH 7.4) with 30 mg (220 u/mg)
crystalline trypsin in a total volume of 5 ml.   The gels
were then washed 3 times with 50 ml of 0.1 M sodium phos-
phate (pH 7.4).

Gel weight	Net corticosterone
mg	*µg ± 10%*
untreated gel	
0.70	0.14
3.11	0.64
trypsin digested gel	
1.60	−0.25
3.20	−0.28

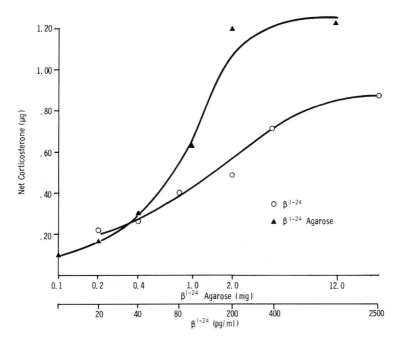

Fig. 1. *Effects of* β^{1-24} *corticotropin and agarose* β^{1-24} *corticotropin on corticosterone formation by trypsin dissociated rat adrenal cells.* From (17).

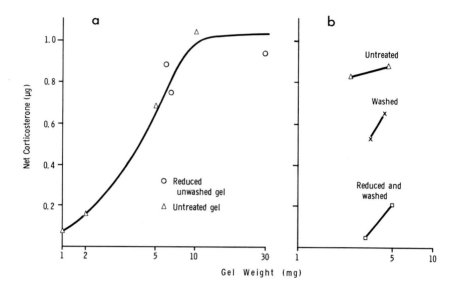

Fig. 2. *a. Composition of agarose-ACTH (porcine) activity of dithionite reduced and control samples, both of which were not washed with desorptive solvents.*

Fig. 2. *b. Agarose-ACTH dithionite reduced and washed with 6 M guanidine HCl and other peptide eluting solvents.*

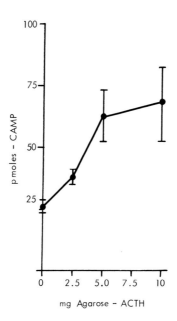

Fig. 3. *Stimulation of cAMP production by agarose* α^{1-24} *corticotropin.* Agarose α^{1-24} corticotropin and 3.5×10^5 cells in 1.0 ml KRBGA-high Ca^{++} medium were incubated 10 min at 37°.

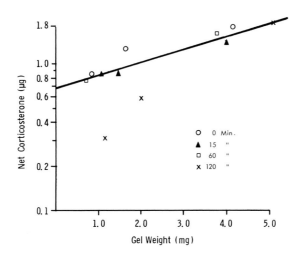

Fig. 4. *The effect of preincubation of agarose* β^{1-24} *corticotropin with adrenal cells on the ability of agarose* β^{1-24} *corticotropin to stimulate corticosteroidogenesis.*

327

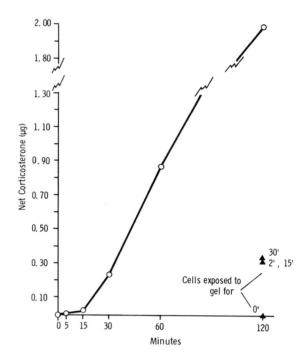

Fig. 5. *The kinetics of agarose* β^{1-24} *corticotropin stimulation of corticosteroidogenesis in free adrenal cells and the effect of early gel removal on cell steroid production.* Two milligrams of agarose β^{1-24} corticotropin were incubated with 180,000 cells in KRBGA-high Ca^{++}.

INSULIN, GLUCOCORTICOID AND ENZYME ACTIVITY

Carolyn D. Berdanier and Lalita Kaul

Introduction

In the mid-sixties, Weber and Singhal (1-4) suggested
that hormones exert their effects on hepatic metabolism by
influencing the synthesis of the enzyme proteins. Hormone
action could thus be explained on the basis of its effects
on the induction or suppression of the synthesis of key rate
limiting enzymes. Accordingly, it was suggested that insulin
served to suppress the synthesis of the gluconeogenic enzymes
while inducing the synthesis of the glycolytic enzymes.
Conversely, it was hypothesized that glucocorticoid suppressed
the synthesis of the glycolytic enzymes while enhancing the
synthesis of the gluconeogenic enzymes.
    Wool *et al.* (5,6) studied the *in vitro* synthesis of
muscle protein with and without insulin. They suggested that
insulin promotes protein synthesis intracellularly by enhancing the formation of a "translation factor" which
facilitates the translation of stable template RNA. Other
studies showing the correction by insulin of the negative
nitrogen balance in the diabetic as well as an enhancement
of tissue protein synthesis have also been reported (7-14).
Unfortunately, the foregoing studies utilized experimental
designs which did not differentiate between the effect of
insulin on amino acid uptake by the cell and an effect of
insulin at an intracellular site. A subsequent report (15)
indicates that the primary action of insulin (at least in
the muscle cell) is to facilitate the influx of amino acids
into the cell. Similarly, the effect of insulin on glucose
metabolism in mammary organ culture also appears to be
primarily concerned with the influx of glucose across the
cell membrane rather than a direct effect of insulin on
protein synthesis (16,17).
    In contrast to these reports, Cahill (18,19) has shown
that the liver does not require insulin for the diffusion of

glucose across the cell wall. Cuatracasas (20,21) has recently reported that insulin is firmly bound to the liver cell membrane. Since insulin is not required for the diffusion of glucose across the liver cell membrane, the question arises as to the biological significance of this binding. Indeed, the understanding of the mechanism of insulin action on liver metabolism and in particular the effect of insulin on glucose-6-phosphate dehydrogenase (G6PD) and malic enzyme (ME) is uncertain. In starved-refed animals it is thought that the increase in G6PD and ME activities is due to *de novo* RNA synthesis (22-24). The increase in enzyme activities (*i.e.* the "overshoot") has not been shown to be due to insulin (25) but rather to an increased food intake of these animals. Other studies using *ad libitum*-fed rats have indicated that daily supplemental doses of insulin increase the activities of G6PD and ME (26-28). An insulin-glucocorticoid antagonistic effect on G6PD and ME activity in *ad libitum*-fed rats (26) indicates that the control of these two enzymes may rest with both hormones. In view of these findings we decided to reinvestigate the effects of insulin and glucocorticoid on the activity of G6PD (D-glucose 6-phosphate:NADP oxidoreductase; EC 1.1.1.49) and ME (malic decarboxylating oxidoreductase; EC 1.1.1.40). We found that G6PD activity was greatest in the presence of insulin and in the relative absence of glucocorticoid; ME activity appeared to be unaffected by glucocorticoid but affected by insulin.

Materials and Methods

Two studies, each utilizing 80 male Wistar rats[1], weighing 170-200 g, were conducted. In the first study half the animals had 70% of their pancreas removed via a dorsal incision while the remaining animals were subjected to an identical operation without endocrine removal. In the second study, half of the animals were bilaterally adrenalectomized via a dorsal incision and again the remaining animals were subjected to a sham operation. Approximately one week was allowed for the recovery of the animals during which time they were fed Purina Chow. The animals were housed in wire mesh cages in a termperature-humidity controlled room having equal periods of light and dark. After the equilibra-

---

[1]*Purina Laboratory Animals, Vincentown, New Jersey.*

tion period the animals were placed on a 66.5% glucose diet[2]. Food intakes and body weight gains were determined weekly and were found to be unaffected by endocrinectomy. Adrenalectomized animals were given 0.9% NaCl in their drinking water. Half of the controls and half of the endocrinectomized animals of each experiment were given daily (9 am) subcutaneous injections of the appropriate hormone (pancreatectomized animals and their controls received 400 μU/kg/day of protamine zinc insulin; adrenalectomized animals and their controls received 0.3 mg/kg/day of glucocorticoid)[3]. After three weeks the animals were anesthesized with sodium amobarbital (90 mg/kg), the abdominal cavity opened and the liver exised, blotted, chilled and weighed. The carcasses were then examined to determine the extent of pancreatic regeneration or for the completeness of adrenal removal. One gram of liver was homogenized in 9.0 ml cold 0.14 M KCl (pH 7.4), and the crude homogenate was centrifuged at 20,000 x g at 0 to 5° for 30 min. The resultant supernatant fraction was drawn off and used at appropriate dilutions for the determination of G6PD and ME (29).

Results

The effects of partial pancreatectomy and insulin replacement on the activities of G6PD and ME enzyme are presented in Table I. The activities of both enzymes were lower in pancreatectomized animals than in sham operated animals. Insulin replacement in the pancreatectomized animals restored the activities of these enzymes to the levels observed in the sham operated animals. Additional insulin given to the sham operated animals did not produce further increases in the activities of the enzymes in these animals. Starvation had the usual expected lowering effect on the relative liver size, liver weight, and enzyme activity. Curiously, insulin supplementation of the starved pancreatec-

---

[2]*Composition of diet: Glucose, 66.5%; Casein, 18%; Mineral mix, 4%; Vitamin mix, 2.2%; hydrogenated vegetable oil, 5.0%; l-cystine, 0.3%; non-nutritive fiber, 4%.*

[3]*Protamine zinc insulin was purchased from Eli Lilly Co., Indianapolis, Ind; glucocorticoid (corticosterone) was purchased from Calbiochem, Los Angeles, Calif.*

tomized animals and the starved sham operated animals resulted in nearly normal (*i.e.* levels only slightly less than
those of the sham *ad libitum* group) G6PD and ME activity.
This may indicate a role for insulin in either the activation
or *de novo* synthesis of these enzymes. No differences in
the effect of starvation on ME activity were observed between
the sham operated and the pancreatectomized animals.

As in Experiment 1, starvation of both adrenalectomized
and sham operated animals resulted in lower relative liver
sizes, lower liver weights, and decreased G6PD and ME
activities (Table II). Adrenalectomy resulted in slightly
lighter livers in the non-starved animals but did not affect
the liver weights of the starved animals. Adrenalectomy
per se did not affect the activities of G6PD and ME but
supplementation with glucocorticoid of both the sham operated
and adrenalectomized animals served to lower G6PD activity.
The lowering effect of glucocorticoid was not statistically
significant in the adrenalectomized group due to the large
variability in the responses of the animals within the group,
however, the lowered G6PD activity in the sham operated
animals was significant. Glucocorticoid seemed to have no
effect on ME activity except when combined with starvation
in the sham operated animal. The activity of ME was lower
in this group than in either the starved adrenalectomized
animals or the *ad libitum*-fed animals given the glucocorticoid. Starvation plus glucocorticoid also had the greatest
lowering effect on liver weight, relative liver size, and
G6PD activity.

Discussion

The results of these studies indicate that the main-
tenance of G6PD and ME activity is a function of both
insulin and glucocorticoid. That insulin enhances the
activities of these two enzymes is well known (22-28); however, the mechanism by which it exerts its effect is unknown.
Possibly the action of insulin is related to its binding to
the liver cell membrane. The work of Cuatrecasas and Kono
(30,31) demonstrated that insulin is firmly bound to the
exterior of the cell membrane and thus is unlikely to enter
the cell. These observations then suggest that the binding
of insulin to the membrane causes the release or activation

of a secondary messenger which could then serve to increase the activities of the enzymes. Since insulin is known to affect a variety of enzymes this secondary messenger must either affect the initial entry of glucose into the pathways of intermediary metabolism or serve as an activator of these enzymes. Possibly this secondary messenger does both. Bessman (32) has suggested the existence of a secondary substance which is released when the insulin is bound to the receptor site and which binds hexokinase to the mitochondria thus facilitating the entry of glucose into the glycolytic pathway. This view is supported by Borreback and Spydevold (33) who found that the stimulation of hexokinase binding to mitochondria could only be observed in whole cells. This observation is in accord with the many observations that the effects of insulin require relatively intact tissue.

Weber (34) has suggested that the increase in blood levels of insulin leads to a fall in hepatic cyclic AMP level. Although he does not state this, one might assume that this fall is a consequence of the binding of insulin to the cell membrane. The decrease in cyclic AMP level and subsequent inactivation of liver lipase should result in a lowering of free fatty acids. Since free fatty acids are known to inhibit glycolysis, increases in glucose metabolizing enzymes with decreases in free fatty acid levels can be expected. The universality of cyclic AMP and its responsiveness to various hormones makes this explanation quite attractive.

Glucocorticoid also enhances the release of free fatty acids and perhaps the control of G6PD can be explained on this basis. Glucocorticoid appears to affect G6PD activity in the relative absence of insulin. It is thought that glucocorticoid penetrates the cell membrane, is bound to either a cytosolic factor or to the nuclear membrane, and enhances RNA synthesis (35,36). It is possible that glucocorticoid might interfere with the action of the secondary messenger thus accounting for its action with respect to free fatty acid release; however, cyclic AMP does not appear to be involved in any of the changes in metabolism associated with glucocorticoid (36). It is evident that G6PD activity in these studies is maximal under conditions of minimal glucocorticoid release, *i.e.* adrenalectomy and minimal under conditions of maximal glucocorticoid release *i.e.* starvation or starvation plus glucocorticoid administration. This is in conflict with the findings of Freedland (26) who reported that cortisol injected-glucose-fed rats had twice as much

G6PD and ME activity as did non cortisol injected controls. In his experiments, Freedland used hydrocortisone (cortisol) the chief glucocorticoid in man; we used corticosterone the principal glucocorticoid in the rat. In addition Freedland used 16 times as much glucocorticoid as we did and made his observations after 5 days of treatment whereas our experiments were of 21 days duration. It may well be that Freedland's study and ours are not comparable.

Summary

Hepatic NADP-linked G6PD and ME activities were determined in glucose fed and 16 hour starved male Wistar rats. Removal of the adrenals did not affect enzyme activity however glucocorticoid replacement served to lower G6PD but not ME activity. Partial pancreatectomy lowered the activity of both enzymes. Insulin replacement restored the activities to normal. It is suggested that insulin when bound to the cell membrane causes the release of a secondary substance which activates the enzymes. Glucocorticoid may act by interfering with this substance.

Presented by Carolyn D. Berdanier.

References

1. Weber, G. and R. L. Singhal. Insulin:inducer of phosphofructokinase. The integrative action of insulin at the enzyme biosynthetic level. Life Sci. 4: 1993-2002 (1965).
2. Weber, G., R. L. Singhal and S. K. Srivastava. Insulin: suppressor of biosynthesis of hepatic gluconeogenic enzymes. Proc. Natl. Acad. Sci. 53: 96-104 (1965).
3. Weber, G., R. L. Singhal and S. K. Srivastava. Action of glucocorticoid as inducer of insulin as suppressor of biosynthesis of hepatic gluconeogenic enzymes. Advan. Enzyme Regulation 3: 43-75 (1965).
4. Singhal, R. L. and G. M. Ling. Metabolic control mechanisms in mammalian systems. IV Androgenic induction of hexokinase and glucose 6-phosphate dehydrogenase in rat seminal vesicles. Canad. J. Physiol. and Pharm. 47: 233-239 (1969).

5. Wool, I. G., W. S. Stirewalt, K. Kurihara, R. B. Low, P. Baily and D. Oyer. Effect of insulin on the synthesis of sarcoplasmic and ribosomal proteins of muscle.

6. Wool, I. G. and K. Kurihara. Determination of number of active muscle ribosomes: Effect of diabetes and insulin. Proc. Nat. Acad. Sci. 58: 2401-2407 (1967).

7. Mirsky, I. A. Influence of insulin on the protein metabolism of nephrectomized dogs. Am. J. Physiol. 124: 569-575 (1938).

8. Forker, L. L., I. L. Chaikoff, C. Enterman and H. Tarver. Formation of muscle protein with diabetic dogs, studied with S^{35} methionine. J. Biol. Chem. 188: 37-43 (1951).

9. Sinex, F. M., J. Macmullen and A. B. Hastings. Effect of insulin on the incorporation of C^{14} into the protein of rat diaphragm. J. Biol. Chem. 198: 615-620 (1952).

10. Krahl, M. E. Incorporation of C^{14} amino acids into peptides by normal and diabetic rat tissues. Science 116: 524-526 (1952).

11. Krahl, M. E. Incorporation of C^{14} amino acids into glutathione and protein of normal and diabetic rat tissues. J. Biol. Chem. 200: 99-105 (1953).

12. Herrera, M. G. and A. E. Renold. Hormonal effects on glycine metabolism in rat epididymal adipose tissue. Biochim. Biophys. Acta 44: 165-170 (1960).

13. Necheles, T. An *in vitro* effect of insulin and thyroxine on incorporation of amino acids into protein of rabbit bone marrow. Fed. Proc. 20: 67 (1961).

14. Bransome, E. D., Jr. and W. J. Reddy. The effect of insulin on the incorporation *in vitro* of amino acids into rat adrenal protein and nucleic acids. Biochim. Biophys. Acta 76: 641-647 (1963).

15. Goldstein, S. and W. J. Reddy. Insulin and protein synthesis in muscle. Arch. Biochem. Biophys. 140: 181-189 (1970).

16. Martin, R. J. and R. L. Baldwin. Effects of insulin on isolated rat mammary cell metabolism: glucose utilization and metabolic patterns. Endocrinology 89: 1263-1269 (1971).

17. Green, C. D., J. Skarda, J. M. Barry. Regulation of glucose 6-phosphate dehydrogenase formation in mammary organ culture. Biochim. Biophys. Acta 244: 377-387 (1971).

18. Cahil, G. F., Jr., J. Ashmore, A. E. Renold and A. B. Hastings. Blood glucose and the liver. Am. J. Med.

26: 264-282 (1959).

19. Cahill, G. F., Jr., J. Ashmore, A. S. Earle and S. Zotter. Glucose penetration into the liver. Am. J. Physiol. 192: 491-496 (1958).

20. Cuatrecasas, P., B. Desbuquois and F. Krug. Insulin-receptors interaction in liver cell membranes. Biochem. Biophys. Res. Comm. 44: 333-339 (1971).

21. Cuatrecasas, P. Isolation of the insulin receptor of liver and fat cell membranes. Proc. Nat'. Acad. Sci. 69: 318-322 (1972).

22. Tepperman, H. M. and J. Tepperman. Role of hormones in glucose 6-phosphate dehydrogenase adaptation of rat liver. Am. J. Physiol. 202: 401-406 (1962).

23. Szepesi, B. and R. A. Freedland. Differential requirement for *de novo* RNA synthesis in the starved-refed rat; inhibition of the overshoot by 8-azaquinine after refeeding. J. Nutr. 99: 449-458 (1969).

24. Szepesi, B. and C. D. Berdanier. Time course of the starved-refeed response in rats: the possible role of insulin. J. Nutr. 101: 1563-1574 (1971).

25. Rudack, D., E. M. Chrisholm and D. Holten. Rat liver glucose 6-phosphate dehydrogenase. J. Biol. Chem. 246: 1249-1254 (1971).

26. Freedland, R. A., T. L. Cunliffe, J. G. Zinkl. Effect of insulin on enzyme adaptations to diets and hormones. J. Biol. Chem. 22: 5448-5451 (1966).

27. Novello, F., J. A. Gumaa, and P. McLean. The pentose phosphate pathway of glucose metabolism. Biochem. J. 111: 713-725 (1969).

28. Berdanier, C. D., B. Szepesi, S. Diachenko and P. Moser. Effect of tolbutamide and exogenous insulin on the metabolic responses of rats. Proc. Soc. Exp. Biol. Med. 137: 861-867 (1971).

29. Freedland, R. A. Effect of progressive starvation on rat liver enzyme activities. J. Nutr. 91: 489-495 (1967).

30. Cuatrecasas, P. The nature of insulin-receptor interactions. In: I. B. Fritz (Editor), (1972), pp. 137-169.

31. Kono, T. The insulin receptor of fat cells: the relationship between the binding and physiological effects of insulin. In: I. B. Fritz (Editor), Insulin Action, (1972), pp. 171-204.

32. Bessman, S. P. Hexokinase acceptor theory of insulin action. Israel J. Med. Sci. 8: 344-351 (1972).

33. Borrebaek, B. and O. Spydevold. The effects of insulin and glucose on mitochondrial-bound hexokinase activity of rat epididymal adipose tissue. Diabetologia 5: 42-47 (1969).
34. Weber, G. Integrative action of insulin at the molecular level. Israel J. Med. Sci. 8: 325-340 (1972).
35. Kenny, F. T., D. L. Greenman, W. D. Wicks and W. L. Albritton. RNA synthesis and enzyme induction by hydrocortisone. Advances in Enzyme Regulation 3: 1-10 (1965).
36. Lang, N. Steroid hormones and enzyme induction. In: R. M. S. Smellie (Editor), The Biochemistry of Steroid Hormone Action, (1971), pp. 85-100.
37. Weber, G., R. L. Singhal, N. B. Stamm, E. A. Fisher and M. A. Mentendiek. Regulation of enzymes involved in gluconeogenesis. Advances in Enzyme Regulation 2: 1-38 (1964).

TABLE I

EFFECT OF PANCREATECTOMY AND INSULIN ON THE ACTIVITIES OF
GLUCOSE 6 PHOSPHATE DEHYDROGENASE AND MALIC ENZYME

Treatment	Relative liver size[a]	Liver Weight	Enzyme[b]	
			G6PD	ME
		g	*units/100 g body weight*	
Pancreax, *ad libitum*	4.37±.18[c]	13.4±.4	31.2±1.5	23.6±2.2
Pancreax, 16 h starved	3.54±.26	10.2±.7	15.7±1.3	15.8±1.8
Pancreax, *ad libitum*, + insulin	3.88±.11	13.1±.4	48.9±2.9	27.2±2.4
Pancreax, 16 h starved, + insulin	3.21±.12	10.1±.5	41.3±2.8	25.5±1.3
Sham, *ad libitum*	3.96±.06	12.8±.3	52.1±6.0	31.1±1.3
Sham, 16 h starved	3.07±.06	9.3±.3	29.0±2.2	19.6±2.3
Sham, *ad libitum*, + insulin	4.05±.09	13.4±.7	47.2±3.2	30.6±3.0
Sham, 16 h starved, + insulin	3.15±.03	9.3±.2	36.2±3.5	22.1±2.1

[a]*Relative liver size = liver weight/body weight X 100.*

[b]*Abbreviations used: G6PD - glucose 6 phosphate dehydrogenase; ME - malic enzyme. One unit of enzyme activity equals the amount of enzyme which can produce 1 μmole of measured product per minute under the conditions of the assay.*

[c]*Standard error of the mean for 10 rats.*

TABLE II

EFFECT OF ADRENALECTOMY AND GLUCOCORTICOID ON THE ACTIVITIES OF
GLUCOSE 6 PHOSPHATE DEHYDROGENASE AND MALIC ENZYME

Treatment	Relative Liver Size[a]	Liver Weight	Enzyme[b]	
			G6PD	ME
		g	units/100 g body weight	
Adrenx, *ad libitum*	4.00±.13[c]	12.6±.8	45.4±5.9	22.3±2.7
Adrenx, 16 h starved	3.14±.06	9.1±.5	27.2±3.1	16.8±1.9
Adrenx, *ad libitum*, + GC[d]	3.88±.09	12.2±.6	35.7±5.5	24.1±2.9
Adrenx, 16 h starved, + GC	3.00±.15	9.0±.6	20.9±3.4	16.1±2.4
Sham, *ad libitum*	4.19±.07	14.4±.3	43.5±5.8	26.1±2.4
Sham, 16 h starved	3.24±.06	10.5±.3	28.7±2.0	18.7±1.1
Sham, *ad libitum*, + GC	4.66±.12	15.1±.6	30.9±1.2	22.5±1.3
Sham, 16 h starved, + GC	3.09±.14	8.7±1.1	9.23±1.40	11.2±3.4

[a]*Relative liver size = liver weight/body weight X 100.*

[b]*Abbreviations used: G6PD - glucose 6 phosphate dehydrogenase; ME - malic enzyme. One unit of enzyme activity equals the amount of enzyme which can produce 1 μmole of product per minute under the conditions of the assay.*

[c]*Standard error of the mean for 10 rats.*

[d]*GC - glucocorticoid.*

INSULIN AND THE MAMMARY EPITHELIAL CELL MEMBRANE

Yale J. Topper and Takami Oka

Insulin has been covalently linked to sepharose beads by Cuatrecasas (1), and some of these preparative methods were described by Dr. Katzen in Chapter 9. The resulting complexes have been shown to possess many of the biological properties of the free, soluble hormone (1-4). Several lines of evidence, including the use of I^{125}-insulin-sepharose by Katzen, indicate that this particulate form of insulin produces these effects without the release of free hormone from the complex. Perhaps the most compelling evidence against such release is the observation that insulin-sepharose, but not free insulin, increases the rate of accumulation of α-aminoisobutyric acid (AIB) by mammary epithelial cells from virgin mice (4). It has been concluded that insulin can effect intracellular processes by impinging on the cell membrane.

Several studies (5-7) have shown that insulin binds tightly to certain target cells. In the case of fat cells the dissociation constant is about 5.0×10^{-11} M (5). This tight binding has, in fact, been used as a marker in the isolation of insulin-receptors from appropriate cell membranes (8,9). The elegant work described by Dr. Katzen in Chapter 9 is another case in point. It has been surmised that tight binding to the receptors is involved in the manifestation of the biological effects of the hormone. Results of the present studies with insulin-sepharose question the dependency of these biological effects upon tight binding.

Mammary epithelial cells from pregnant mice have been shown to respond to insulin in several ways, including an enhanced rate of accumulation of AIB (10). Insulin-sepharose also increases this rate (4). The results presented in Fig. 1 demonstrate that 1) sepharose does not alter the rate of AIB accumulation; 2) insulin and insulin-sepharose increase the rate to about the same extent; and 3) the effect is no greater in the presence of both forms of the hormone than in the presence of each alone. It appears, therefore, that insulin and insulin-sepharose produce this augmentation by the same mechanism.

While free insulin obviously cannot be visualized in the light microscope, insulin-sepharose beads can be so seen. This provides an opportunity to determine whether the mammary cells and the particulate-bound hormone bind to each other when the effect on AIB accumulation is manifesting itself. Figures 2A and 2B illustrate the virtual lack of visible binding between the cells and either sepharose or insulin-sepharose. The pattern was the same immediately after the mixed suspensions were made, and after shaking for periods of 15, 30, and 45 minutes. Also, increasing the concentration if insulin-sepharose by a factor of three did not alter the appearance of the suspension. Moreover, almost no binding was visible even when shearing of the sample was reduced by setting two cover slips on each side of the slide such that the cover slip over the sample was bridged.

The present results indicate that mammary epithelial cells and insulin-sepharose effectively interact without binding tightly to each other. This is not to say that contact between them is unnecessary. But *transient* contact resulting from collisions that occur during shaking is sufficient for elicitation of the biological effect.

Tight binding of other protein hormones to their target cells occurs. Moreover, microscopic examination has revealed that fat cells bind to insulin-sepharose beads [*see* Chapter 9; *also* (8)].

It remains to be proved, however, whether the tight binding that occurs in these instances is necessary for expression of the observed biological effects. Transient contact may suffice in these cases, too.

Presented by Yale J. Topper

References

1. Cuatrecasas, P. Interaction of insulin with the cell membrane: The primary action of insulin. Proc. Nat. Acad. Sci. USA 63: 450-457 (1969).
2. Turkington, R. W. Stimulation of RNA synthesis in isolated mammary cells by insulin and prolactin bound to sepharose. Biochem. Biophys. Res. Communs. 41: 1362-1367 (1970).
3. Blatt, L. M. and K. H. Kim. Regulation of hepatic glycogen synthetase: Stimulation of glycogen synthetase in an *in vitro* liver system by insulin bound to sepharose. J. Biol. Chem. 246: 4895-4898 (1971).
4. Oka, T. and Y. J. Topper. Insulin-sepharose and the dynamics of insulin action. Proc. Nat. Acad. Sci. USA 68: 2066-2068 (1971).
5. Cuatrecasas, P. Insulin-receptor interactions in adipose tissue cells: Direct measurement and properties. Proc. Nat. Acad. Sci. USA 68: 1264-1268 (1971).
6. Freychet, P., J. Roth and D. M. Neville, Jr. Monoiodo-insulin: Demonstration of its biological activity and binding to fat cells and liver membranes. Biochem. Biophys. Res. Communs. 43: 400-408 (1971).
7. Kono, T. and F. W. Barham. The relationship between the insulin-binding capacity of fat cells and the cellular response to insulin. J. Biol. Chem. 246: 6210-6216 (1971).
8. Cuatrecasas, P. Properties of the insulin receptor isolated from liver and fat cell membranes. J. Biol. Chem. 247: 1980-1991 (1972).
9. Soderman, D. D., J. Germershausen and H. M. Katzen. Specific binding of insulin-sepharose to isolated fat cells and affinity chromatography of receptor-containing membranes. Federation Proc. 31: 486 Abs. (1972).
10. Friedberg, S. H., T. Oka and Y. J. Topper. Development of insulin-sensitivity by mouse mammary gland *in vitro*. Proc. Nat. Acad. Sci. USA 67: 1493-1500 (1970).
11. Bray, G. A. A simple efficient liquid scintillator for counting aqueous solutions in a liquid scintillation counter. Anal. Biochem. 1: 279 (1960).

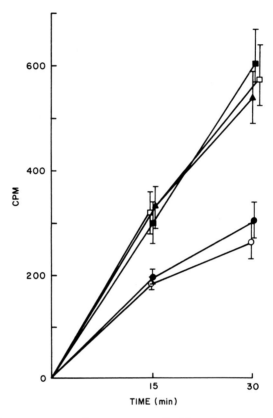

Fig. 1: *Time course of AIB accumulation by mammary epithel-ial cells.* Abdominal mammary glands from 6 midterm C3H/HeN mice in their first pregnancy were pooled and treated with collagenase as described previously (4). The resulting epithelial cells were equally divided into Erlenmeyer flasks containing 3.5 ml of Medium 199 (Microbiological Associates, Inc., Bethesda, Md.), 2.5% bovine serum albumin (CalBiochem, San Diego, Calif.), and non-isotopic α-aminoisobutyric acid (7.5 μg/ml). Each flask was shaken (90 cycles/min) for 45 min. at 37^0. Then 30 μCi of [^{3}H]α-aminoisobutyric acid (817 mC/mM, ICN Chemical and Radioisotope Division, Irvine, Calif.) and one of the substances listed below were added. Shaking was continued and five 300 μl samples containing approximately 4.2×10^4 cells were collected from each flask at 15 min and 30 min after the addition of the isotope and the appropriate agent. Radioactivity of the samples was

344

determined as follows: the cells were collected on a Millipore filter, washed with Medium 199 and 0.15 M NaCl, and
placed in a vial containing 300 μl of distilled water. After
soaking overnight, 10 ml of Bray's (11) scintillation fluid
was added to each vial and the samples were counted in a
liquid scintillation counter. The experimental systems
used in this study were as follows: a) cells only 0; b)
cells plus sepharose-4B (Pharmacia) (●); c) cells plus
soluble pork insuli plus sepharose-4B (Δ); d) cells plus
pork insulin-sepharose-4B complex (□); e) cells plus soluble
pork insulin plus pork insulin-sepharose-4B complex (■).
The concentration of the soluble and particulate hormone
in each case was 10μg per ml. Soluble pork insulin was a
gift from Eli Lilly Co. and insulin-sepharose was kindly
provided by Dr. P. Cuatrecasas at John Hopkins University
(Baltimore, Md.). Each point is the mean ± SEM of 5 determinations.

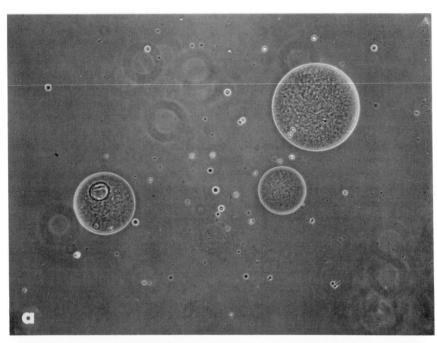

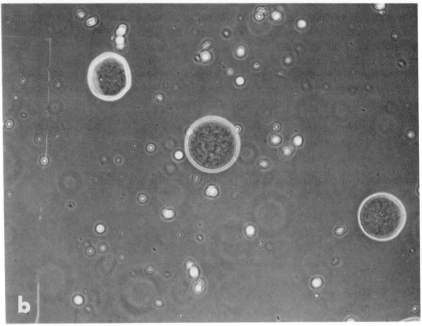

346

Fig. 2: *Microscopic appearance of mixtures of cells and sepharose or insulin-sepharose beads.* The experimental procedure was similar to that described in the legend to Fig. 1. In a typical experiment the concentration of sepharose or insulin-sepharose beads was about 2.2×10^4 per ml, and the concentration of cells was about 1.4×10^5 per ml. At a given moment less than 1% of the cells were in contact with the insulin-sepharose beads. Essentially identical results were obtained when sepharose beads were used. In each instance about 1200 cells were examined. Photographs were taken under the phase microscope (X 160). A) Mixture of mammary epithelial cells and sepharose-4B beads; B) mixture of cells and insulin-sepharose-4B beads. Note that the beads are much larger than the cells.

GLUCAGON RECEPTOR

Stephen L. Pohl

Introduction

Regulation of metabolism by a hormone is usually studied by monitoring changes in the composition of biological fluids or in the function of some organ system. It has long been recognized that these phenomena represent secondary effects of hormones, and this recognition has led to investigations of the earliest, or primary, actions of hormones on cellular function. The discovery by Sutherland and Rall that some hormones act by stimulating adenylate cyclase and that the resulting increased intracellular concentrations of cyclic 3',5'-adenosine monophosphate (cyclic AMP) mediate the subsequent effects of the hormone has been a major advance toward the goal of elucidating the primary actions of these hormones. The subsequent demonstration that hormone sensitive adenylate cyclase systems are located in plasma membranes of target cells has moved investigations of hormone action to the molecular level and linked these investigations to more general problems of membrane structure and function. Although somewhat ambiguous, the term "receptor" is usually used to designate all of the plasma membrane components which are involved in the actions of a peptide hormone, and each hormone probably has its own receptor.

During the past four years, studies with purified hormones and plasma membranes have provided considerable information regarding the nature of adenylate cyclase systems. One such preparation, the glucagon sensitive adenylate cyclase in plasma membranes from rat liver parenchymal cells, has proved particularly fruitful. This system has been described in great detail (1-10) and has recently been reviewed elsewhere (11,12). The purpose of this paper will be to summarize the important features of the liver membrane system, to raise certain questions about current methods of approaching the problem of hormone-receptor interaction, and to introduce alternative ways of investigating hormone sensitive systems.

Results and Discussion

Organization of Hormone Sensitive Adenylate Cyclase Systems

As illustrated in Fig. 1, adenylate cyclase systems in mammalian cells are thought to be located in plasma membranes of target cells for specific hormones. A catalytic site which converts ATP to cyclic AMP is located on or near the intracellular surface of the membrane. A divalent cation is required for activity. A regulatory subunit is located on or near the extracellular surface. This distinct molecular entity interacts specifically with hormone molecules circulating in the extracellular fluid, and, as a consequence of this interaction, the activity of the catalytic site is increased.

The Liver Plasma Membrane Adenylate Cyclase System

Plasma membranes can be isolated from rat liver by a combination of differential and density gradient centrifugation (13). The membranes are free from significant contamination by other organelles and have been characterized extensively regarding composition and enzyme content (14). They can be obtained in gram quantitites and are stable indefinitely in liquid nitrogen (2). For these reasons, liver plasma membranes provide an ideal biological material for studies of hormone receptors.
The catalytic site of the liver plasma membrane has been studied by measuring adenylate cyclase activity according to the method of Krishna *et al*. (15). The enzyme is firmly bound to the membrane and requires magnesium for activity. The activity of the enzyme is increased specifically by glucagon (2) with a dose-response relationship which is very similar to that for glucagon on cyclic AMP levels in the isolated perfused rat liver (16). Fluoride ion stimulates the same enzyme but through a mechanism which is distinctly different from that of glucagon (3).
An attempt has been made to observe the initial interaction between glucagon and the receptor system by labeling the hormone with ^{125}I and measuring binding to the membranes (4). The binding is specific for glucagon, and the concen-

tration dependence of binding is identical to that of glucagon stimulated adenylate cyclase activity. Both binding
and glucagon stimulated adenylate cyclase activity are
markedly reduced by treating the membranes with trypsin,
detergents, phospholipase or urea. All of these findings
suggest that the observed binding is the initial step in
the activation of adenylate cyclase by glucagon. The extent and reversibility of binding is profoundly influenced
by the presence or absence of nucleotides, particularly GTP,
in the assay medium (5).

A third property of the liver plasma membrane is the
ability to alter the glucagon molecule so that it no longer
binds to membranes or activates adenylate cyclase (9). This
inactivation process is rapid and specific for glucagon and
is also susceptible to the destructive effects of trypsin,
phospholipase A, detergents, and urea. The inactivation
site is clearly distinct from the binding site since active
glucagon can be extracted from the membranes with urea (4).
A definite relationship between inactivation of glucagon
and stimulation of adenylate cyclase has not been established
nor has the product of glucagon inactivation been identified.

This brief review of the adenylate cyclase system in
liver membranes illustrates the fact that most of the information obtained to date is descriptive and that very little
has been learned about the actual mechanism of hormone action. The direct approach to this more difficult problem
is to solublize the hormone receptor, separate it from all
other membrane constituents, and study it by conventional
enzymological methods.

*The Solubilization Approach to Study of Hormone
Receptors*

In order to undertake solubilization experiments, it
is necessary to stipulate what is to be solubilized and
what is to be assayed. In the present case it is clear
that solubilization of material with hormone sensitive
adenylate cyclase activity would be an ideal goal. This
problem has been approached using a variety of methods, but
unfortunately with little success. The techniques devised
by Levey (17,18,19) have been successful for solubilizing
the adenylate cyclase of heart muscle, but these methods
have not been applied successfully to other tissues. Also,
the physical state of the heart preparation following
restoration of hormone sensitivity has

351

not been established. Thus, a method for obtaining soluble, hormone sensitive adenylate cyclase from a variety of tissues is not yet at hand.

Since solubilization of hormone sensitive adenylate cyclase poses such severe obstacles, an attractive alternative would appear to be solubilization of specific, saturable hormone binding proteins from membranes. This approach has the theoretical advantage that the integrity of the catalytic site of adenylate cyclase need not be preserved. Initial reports of successful solubilization of hormone binding substances appear in this volume and elsewhere (20). However, this approach requires the assumption that the observed binding sites are, in fact, the structures involved in the first step of the chain of events which leads to hormone action, and this point has not yet been proven.

In the case of the glucagon sensitive liver membrane system, all correlations between glucagon binding and activation of adenylate cylcase appear perfect until one compares the kinetics of the two processes. Under all conditions so far examined, the binding of glucagon is a relatively slow process. Approximately 30% of the total binding occurs in the first minute of incubation, but then binding continues at a progressively slower rate until a maximum is achieved at 10 to 20 minutes (4). The degree of maximal binding depends at least in part on simultaneous inactivation of the hormone by the membranes (9). Glucagon stimulated adenylate cyclase activity, on the other hand, is linear with time during the first 10 minutes of incubation and there is no detectable lag in the onset of the glucagon effect (2). Thus, during the first 10 minutes of incubation, glucagon binds to liver membranes at a variable rate but adenylate cyclase activity does not change.

Although these kinetic observations make the significance of glucagon binding somewhat questionable, a variety of models can be proposed to explain the data. Recently, however, an independent series of experiments, performed principally by Birnbaumer, casts additional doubt on the significance of hormone binding. Both by experiments involving alteration of the glucagon concentration in an adenylate cyclase assay and by use of a competitive inhibitor of glucagon, des-His-glucagon (*see* below), it was established that activation of adenylate cyclase by glucagon is a rapidly reversible process (8). Glucagon stimulates adenylate cyclase fully within seconds, and des-His-glucagon

reduces glucagon stimulated activity to the unstimulated
level within 30 seconds. Given this rapid reversibility by
a competitive inhibitor, des-His-glucagon must displace
glucagon from all glucagon binding sites which are involved
in adenylate cyclase activation. However, in an experiment
in which identical tubes were used for measurement of binding and of adenylate cyclase, des-His-glucagon completely
reversed the stimulation of adenylate cyclase by glucagon
but displaced only about 15% of the glucagon bound to the
membranes (21). Thus, glucagon bound to the membranes
failed to stimulate adenylate cyclase under conditions in
which glucagon in the medium could stimulate the enzyme.

Because of the specificity and membrane location of
peptide hormone binding sites, it seems almost certain that
this observed binding is biologically significant. However,
the role of binding need not be directly involved in hormone
action. For example, the membrane binding sites may serve
to concentrate peptide hormones in the region of a separate
true receptor in the membrane. As studies of hormone binding progress, it will be necessary to view the results crit-
ically until the significance of binding is understood.

An Alternative Approach to the Receptor Problem

Until suitable methods become available for solubilization of hormone receptors, an attempt to obtain mechanistic
information can be made using intact membranes. In order
to devise appropriate experiments, it is useful to formulate
a minimal set of questions which must be answered in order
to understand the mechanism of action of a polypeptide hormone on the adenylate cyclase receptor system. These are:
1) What is the primary and three dimensional structure of
the hormone in the extracellular fluid? 2) What is the
structure of the receptor? 3) What are the forces of interaction between hormone and receptor? 4) What structural
changes occur in both hormone and receptor as a consequence
of their interaction, and how do these structural changes
lead to an alteration of adenylate cyclase activity?

The Structure of Glucagon

Glucagon is a relatively simple polypeptide hormone
consisting of a single chain of 29 amino acids. The
sequence is identical for bovine, porcine and human glucagons
(22,23). All naturally occurring L-amino acids are present

353

except cysteine, cystine, proline, and isoleucine. Both termini are free, and no unusual amino acids are present.

The amount of primary structure of glucagon required for biological activity has been investigated in several ways. Spiegel and Bitensky have shown that glucagon treated with cyanogen bromide is biologically active (24). Cyanogen bromide cleaves two amino acid residues from the carboxy terminus of the peptide and converts the third amino acid, methionine, to homoserine. However, synthetic [1–23]-glucagon is biologically inactive (24). Therefore, at least two and no more than six amino acids can be removed from the carboxy terminal portion of the peptide without loss of biological activity. Removal of the amino terminal amino acid, histidine, from glucagon has been accomplished in a number of laboratories by one step Edman degradation. The resulting peptide, des–His–glucagon, is biologically inactive (25,27). In addition, Rodbell *et al.* have presented evidence that des–His–glucagon is a competitive inhibitor of glucagon stimulated adenylate cyclase (10). However, Lande *et al.* (27) have called attention to the fact that the presence of the N-phenylisothiocarbamyl derivative of the single lysine residue in glucagon was not rigorously excluded in the studies of Rodbell *et al.* Thus, the amino terminal histidine of glucagon is required for biological activity of the peptide but may not be required for binding of the hormone to its receptor. It should be noted that the conclusions described above regarding the reversibility of adenylate cyclase activation by glucagon remain valid even if the des–His–glucagon preparations used to establish this point had altered lysine residues.

Higher structure of glucagon has been studied by a variety of techniques including UV absorption and fluorescence spectroscopy, circular dichroism, nuclear magnetic resonance, sedimentation equilibrium and x-ray crystallography (28). At concentrations of the order of 10^{-4}M, glucagon probably exists in a compact globular structure. Unfortunately, the concentrations of glucagon required for these physical techniques are five to seven orders of magnitude higher than the concentrations of the hormone *in vivo*. Consequently, the information obtained in these studies may have little bearing on the mechanisms of action of glucagon on its receptor.

Structure of the Glucagon Receptor

Very little is known of the structure of the glucagon receptor in the liver plasma membrane. Sensitivity to both lipolytic and proteolytic enzymes indicates that it probably is a lipoprotein, but carbohydrate and metal ion content have not yet been established.

Although it seems unlikely that the receptor structure can be determined without isolation and purification, it may be possible to obtain some structural information with intact membranes. If the forces of interaction between hormone and receptor can be established (*see* below), the existence of classes of structure at specific locations in the receptor can be inferred; for example, a negatively charged group to complement a positively charged group on the hormone or an acceptor for a hydrogen bond formed by a hydroxyl group on the hormone may be present. In addition, the use of specific probes such as phospholipase A (*see* below) can be expected to give structural information about the receptor.

The Forces of Interaction Between Hormone and Receptor

Since both glucagon and the glucagon receptor represent distinct chemical entities, it must be possible ultimately to describe their interaction in terms of a set of chemical forces. These include formation of covalent, electrostatic, and hydrogen bonds and hydrophobic interactions. Furthermore, because of the size of the glucagon molecule and the great specificity of the system for glucagon, it is reasonable to postulate that these forces of interaction are multiple in both number and kind. Formation of a covalent bond between glucagon and its receptor can be safely excluded because of the rapid reversibility of glucagon stimulated adenylate cyclase by des-His-glucagon (*see* above) and the susceptibility of the system to relatively low concentrations of urea (2,4).

The amino acid sequence of glucagon can be divided roughly into three parts (10). The segment of the peptide representing the first one-third from the amino terminus contains mainly polar but uncharged amino acids including two serine, two threonine, one histidine, and one glutamine. The middle one-third of the sequence contains a large number of residues which are charged at neutral pH including three aspartic acids, two arginines, and one lysine. The third of the sequence at the carboxy terminus is intensely hydrophobic, containing phenylalanine, valine, tryptophan,

leucine and methionine. Thus, it is clear that the potential
exists for formation of many different bonds between glucagon and its receptor. Sorting out these possibilities
would be nearly unapproachable were it not for the simila-
rity between glucagon and another peptide hormone, secretin
(29). Both glucagon and secretin activate adenylate cyclase
in the adipocyte plasma membrane but do so through different
receptors (30). Proof of the existence of different receptors is based on the demonstration that des-His-glucagon is
a competitive inhibitor of glucagon- but not secretin-stimu-
lated adenylate cyclase in the fat cell membrane (31), and,
conversely, des-His-secretin is a competitive inhibitor of
secretin- but not glucagon-stimulated adenylate cyclase (32).
Secretin does not stimulate adenylate cyclase in liver plasma
membranes (2).

Secretin is also a single chain polypeptide but has
27 instead of 29 amino acids (29). Fourteen of these residues in sequence are identical to the corresponding amino
acids in glucagon. In addition, six amino acid pairs in
the two peptides are very similar; for example, aspartic
acid in glucagon and glutamic acid in secretin at position
nine and valine in glucagon and leucine in secretin at
position 23 (11,12). Thus, there are only seven major differences in the sequences of the two peptides. These are at
positions 3, 10, 13, 14, 17, 21, and 25, mainly in the central portion of the peptides. Two of the differences, at
positions 10 and 13, involve tyrosine in glucagon and leucine in secretin, and four of the differences involve changes
in net charge. Thus, there is ample reason for suspecting
that both hydrogen bonds and electrostatic forces are involved in the interactions between these peptide hormones
and their receptors and that these interactions determine
the specificity. However, there is as yet no direct experimental support for this contention.

An attractive hypothesis which has been approached
experimentally is that the carboxy end of the glucagon peptide is involved in a hydrophobic interaction with a site
on the plasma membrane. Several kinds of evidence support
this hypothesis. First, this region of the glucagon peptide
binds detergents and phospholipids (33). Second, the membranes can be modified with detergents or lipases in such
a way that adenylate cyclase remains intact as judged by its
ability to respond to stimulation by fluoride ion but is
unresponsive to glucagon stimulation (3). Third, part of
this loss of glucagon sensitivity can be restored by incuba-

ting the treated membranes in dispersions of phospholipids (7,34).

These studies with phospholipase A have recently been extended to provide more information about the glucagon-receptor interaction. The effects of a highly purified phospholipase A obtained from *Crotalus adamanteus* (35) on adenylate cyclase are illustrated in Fig. 2. In this experiment, the lower glucagon concentration gives half-maximal stimulation and the higher concentration gives maximal stimulation of the enzyme. Relatively high concentrations of the phospholipase nearly abolish all adenylate cyclase activity. Lower concentrations, however, do not affect the basal or NaF stimulated activities but render the adenylate cyclase unresponsive to glucagon. At even lower concentrations of the lipase, the activity given by 10^{-6} M glucagon is reduced, but 4×10^{-9} M glucagon no longer gives any stimulation of the enzyme. This last effect was explored further by digesting the membranes with phospholipase A at 1 µg/ml for a shorter time. After this treatment, the apparent affinity of adenylate cyclase for glucagon is reduced with only a small decrease in the maximal glucagon stimulated activity (Fig. 3). Finally, under certain conditions, the effects of phospholipase A can be partially prevented by pretreatment of the membranes with glucagon (Table I). Taken together, these observations indicate that there is a direct hydrophobic interaction between glucagon and membrane phospholipids, that this interaction provides part of the force for but not the specificity of the binding, and that it is not required for action of the hormone on the receptor.

Structural Changes Consequent to Interaction Between Hormone and Receptor

It is evident that changes in structure must occur in glucagon, the receptor, or both, consequent to their interaction in order for a signal to be generated. The possibilities include formation or breakage of covalent bonds and conformational changes. There appears to be a covalent change in the glucagon molecule consequent to interaction with plasma membranes resulting in inactivation of the hormone (9), but the relationship of this process to the receptor has not been established. Evidence for a conformational change in glucagon upon binding of the peptide to detergents and phospholipids has been presented (33), but this system is not necessarily a valid model for events occurring at the receptor. There is as yet no information regarding any structural changes occurring in the receptor upon interaction with glucagon.

Coupling of the Hormone Receptor Interaction to Adenylate Cyclase Activation

The most provocative but least well understood aspect of the glucagon receptor problem is the mechanism by which the structural changes consequent to the interaction of glucagon with the receptor leads to an increase in the activity of adenylate cyclase. Attractive possibilities include phosphorylation of some site on the membrane, by analogy to the Na, K-dependent ATPase in plasma membranes, or a conformational change such as those occurring in enzymes with allosteric regulatory sites. In additon, lipids may be involved in this coupling process since the system as a whole operates to transmit information across a lipid barrier. Unfortunately, there is no experimental evidence bearing directly upon these possibilities. It has been shown recently that nucleoside di- or tri-phosphates are required for coupling of the glucagon-receptor interaction to adenylate cyclase activation (6,8).

The observation that des-His-glucagon is a competitive inhibitor of glucagon, if substantiated, may provide powerful tools for studying the nature of the coupling process. Models have been developed in other systems for the participation of histidine in active sites. Since a histidine interacts with a nearby serine to produce a uniquely reactive hydroxyl group in chymotrypsin and other endopeptidases [for review see (36)], it may be possible to identify such uniquely reactive groups specific for glucagon in the plasma membrane. In hemoglobin, histidines form complexes with heme iron [for review see (36)]; it may also be possible to identify membrane bound cations with which the glucagon histidine interacts causing changes in reactivity.

Summary

The glucagon sensitive adenylate cyclase system in plasma membranes from rat liver parenchymal cells is an attractive and highly advanced model for the primary interactions of polypeptide hormones with their receptors. However, it should be clear that nearly all of the information regarding this system obtained so far is descriptive and that the direction of further research on this problem must turn to actual mechanisms. Solubilization, while the most obvious and perhaps the only approach which can lead to a complete understanding of the system, is presently beset by several theoretical and practical difficulties. The purpose of this paper has been to point out that some meaningful mechanistic information can be obtained using intact membranes. It is even possible that these studies may lead to an intimate understanding of primary action of a peptide hormone on its target cell.

Presented by Stephen L. Pohl

References

1. Pohl, S. L., L. Birnbaumer and M. Rodbell. Glucagon-sensitive adenyl cyclase in plasma membrane of hepatic parenchymal cells. Science 164: 566 (1969).
2. Pohl, S. L., L. Birnbaumer and M. Rodbell. The glucagon-sensitive adenyl cyclase system in plasma membranes of rat liver. I. Properties. J. Biol. Chem. 246: 1849 (1971).
3. Birnbaumer, L., S. L. Pohl and M. Rodbell. The glucagon-sensitive adenyl cyclase system in plasma membranes of rat liver II. Comparison between glucagon- and fluoride-stimulated activities. J. Biol. Chem. 246: 1857 (1971).
4. Rodbell, M., H. M. J. Krans, S. L. Pohl and L. Birnbaumer. The glucagon-sensitive adenyl cyclase system in plasma membranes of rat liver III. Binding of glucagon. Method of assay and specificity. J. Biol. Chem.246: 1861 (1971).
5. Rodbell, M., H. M. J. Krans, S. L. Pohl and L. Birnbaumer. The glucagon-sensitive adenyl cyclase system in plasma membranes of rat liver. IV. Effects of guanyl nucleotides on binding of ^{125}I-glucagon. J. Biol. Chem. 246: 1872 (1971).
6. Rodbell, M., L. Birnbaumer, S. L. Pohl and H. M. J. Krans. The glucagon-sensitive adenyl cyclase system in plasma membranes of rat liver. V. An obligatory role of guanyl nucleotides in glucagon action. J. Biol. Chem. 246: 1877 (1971).

7. Pohl, S. L., H. M. J. Krans, V. Kozyreff, L. Birnbaumer and M. Rodbell. The glucagon-sensitive adenyl cyclase system in plasma membranes of rat liver VI. Evidence for a role of membrane lipids. J. Biol. Chem. 246: 4447 (1971).

8. Birnbaumer, L., S. L. Pohl, M. Rodbell and F. Sundby. The glucagon-sensitive adenylate cyclase system in plasma membranes of rat liver VII. Hormonal stimulation: reversibility and dependence on concentration of free hormone. J. Biol. Chem 247: 2038 (1972).

9. Pohl. S. L., H. M. J. Krans, L. Birnbaumer and M. Rodbell. Inactivation of glucagon by plasma membranes of rat liver. J. Biol. Chem. 247: 2295 (1972).

10. Rodbell, M., L. Birnbaumer, S. L. Pohl and F. Sundby. The reaction of glucagon with its receptor: evidence for discrete regions of activity and binding in the glucagon molecule. Proc. Nat. Acad. Sci. USA 68: 909 (1971).

11. Pohl, S. L., L. Birnbaumer and M. Rodbell. Glucagon-sensitive adenyl cyclase: a model for receptors in plasma membranes. In: C. K. Cain (Editor), Annual Reports in Medicinal Chemistry, 1970. Academic Press, New York (1971), p. 233.

12. Rodbell, M., L. Birnbaumer, S. L. Pohl and H. M. J. Krans. Regulation of glucagon action at its receptor. In: M. Margoulies and F. C. Greenwood (Editors), Structure-Activity Relationships of Protein and Polypeptide Hormones. Excerpta Medica, Amsterdam (1971), p. 199.

13. Neville, D. M., Jr. Isolation of an organ specific protein antigen from cell-surface membrane of rat liver. Biochim. Biophys. Acta 154: 540 (1968).

14. Emmelot, P., C. J. Bos, E. L. Benedetti and P. H. Rumke. Studies on plasma membranes I. Chemical composition and enzyme content of plasma membranes isolated from rat liver. Biochim. Biophys. Acta 90: 126 (1964).

15. Krishna, G., B. Weiss, B. B. Brodie. A simple, sensitive method for the assay of adenyl cyclase. J. Pharm. Exp. Ther. 163: 379 (1968).

16. Exton, J. H., G. A. Robison, E. W. Sutherland and C. R. Park. Studies on the role of adenosine 3',5'-monophosphate in the hepatic actions of glucagon and catecholamines. J. Biol. Chem. 246: 6166 (1971).

17. Levey, G. S., Solubilization of myocardial adenyl cyclase. Biochem. Biophys. Res. Commun. 38: 86 (1970).

18. Levey, G. S. Restoration of glucagon responsiveness of solubilized myocardial adenyl cyclase by phosphatidyl-serine. Biochem. Biophys. Res. Commun. 43: 108 (1971).
19. Levey, G. S. Restoration of norepinephrine responsiveness of solubilized myocardial adenylate cyclase by phosphatidylinositol. J. Biol. Chem. 246: 7405 (1971).
20. Cuatrecasas, P. Isolation of the insulin receptor of liver and fat-cell membranes. Proc. Nat. Acad. Sci. USA 69: 318 (1972).
21. Birnbaumer, L. Personal communication.
22. Bromer, W. W., M. E. Boucher and J. E. Koffenberger Jr. Amino acid sequence of bovine glucagon. J. Biol. Chem. 246: 2822 (1971).
23. Thomsen, J., K. Kristiansen and K. Brunfeldt. The amino acid sequence of human glucagon. FEBS Letters 21: 315 (1972).
24. Spiegel, A. M. and M. W. Bitensky. Effects of chemical and enzymatic modification of glucagon on its activation of hepatic adenyl cyclase. Endocrinology 85: 638 (1969).
25. Sundby, F. Des-histidine glucagon: preparation and chemical, biological and immunological properties. In: R. R. Rodrigues, F. J. G. Ebling, I. Henderson and R. Assan (Editors), Abstracts, VII Congress of the International Diabetes Federation. Excerpta Medica, Amsterdam (1970), ICA No. 209, p. 80.
26. Felts, P. W., M. E. C. Ferguson, K. A. Hagey, E. S. Stitt and W. M. Mitchell. Studies on the structure-function relationship of glucagon. Diabetologia 6: 44 (1970).
27. Lande, S., R. Gorman and M. Bitensky. Selectively blocked and des-histidine-glucagons: Preparation and effects on hepatic adenylate cyclase activity. Endocrinology 90. 597 (1972).
28. Epand, R. M. Conformational properties of cyanogen bromide-cleaved glucagon. J. Biol. Chem. 247: 2132 (1972).
29. Mutt, V. and J. E. Jorpes. Contemporary developments in the biochemistry of the gastrointestinal hormones. Recent. Progr. Hormones Res. 17: 539 (1967).
30. Rodbell, M., L. Birnbaumer and S. L. Pohl. Adenyl cyclase in fat cells III. Stimulation by secretin and the effects of trypsin on the receptors for lipolytic hormones. J. Biol. Chem. 245: 718 (1970).
31. Pohl, S. L. and M. Rodbell. Unpublished observations.
32. Rodbell, M. Personal communication.
33. Bornet, H. and H. Edelhoch. Polypeptide hormone inter-

action I. Glucagon detergent interaction. J. Biol. Chem. 246: 1785 (1971).

34. Rethy, A., V. Thomasi and A. Trevisani. The role of lipids in the activity of adenylate cyclase of rat liver plasma membranes. Arch. Biochem. Biophys. 147: 36 (1971).

35. Wells, M. A. and D. J. Hanahan. Studies on phospholipase A. I. Isolation and characterization of two enzymes from Crotalus adamantus Venom. Biochemistry 8: 414 (1969).

36. Dickerson, R. E. and I. Geis. The structure and action of proteins. Harper and Row, New York (1969).

TABLE I

GLUCAGON-STIMULATED ADENYLATE CYCLASE ACTIVITY

Liver plasma membranes, 4 mg/ml, were incubated in 25 mM Tris-HCl (pH 7.6), and 1 mM CaCl$_2$ for 5 min at 37° in the presence or absence of 10^{-6} M glucagon. Either water or phospholipase A, 5 μg/ml, was then added and incubation was continued for 3 min. The reaction was stopped by adding 2 mM EDTA to the medium, and adenylate cyclase activity in the presence of 10^{-5} M glucagon was determined under standard assay conditions (2). Values are the mean ± S. E. of triplicate determinations.

Glucagon	Control	Phospholipase A	%
		nmoles/mg/10 min	
−	6.21 ± .30	3.57 ± .11	57.4
+	5.38 ± .03	4.31 ± .33	80.2

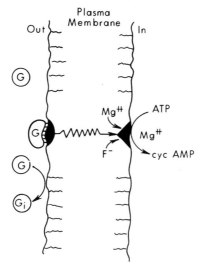

Fig. 1. *Schematic representation of the organization of the glucagon sensitive adenylate cyclase system in plasma membranes from rat liver parenchymal cells.* G = glucagon. G_i = inactivated glucagon.

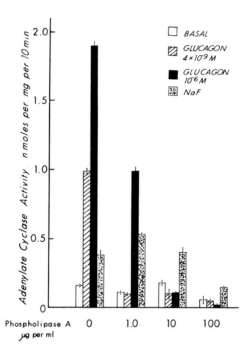

Fig. 2. *Effects of phospholipase A on adenylate cyclase activity in liver plasma membranes.* Liver membranes, 4 mg membrane protein/ml, were incubated in 25 mM Tris-HCl (pH 7.6), 1 mM $CaCl_2$, and varying concentrations of phospholipase A for 5 min at 37°. The phospholipase digestion was then stopped by addition of 2 mM EDTA, and adenylate cyclase activity in the presence of the indicated stimulators was determined under standard assay conditions (2).

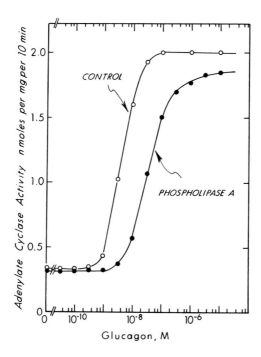

Fig. 3. *Effect of limited digestion of liver plasma membranes with phospholipase A on the glucagon stimulated adenylate cyclase activity.* Liver membranes, 4 mg membrane protein/ml, were incubated in 25 mM Tris-HCl (pH 7.6) and 1 mM $CaCl_2$ for 3 min at $37°$ in the presence or absence of phospholipase A (1 μg/ml). The reaction was stopped by adding 2 mM EDTA to the medium, and adenylate cyclase activity in the presence of varying concentrations of glucagon was then determined under standard assay conditions (2).

HORMONE RECEPTORS, II. BIOLOGICAL ACTIVITY OF AGAROSE-
GLUCAGON, AND ISOLATION OF GLUCAGON-BINDING PROTEINS FROM
SOLUBILIZED LIVER PLASMA MEMBRANES BY GEL AND AFFINITY
CHROMATOGRAPHY

Melvin Blecher, Nicholas A. Giorgio, Jr. and Carl B. Johnson

Introduction

We have recently (1,2) described the chemical synthesis
and several biological activities of glucagon and norepinephrine covalently bound to beads of 4% agarose. The binding
to agarose-glucagon of liver cell membrane particles containing glucagon receptors (3) and the stimulation of liver and
fat cell plasma membrane adenylate kinase by agarose-glucagon
and agarose-norepinephrine (1,2) suggested employment of
these gel derivatives for the isolation of glucagon and norepinephrine receptors from solubilized plasma membranes, in
the fashion used by others (4) for isolating various ligand-
binding proteins. We describe in this paper our recent ex-
periences in the identification and isolation of glucagon-
binding proteins from detergent-solubilized rat liver plasma
membranes, and the further purification of such proteins by
affinity chromatography.

Results and Discussion

^{125}I-glucagon was used to tag membrane glucagon receptors and to identify glucagon-binding proteins in solubilized
membrane preparations. Porcine glucagon (a gift from the
Lilly Research Laboratories) was lightly radioiodinated
(average of 0.75 to 1.8 atoms of iodide per mole of glucagon)
and purified by the procedures described by Rodbell *et al.*
(5), modified to halve the ratio of chloramine-T to hormone
and to elute iodoglucagon from the cellulose column with
50% aqueous ethanol instead of with a solution of serum
albumin at pH 10. These preparations of ^{125}I-glucagon,
which were comparable to native glucagon in activating

membrane adenylate cyclase, yielded a single ninhydrin positive radioactive spot upon chromatography on thin, layers of
cellulose (5), and were totally excluded by beads of Sephadex G-10; however, electrophoresis on polyacrylamide gel
revealed heterogeneity in the preparation. The results of
gel electrophoresis, in which tracer amounts of ^{125}I-gluca-
gon were co-electrophoresed with carrier, native glucagon,
are shown diagramatically in Fig. 1. The two, fast-moving
bands (A and B) accounted for the bulk of the Coomassie
blue-staining polypeptide and about 77% of the total radioactivity. The more rapid migration of these materials to
the anode may be attributable both to the presence of the
more-electronegative desamidoglucagons (7) and to the increased ionization of the iodotyrosyl hydroxyl groups (8).
Small amounts of two additional polypeptides, a sharp band
(C) and a lightly-stained, diffuse band (D), accounted for
the remainder of the radioactivity. Because of the coinci-
dence of radioactivity (from ^{125}I-glucagon) with bulk polypeptide (from carrier glucagon), it seemed clear that the
multiple bands were not artifacts of the iodination procedure, but were indigenous to the samples of porcine glucagon employed. Bromer *et al.* (7) have recently demonstrated
the presence of multiple (at least seven) components, including glucagon and mono- and di-desamidoglucagons, in our
preparations of crystalline porcine and bovine glucagon.

In Table I are outlined the procedures we have employed
for the solubilization of rat liver plasma membranes and
for the identification and isolation of glucagon-binding
proteins. A preliminary incubation of membranes [5-to-15
mg protein, prepared according to Neville (9) and stored at
-80^{6}] with ^{125}I-glucagon tagged the glucagon receptors.
Membranes were then solubilized with the nonionic detergent
Lubrol-PX (ICI America, Stamford, Conn.). Five-tenths
percent, 1.0% and 2.0% detergent solubilized about 45%, 60%
and 70%, respectively, of membrane protein; brief (15 sec)
sonication slightly improved the solubilization yield.
Ultracentrifugation at 104,5000 x g for 1.5 hours removed
insoluble membrane material; over 90% of the radioactivity
remained in the soluble phase. Gel filtration of the supernatant fluid on 4-to-8 % agarose separated free from protein-
bound ^{125}I-glucagon. In the experiment shown in Fig. 2,
membrane protein, solubilized in 0.5% Lubrol-PX in the
presence of ^{125}I-glucagon, was chromatographed on 8% agarose
in the presence of 0.5% Lubrol. Under these conditions,
75% of the protein (peak I) eluted with the void volume (V_o)

of the column, and the remainder of the protein was distributed between two included peaks (II and III). Radioactive glucagon emerged in three fractions: about 60% of the total was coincident (peak A) with the major protein peak (I); unbound ^{125}I-glucagon (peak C at the V_t of the column) accounted for 17% of the total radioactivity. The material of peak B, which accounted for the remainder of the radioactivity, contained glucagon in a form not previously described. It is likely that this was glucagon associated with micelles of Lubrol. Reference to the molecular weight calibration curve for this column indicated that the approximate molecular weight of the material in peak B was 100,000. Micellar molecular weights for lysolecithin of 92,000-95,000 have been reported (10), and the association of 8 moles of glucagon per mole of micellar lysolecithin, to yield particles of molecular weight 120,000, has recently been observed (H. Edelhoch, NIH, unpublished experiments). As a control, ^{125}I-glucagon was carried through the entire procedure, but in the absence of membrane material; the formation of micellar (peak B') and monomeric (peak C') was again observed (Fig. 2), showing that membrane components were not responsible for the formation of two forms of glucagon.

Proof that the detergent was responsible for the production of polymeric glucagon was obtained by chromatographing ^{125}I-glucagon on 6% agarose, first in the presence and then in the absence, of 0.5% buffered Lubrol-PX (Fig. 3) or of Triton X-100 (data not shown). In the presence of detergent both high molecular weight (peak A) and native (peak B) glucagons appeared. Chromatography of another sample of radioglucagon on the same column, following removal of detergent from the system, produced essentially only (94% of the total) monomeric, native glucagon, at the V_t of the column.

It is clear from the foregoing that ligands may become associated with high molecular weight micelles of detergents used to solubilize membranes, and that these ligands may behave on gel filtration columns as though associated with high molecular weight membrane proteins. It is imperative, therefore, that one not merely follow the elution pattern of the ligand, but that protein determinations be performed as well. However, even when such care is taken, the presence of micellar ligand may make difficult the identification of binding proteins. For example, in the experiment shown in Fig. 2, micellar ^{125}I-glucagon may have obscured binding of monomeric radioglucagon to proteins in peaks I and II.

For affinity chromatography we have used glucagon coupled in diazo linkage to a 22 Å extension of 4% agarose (Fig. 4). The pH of the coupling reaction determined to which amino acid residues of glucagon derivitization occurred, *i.e.* the single N-terminal histidyl and/or the tyrosyls at positions 10 and 13 (11). One preparation of agarose-glucagon was coupled at pH 8. Although, theoretically, only the histidyl residue should have been involved in the re-action (11-13), Krug *et al.* (3) found by amino acid analysis that, at pH 8, the tyrosyl residues also participated in the coupling reaction. In a second preparation of agarose-glucagon, in which diazo coupling was accomplished at pH 5, we found by amino acid analysis that only the histidyl residue was derivitized, and that about 145 µg of glucagon were bound per ml of agarose, packed volume.

Both preparations of agarose-glucagon activated rat liver plasma membrane adenylate kinase. The effect of agarose-(His, Tyr) glucagon on this enzyme complex is com-pared with that of native glucagon in Fig. 5. The concen-tration-activity relationships of agarose-glucagon and native glucagon were the same and typical of hormone effects in general. The abilities of agarose-(His, Tyr) glucagon and agarose-(His) glucagon to activate plasma membrane adenylate kinase are compared in Table 2; the activity of the former was more than twice that of the latter. This difference may be a reflection of the relative involvement of the histidyl residues in both preparations of agarose-glucagon; the involvement was total in the pH 5 preparation, only partial in the pH 8 preparation. Since deshistidine glucagon did not activate liver plasma membrane adenylate kinase, although it did bind to the membranes (14), it is clear that the histidyl residue is required for this bio-logical activity. If derivitization of the histidyl resi-dues attenuates biological activity, it is likely that the pH 8 preparation was more active because fewer histidyl residues were involved in the diazo reaction. An alternate explanation for the difference between the activities of the two gel derivatives is based upon a possible effect of pH upon the amount of glucagon coupled to the gel in the diazo reaction; data presently available do not permit an evalu-ation of this hypothesis.

For affinity chromatography, the membrane solubilization procedures described in Table I were scaled up four-fold, but in the absence of glucagon. Following chromatography on Bio-Gel A (1.5m), the glucagon-binding fractions (*cf.* Fig. 2, peak I) were pooled and dialyzed to reduce the concentration of Lubrol and the ionic strength. Although the detergent concentration in the affinity chromatography experiment of Fig. 6 was 0.1%, subsequent experience suggested that the concentration of Lubrol-PX could be reduced to as low as 0.02% without significant precipitation of proteins. It is of interest in this connection that Cuatracasas (15) has reported that 0.05% Triton X-100 was the lower limit to which solubilized rat liver plasma membranes could be taken without significant precipitation of insulin-binding proteins.

Identical amounts of a dialyzed, glucagon-binding fraction were chromatographed simultaneously on paired columns with 4% agarose as a control and agarose-(His, Tyr) glucagon for affinity chromatography. As shown in Fig. 6, when applied to the control column, no retention or fractionation of protein occured. In contrast, on the agarose-glucagon column fractionation of the protein occurred into two major peaks, the first being eluted with one column volume of starting buffer (0.1% Lubrol-PX in 1 mM Tris buffer, pH 7.6) and the second with 4-to-5 column volumes of this buffer. All of the protein applied to the column was accounted for by these two fractions, and neither increasing the ionic strength of the buffer with 1 M NaCl nor application of 5 M urea eluted additional 280 nm absorbing material.

It is clear from these results that affinity of the glucagon-binding proteins in this preparation for agarose-glucagon was not great, since all proteins were eluted by the starting, low ionic strength buffer. It is also clear that, under these conditions, relatively little purification of glucagon-binding proteins had been achieved, since so much extraneous protein was also retained by the column. This behavior is reminiscent of one observed by Krug *et al.* (3) in studies of the adsorption of particulate liver cell membranes to beads of agarose-glucagon. About 60% of the membrane particles applied to the column was retained by the gel, and it was suggested that such behavior could be explained if 60% of the particles contained glucagon receptors (3). In the present instance (Fig. 6), the retention of so much protein by agarose-glucagon could have occurred if glucagon-binding proteins were still strongly associated with other, high molecular weight membrane proteins; it should be recalled (Fig. 2) that all of these proteins had molecular weights exceeding 1.5 million. This hypothesis is supported by experiments to be described in Figs. 8 and

371

9 in which 2% Lubrol-PX was used to solubilize liver plasma membranes. Under these conditions, glucagon-binding proteins were better dissociated from other membrane proteins. A similar observation was made by Cuatracasas (15) in which solubilization of membranes in 1 to 2% Triton X-100 dissociated insulin-binding proteins from other membrane proteins.

Glucagon-binding capacities of affinity chromatography fractions were determined by an adaptation of the technique of Hummel and Dryer (16). In this technique, the ligand (^{125}I-glucagon) was incorporated into the buffer used for gel filtration. A sample of glucagon-binding protein was placed on the Sephadex G-50 column, and elution began with the ligand-buffer solution. The radioglucagon which is bound to the binding protein is, like the protein, excluded from the gel beads; this appeared in the void volume as a peak of radioactivity (Fig. 7). For mass to be conserved, the excess of radioactivity must be matched by a corresponding deficiency; this appeared as a trough at the V_t of the column (Fig. 7). The peak and trough should be, and was, separated by a plateau of radioactivity similar to that of the ligand-buffer solution. The number of moles of glucagon bound to the protein was calculated from the area under the peak of radioactivity and the specific radioactivity of the glucagon. The binding capacities of several of these affinity chromatography fractions are given in Table III. For comparison, Table III also lists binding capacities obtained by others for glucagon with particulate liver membranes, and for insulin with particulate and solubilized liver membranes. Despite the variety of systems and the differences in methods used to assay for binding capacity, all binding capacity values are remarkably similar, which reinforces the belief that these values are physiologically meaningful.

In an attempt more completely to dissociate glucagon-binding proteins from other membrane proteins, liver plasma membranes were solubilized in 2% Lubrol-PX in the absence of radioglucagon. The clarified membrane extract was then chromatographed on a column of 6% agarose equilibrated with monomeric ^{125}I-glucagon (isolated by Sephadex G-50 chromatography) in 0.1% Lubrol-PX. It was anticipated that the equilibrium between free and protein-bound ^{125}I-glucagon would be shifted in the direction of association if glucagon were present throughout the gel filtration system. In the present experiment (Fig. 8), the membrane proteins were fractionated into two peaks; the bulk of the protein was represented by the material emerging just after the void volume, and a small amount of protein eluted just ahead of the V_t of the column. The ^{125}I-glucagon also emerged in two fractions, both of which were coincident with the protein peaks. In preparation for affinity chromatography, fractions containing high molecular weight proteins with glucagon-binding activity (Fig. 7, fractions 6 to 9 ml) were pooled and dialyzed for three days to remove bound radioglucagon and to reduce the concentration of Lubrol-PX to 0.02%.

Aliquots (240 μg protein) of the dialysate were applied to a column of agarose-(His)glucagon equilibrated with buffered 0.02% Lubrol (Fig. 9). Of the protein applied to the column, about 160 μg were eluted by the starting buffer between the V_o and V_t of the column. The remainder of the protein was strongly bound by the agarose-glucagon, but was eluted by 5 M urea buffered at pH 6.0. Although this procedure greatly improved the separation and purification of glucagon-binding proteins, compared to earlier procedures (Figs. 2 and 6), it is apparent that extraneous protein remained associated with the glucagon-binding material. We are presently attempting to improve the purification, and to develop a faster and more-facile binding assay that will lend itself to multiple determinations during the course of the purification procedures.

Summary

Rat liver plasma membranes, pre-labeled with ^{125}I-glucagon, were solubilized with the nonionic detergent Lubrol-PX; glucagon-binding proteins were identified and isolated by gel filtration. Alternately, glucagon-binding proteins were isolated from solubilized membrane preparations by chromatography on Hummel-Dryer columns in the presence of ^{125}I-glucagon.

Several agarose-glucagon derivatives, capable of activating rat liver plasma membrane adenylate cyclase, were used to further purify glucagon-binding proteins from crude gel filtration fractions. Proteins were obtained with a capacity for binding glucagon (0.5 to 0.75 pmoles/mg protein) similar to those reported by others for the binding of glucagon by liver membrane particles, and for the binding of insulin to plasma membrane particles and to detergent-solubilized membrane proteins.

Presented by Melvin Blecher. The work was supported by research grants to Melvin Blecher from the National Institutes of Health (AM-05475) and the Washington Heart Association. The data are taken from a Ph.D. Thesis to be submitted by C. B. Johnson to the Graduate School of Georgetown University. We thank Dr. Martin Rodbell (NIH) for providing us with details on modifications of the purification procedure reported in reference (5). We are indebted to Dr. Fred Downs, New York Medical College, for performing the amino acid analyses.

References

1. Johnson, C. B., M. Blecher and N. A. Giorgio, Jr. Hormone receptors. Activation of rat liver plasma membrane adenylate cyclase and fat cell lipolysis by agarose-glucagon. Biochem. Biophys. Res. Commun. 46: 1035 (1972).
2. Johnson, C. B., M. Blecher and N. A. Giorgio, Jr. Activation of plasma membrane adenylate cyclase by agarose-glucagon and agarose-norepinephrine. Federation Proc. 31: 439 Abs (1972).
3. Krug, F., B. Desbuquois and P. Cuatrecasas. Glucagon affinity absorbents: selective binding of receptors of liver cell membranes. Nature New Biology 234: 268 (1971).
4. Cuatrecasas, P. and C. B. Anfinsen. Affinity chromatography. Ann. Rev. Biochem. 40: 259 (1971).
5. Rodbell, M., H. M. Krans, S. L. Pohl and L. Birnbaumer. The glucagon sensitive adenyl cyclase of rat liver plasma membranes. III Binding of glucagon: method of assay and specificity. J. Biol. Chem. 246: 1861 (1971).
6. Giorgio, N.A., Jr. A. T. Yip, J. Fleming and G. W. E. Plaut. Diphosphopyridine nucleotide-linked isocitrate dehydrogenase from bovine heart. J. Biol. Chem. 245: 5469 (1970).
7. Bromer, W. W., M. E. Boucher, J. M. Patterson, A. H. Peker and B. H. Frank. Glucagon structure and function. I Purification and properties of bovine glucagon and monodesamidoglucagon. J. Biol. Chem. 247: 2581 (1972).

8. Swan, J. C. and G. G. Hammes. Self-association of glucagon. Equilibrium studies. Biochemistry 8: 1 (1969).
9. Neville, D.M., Jr. Isolation of an organ specific antigen from cell surface membrane of rat liver. Biochim. Biophys. Acta 154: 540 (1968).
10. Perrin, J. H. and L. Saunders. The micellar size and shape of lysolecithin. Biochim. Biophys. Acta 84: 216 (1964).
11. Cuatrecasas, P. Protein purification by affinity chromatography. Derivatizations of agarose and polyacrylamide beads. J. Biol. Chem. 245: 3059 (1970).
12. Brown, R. D., H. C. Duffin, J. C. Maynard and J. H. Ridd. The mechanism of coupling of diazonium salts with heterocyclic compounds. J. Chem. Soc. (London) 3937 (1953).
13. Waley, S.G., Mechanisms of organic and enzymatic reactions. Oxford Univ. Press, Oxford, 1962, p. 324.
14. Rodbell, M., L. Birnbaumer, S. L. Pohl and F. Sundby. The reaction of glucagon with its receptor: evidence for discrete regions for activity and binding in the glucagon molecule. Proc. Nat. Acad. Sci. 68: 909 (1971).
15. Cuatrecasas, P. Properties of insulin receptor isolated from liver and fat cell membranes. J. Biol. Chem. 247: 1980 (1972).
16. Hummell, J. P. and W. J. Dryer. Measurement of protein binding phenomena by gel filtration. Biochim. Biophys. Acta 63: 530 (1962).
17. Freychet, P., J. Roth and D. M. Neville, Jr. Insulin receptors in liver: specific binding of [^{125}I]-insulin to the plasma membrane, and its relation to insulin bioactivity. Proc. Nat. Acad. Sci. 68: 1833 (1971).

TABLE I

ISOLATION OF GLUCAGON-BINDING PROTEINS FROM LIVER PLASMA MEMBRANES

1. Receptors tagged by pretreatment of membranes with ^{125}I-glucagon.

2. Membranes extracted with detergent (Lubrol-PX or Triton X-100, 0.5 - 2.0%) in 0.2 M dithiothreitol - 50 mM Tris (pH 7.6) ± sonication. Clarified by ultra-centrifugation ($4°$; > 100,000 x g; 1.5 to 2 hours).

3. Aliquot of supernatant fluid chromatographed on agarose (4 to 8%) with detergent (0.1 to 0.5%) - 50 mM Tris. Eluates analyzed for A_{280}, protein and ^{125}I.

4. For preparative work, steps 2 and 3 scaled up, and glucagon-binding fractions pooled and dialyzed to reduce ionic strength and [detergent].

5. Dialysate clarified by centrifugation, then chromatographed on agarose-glucagon column with detergent (0.02 to 0.1%) - 1 mM Tris. Elution also with high ionic strength buffers and/or urea. Eluates analyzed for A_{280} and protein.

6. Protein fractions analyzed for binding capacity with ^{125}I-glucagon.

TABLE II

GLUCAGON EQUIVALENCY OF AGAROSE-GLUCAGON PREPARATIONS

Glucagon equivalencies were determined by comparison of agarose-glucagon preparations with native glucagon in the activation assay for rat liver plasma membrane adenylate cyclase (1).

Gel preparation	Glucagon equivalency
	µg glucagon/ml gel (packed vol.)
Sepharose-4B-(His, Tyr) glucagon	2.04 ± 0.46
Sepharose-4B-(His) glucagon	0.80 ± 0.08

377

TABLE III

BINDING CAPACITIES OF PARTICULATE AND SOLUBILIZED RAT LIVER
MEMBRANES FOR GLUCAGON AND INSULIN

Hormone	Binding preparation	Binding capacity *pmoles/mg protein*	Reference
^{125}I-glucagon	18 ml eluate fraction from affinity chromatography (Fig. 5)	0.75	Present study
	20 ml eluate fraction	0.26	
	22 and 24 ml eluate fraction	0.14	
	26 ml eluate fraction	0.51	
^{125}I-glucagon	Liver cell membranes	0.67	3
^{125}I-glucagon	Liver plasma membranes	0.1-1.1	5
^{125}I-insulin	Liver plasma membranes	0.15	17
^{125}I-insulin	Solubilized liver cell membranes	0.20-0.26	15

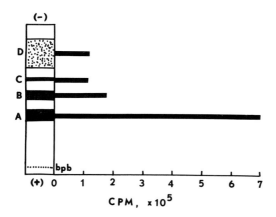

Fig. 1. *Co-electrophoresis of crystalline native glucagon and purified* ^{125}I*-glucagon on 7.5% polyacrylamide gel at pH 8.3 (6).* Following electrophoresis, proteins were stained by Coomassie Blue.

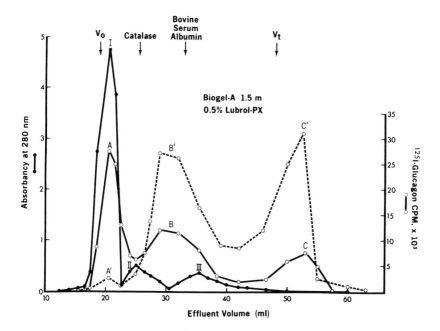

Fig. 2. *Isolation of a solubilized, rat liver plasma membrane glucagon-binding fraction by filtration on Bio-Gel-A (1.5m).*

379

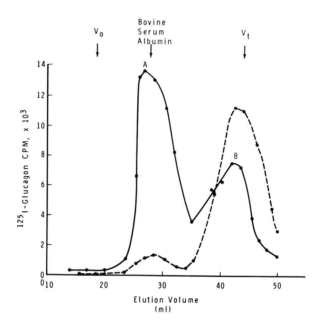

Fig. 3. *Effect of detergent on the behavior of* ^{125}I-*gluca-gon on a gel filtration column of Sepharose-6B*. Radiogluca-gon was chromatographed first in the presence (●—●) and then in the absence (o—o) of 0.5% Lubrol-PX.

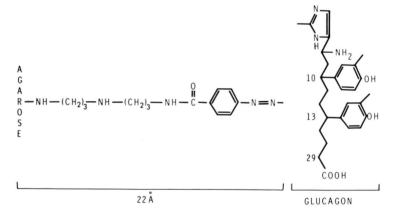

Fig. 4. *Schematic view of structures of Sepharose-4B-glucagon derivatives.*

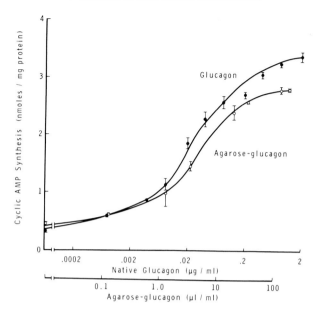

Fig. 5. *Effects of native glucagon (●) and Sepharose-4B-(His, Tyr) glucagon (o) on the adenylate cyclase activity of rat liver plasma membranes.* Taken from ref. 1.

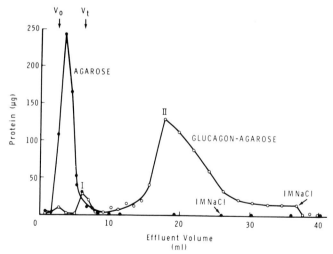

Fig. 6. *Affinity chromatography of glucagon-binding proteins on a control column of Sepharose-4B (●) and on a column of Sepharose-4B-(His, Tyr) glucagon (o).*

381

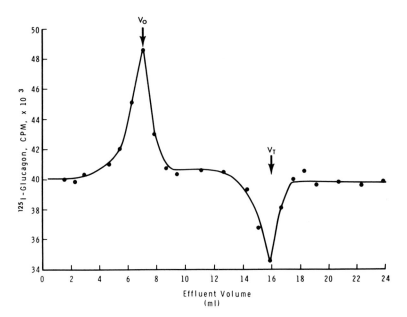

Fig. 7. *Chromatography of a partially-purified glucagon-binding protein fraction (200 μg protein) on a Hummel-Dryer column of Sephadex G-50 equilibrated with monomeric* [125]*I-glucagon in 0.1% Lubrol-PX - 1 mM Tris buffer (pH 7.6).*

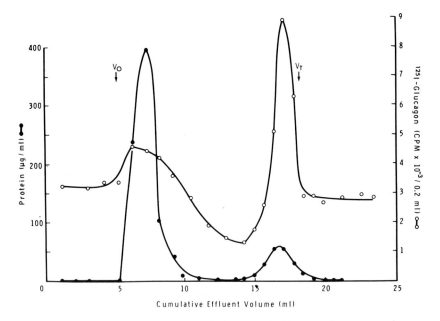

Fig. 8. *Chromatography of solubilized liver plasma membranes on a column of Sepharose-6B equilibrated with monomeric* [125]*I-glucagon in 0.1% Lubrol-PX in 50 mM Tris buffer (pH 7.6).*

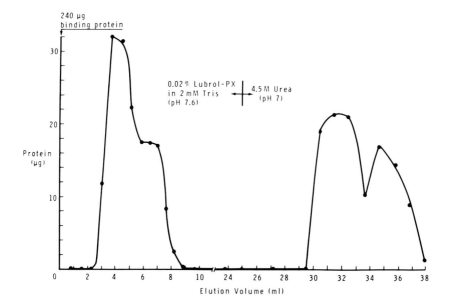

Fig. 9. *Affinity chromatography of a glucagon-binding protein fraction on Sepharose-4B-(His) glucagon equilibrated with 0.02% Lubrol-PX in 2 mM Tris buffer, (pH 7.6).* At the arrow, the eluting buffer was changed to include 4.5 M urea.

STUDIES ON FACTORS AFFECTING THE ADENYLATE CYCLASE SYSTEM OF RAT ERYTHROCYTES

Herbert Sheppard and Charles R. Burghardt

Introduction

Our attention was focused on the adenylate cyclase system because it represented a hormone-stimulated *coupled* system at a molecular level. Within the structure of this system lay buried the elements contributing to the exquisite specificity of hormone action. Involved in the coupling is a receptor molecule, whose exploration has already been discussed, in some type of relationship with a catalytic unit, the adenylate cyclase. Such a system seemed to offer excellent possibilities for understanding the *functional* relationships existing between components of the membrane. Once having decided to look at this system it was necessary to choose a suitable source. I convinced myself that I wanted a system which was readily obtainable, easily prepared and relatively free from other intracellular membranes. The non-nucleated mammalian erythrocyte seemed to meet these requirements but the report by Klainer *et al.* (1) indicated that adenylate cyclase was absent from the erythrocyte of the dog, though present in the nucleated erythrocyte of birds. While I was discouraged from the start, this was a time when bits of information picked up along the way proved helpful. I recalled that some years earlier I was surprised to learn that dog and cat erythrocytes have high internal Na^+ concentrations and therefore, are probably deficient in a Na^+, K^+-ATP-ase. It was reasoned, therefore, that a deficiency in one enzyme associated with ATP metabolism could be associated with the deficiency of another, in this case, adenylate cyclase. We, therefore, compared the pump-deficient cat and dog erythrocytes with the pump-containing rat, mouse and human erythrocytes for adenylate cyclase activity (2). We were very excited to find that the erythrocyte ghosts of the rat and mouse had an active adenylate cyclase while that of the dog and cat had none. A good correlation between the presence of the cyclase and the sodium pump began to emerge but, as is so often the case, man proved to be uncooperative. No adenylate cyclase could be found.

Results

ATP Metabolism

Further work with these ghosts showed that a lack of adenylate cyclase was not related to ATP metabolism (Table I). Under basal conditions, less than 40% of the ATP remained at the end of the incubation with erythrocyte ghosts from man, rat and mouse while 50% or more remained with that of dog and cat. In general, norepinephrine (NE) had little effect while fluoride (F) was very inhibitory. Among the major metabolic products the concentration of ADP was greater than that of AMP. Very little 5'-nucleotidase activity was present as evident from the very small amounts of adenosine which was produced.

Effect of Biogenic Amines

It was soon learned that the adenylate cyclase of the rat erythrocyte would respond to catecholamines in a fashion which was typical for β-receptor systems (3,4); i.e. the potency of isoproterenol (ISO) > epinephrine (E) > norepinephrine (NE). Dopamine (DA) was found to activate this system while histamine and serotonin would not. Of the other hormones tested only prostaglandin E_2 was active. It should be noted, however, that no other prostaglandin was tested in this system.

The positive response to DA was at that time unique since no such stimulation was observed with other preparations whether as slices or homogenates. Attempts were made to determine if we were in any way the proud possessors of a system which contained what could be classified as a DA receptor (4). In Fig. 1, it can be seen that DA was weaker than NE and seemed to have less intrinsic activity; i.e. it never achieved the same maximum. N-methyl dopamine ($N-CH_3$ DA), another activator of a dopamine receptor (5), was equipotent with NE in stimulating cyclic AMP production. It should be noted that all of these compounds were less stimulatory at higher concentrations and it was possible that the dopamine effect never reached the same maximum because inhibitory factors predominated at the higher concentrations.

In considering the potencies of the various catecholamines the presence of a β-hydroxy group could be correlated with increased activity. One wondered therefore, whether the active site of the receptor would consider the β-hydroxyl as absent if it were in the wrong configuration (*i.e.* dextrorotatory). As seen in Fig. 2, the potency of L(+) isoproterenol was much less than that of the D(-) isomer but was equipotent with N-isopropyl DA. Interestingly, L(+)-epinephrine had the same potency as N-CH$_3$ DA. Thus in the D(-) series the potency of N-isopropyl > N-methyl analogue while in the L(+) series the reverse was true. The maximum activity of the L(+) isomer of ISO and of N-CH$_3$ DA was lower than that of the D(-) analogue and since inhibition was not appreciable at these concentrations the intrinsic activity was definitely reduced.

It is believed that when the catecholamine interacts with receptors a conformational change occurs which induces an activated conformation in the adenylate cyclase. Thus the activation becomes a function of the degree of change which occurs in the receptor. The results would then suggest that the absence of a β-hydroxyl group leads to a less favorable change in the receptor and therefore, a less than maximal activation of the cyclase. Alternatively, however, we could be dealing with two receptors, one for DA and the other for the D(-) isomers of the β-hydroxylated catecholamines. Pharmacologically, a dopamine receptor has been described by Goldberg *et al.* (5) as one which can be activated in the presence of blocking agents of the α-receptors (phentolamine, phenoxybenzamine) and β-receptors (propranolol, dichloroisoproterenol) but blocked by neuroleptic agents (haloperidol, chlorpromazine). In Table II, we demonstrate that all of these classes of blocking agents inhibit the stimulation by N-CH$_3$ DA, NE and E to the same extent (4). Even when haloperidol was combined with low concentrations of phenoxybenzamine the effect of the N-CH$_3$ DA and NE responses were no different. The conclusion was forced on us that DA was acting through a standard β-receptor system on the surface of the ghost and not through a specific DA system. This conclusion was reinforced by the observation that apomorphine, a substance believed to act on a DA receptor (5,6), was not able to stimulate the erythrocyte cyclase. Recently, however, dopamine stimulation of adenylate cyclase in superior cervical ganglia (7) and retina (8) homogenates has been demonstrated. Since these dopamine effects are inhibited by the α-blocking agent phentolamine they may not represent action on a true dopamine receptor. Further work is obviously required to define this receptor at a molecular level.

The inhibitory effect of serotonin seen here has also been reported by Weiss (9) for the pineal gland. This observation may have some physiological relevance since some actions of serotonin can be explained by an inhibition of NE effects (10).

Much of what was observed could be explained by the interaction of these catecholamines with the same macromolecule whose organization in the membrane under the conditions of the experiment permitted only a β-type response. It was necessary to consider the possibility that a modified arrangement of this macromolecule could expose a more specific DA response. It was considered that any such organization should be susceptible to changes in pH and in Fig. 3 we have collected the results of three experiments covering a pH range from 5.8 to 8.4. Maximum stimulation with the catecholamines and F occurred at about pH 7.4 (11) and it is apparent that no difference in response was noted for the two catecholamines. No catecholamine stimulation could be detected below pH 6.4. It was of interest, however, that while fluoride stimulation showed the same maximum and minimum pH response, its effects were never completely lost, even down to a pH of 5.6. This suggests that catecholamine stimulation was completely lost because of an alternation of the interaction with the receptor and/or the coupling of receptor to the cyclase rather than to an inactivation of the catalytic unit.

The nature of the interaction of the catecholamine with the receptor has, of course, been discussed to some extent. Considerations have been given to the possibility that catechol O-methyl transferase (COMT) might serve as a model of the receptor (12) and we had even entertained the notion that COMT might be that receptor. In agreement with a recent report (13), we had found that the rat erythrocyte membrane did possess COMT. However, if COMT were in fact the receptor, then inhibitors such as catechol or L-DOPA, would be expected to inhibit the activation of adenylate cyclase.

388

This did not occur despite the fact that these particular compounds are readily O-methylated (14) and therefore, must be competing with the substrate at the active site of COMT. It is apparent that the concept of identity between COMT and β-receptor is unsupportable. It should also be stated that while the catechol group is necessary for the activation of the cyclase, the inhibitors such as propranolol and dichloro-isoproterenol inhibit quite strongly but contain no catechol moiety. Perhaps access to the catechol binding site of the receptor is blocked unless the compound has a basic nitrogen present. Thus, catechol would not have access because of lack of a nitrogen and L-DOPA would not because of the presence of the negative charge of the carboxy group.

The nature of the interaction of the amino group remains unclear. One could envision interactions of an ionic, a Schiff-base or amide type. However, the latter two could not occur if a tertiary nitrogen was present and we have found that N,N-dimethyl DA is as active as DA. These considerations would therefore, favor a site on the receptor with an anionic group forming a salt linkage with the agonist and placing the catechol in the appropriate position. Thus, a multiple point attachment would be necessary (Fig. 4).

In this model, two cationic centers lie close to an anionic region and one of these is in a salt linkage with the negatively charged group. The cationic amino group of the catecholamine forms a salt linkage at the same time that the phenolic oxygen interacts with the more exposed cationic center (I). This breaks the lower salt linkage and allows the protein to unfold. In this unfolding, the catecholamine rotates, makes contact with the other catechol binding site and activates the adenylate cyclase (II). With a β-hydroxyl group in a D(-) configuration a better activating conformation (III) is obtained. This model is, of course, highly conjectural but can serve as a basis for further work in this area.

Action of Enzymes on Erythrocyte Ghosts

While the above mentioned studies were being carried out, a series of experiments were outlined in an effort to disrupt the membranes by enzymatic means.

Typical results were achieved in Table III by incubating ghosts with neuraminidase (NAm) for removal of sialic acid residues, with phospholipase C (PL-C) for removal of phosphorylcholine, phosphoryserine or phosphorylethanolamine from their respective phospholipids and with trypsin (T) for the splitting of peptide bonds. All were tested at hemolytic doses. Firstly, it is apparent that NAm had very little effect on the basal or F stimulation of adenylate cyclase, but NE stimulation was significantly depressed. PL-C increased the basal and F but not NE stimulated cyclic AMP production. Trypsin, on the other hand, all but eliminated cyclic AMP production in the presence of F and NE. The basal values for all but the PL-C incubation could be accounted for by simply incubating ATP in the buffer. Examination of the ghosts disclosed that those treated with NAm and PL-C were quite normal in appearance while those treated with trypsin changed from a red to a brown and became quite sticky.

The situation with adenosine (Ar) production was quite interesting. A small amount of Ar was produced by the untreated ghosts and, as expected, could be inhibited by F. The Ar production in the presence of NE has never been seen to be significantly different from that under basal conditions and has therefore, been excluded from the tables. In the presence of NAm a significant increase in Ar production was noted. With PL-C, however, almost 19 nmoles of Ar were produced which represents approximately 8% of the ATP in the incubation. The Ar production in the presence of trypsin, however, was significantly reduced. Fluoride consistently inhibited Ar production, though not always completely, in the incubations containing NAm or PL-C.

This rather amazing effect of PL-C on adenosine production prompted some further studies with this enzyme. It is apparent from Table IV that 20 µg of PL-C in the absence of the ghosts produced a small amount of Ar from ATP, and that this too was inhibited by F. For all practical purposes no cyclase activity could be detected, and the recorded counts represent the levels to be found from ATP in the absence of the ghosts. Incubation of the ghosts with boiled PL-C yielded a pattern of activity very much like that obtained with ghosts alone suggesting that the enhanced activities obtained with PL-C can be destroyed by boiling. With unboiled PL-C a definite enhancement of the F stimulatory effect is again seen. The NE effect is not altered after the basal value is subtracted. In this experiment Ar production was even greater than seen earlier (Table III).

The effect of increasing concentrations of PL-C is demonstrated in Table V. In order to eliminate the Ar producing capacity of the PL-C from the cyclase assay, the ghosts were *preincubated* with the enzyme for 30 min at 37°, diluted 14 fold and centrifuged at 20,000 x g for 40 min. The supernatant was discarded and the ghosts were brought to their original volume with Tris buffer. The first thing to be noted was the marked decrease in F and NE stimulation which resulted from preincubation alone. I will return to this point somewhat later. A quick glance down the "basal" column demonstrates a marked increase in cyclic AMP production as evidenced by an increase in counts in that area. Fluoride stimulation increased somewhat and then fell at the higher concentrations. The NE values also rose steadily. With 80 µg and more, the difference from basal was not significant indicating that NE stimulation of the adenylate cyclase could no longer be detected. As seen before, 20 µg of PL-C, significantly enhanced F stimulation even though the enzyme was present only during the preincubation period. In this experiment, we decided to determine the levels of the other adenine nucleotides by chromatographing the extracts on paper in isobutyric:H_2O:concentrated NH_3 (66:33:1).

The results in Fig. 5 demonstrate the extensive breakdown of ATP. As seen earlier, in the absence of PL-C, approximately 32% of the ATP remained intact. Almost 40% of added ATP was converted to ADP and somewhat less than 30% to AMP. With increasing PL-C both ATP and ADP disappeared more rapidly while AMP increased slightly and adenosine almost linearly with amount. With 200 µg of PL-C/incubation, over 35% of the ATP was found as Ar. It is of interest that no adenine could be detected even at these high levels indicating the absence of nucleosidase activity. At this stage we were unable to ascribe this hydrolysis to known enzymes in the membrane and so we have chosen to refer to it as phosphohydrolase activity. The inhibitory action of F was not overwhelmed by the increasing amounts of PL-C although Ar production was able to creep up slightly.

A study of the effect of preincubation time on the stimulation of phosphohydrolase activity demonstrated that those samples which were not preincubated at 37° but were immediately diluted 14 fold and centriguted had as much phosphohydrolase activity as those preincubated for 30 min. This was completely unexpected and suggested that: a) the activation was occurring during centrifugation in the cold or b) no activation was actually occurring during the preincubation but PL-C was being carried over into the final incubation. The latter concept gave rise to the possibility that PL-C was tightly bound to its substrate in the ghost membrane, and carried over into the final incubation. To demonstrate this, 200 µg of PL-C were added to the ghosts and the mixture was immediately diluted 14 fold, centrifuged and washed with 13 volumes of 2 mM Tris-glucose buffer. If no absorption or non-reversible entrapment had occurred, the final incubation would be expected to have 0.05 µg of PL-C. The hydrolytic activity of these PL-C exposed ghosts was compared with that effected by naive ghosts incubated with as much as 0.29 µg of PL-C. Table VI demonstrates that the ghosts exposed to PL-C, prior to washing, retained marked phosphohydrolase activity. The naive ghosts incubated with 0.29 µg of PL-C, produced only slightly more Ar than the ghosts never exposed to PL-C. In agreement with other findings (15) thin layer chromatograms of the lipids demonstrated a decrease in most phospholipids, except sphingomyelin, and an increase in diglyceride formation as a function of incubation time with the PL-C exposed ghosts. Thus, PL-C was tightly-bound to the ghost or entrapped in a fashion which was not readily reversible and consideration was given to the possibility that it was the PL-C in contrast to the membrane enzymes which was producing the large quantities of Ar. It was important, therefore, to evaluate the activity of the PL-C on the membrane-produced hydrolytic products of ATP. The ghosts were incubated with ATP for the regular 30 min after which they were denatured by boiling and separated by centrifugation. The supernatant was then incubated with 16 µg of PL-C for an additional 30 min. The marked rise in Ar production with a comparable loss of 5'-AMP but not ATP or ADP demonstrated the intense 5'-nucleotidase activity contributed by the PL-C. This, however, could not explain the rise in AMP and decrease in ATP and ADP as seen in Fig. 5. It is still possible that the absorption of PL-C results in an activation of other contaminating phosphohydrolases or that the phospholipase action activates the phosphohydrolase activity of the membrane. In this regard, it was noted that preincubation with PL-C for up to 30 min at $37°$ just prior to the addition of ATP-^{14}C yielded time-dependent increases in Ar production over that seen at $1°$. Since preincubation in cold did not yield a time-dependent increase in Ar production, it can be inferred that at $37°$ another component of the Ar producing system is activated. It is possible that this other component actually represents the membrane-bound phosphohydrolase.

Preincubation Effects

Returning to our original concern for the adenylate

cyclase it should be recalled that while PL-C did alter the responsiveness of the system to hormones an even greater change occurred by simply preincubating the ghosts in hypotonic Tris or phosphate buffer.

Most of the studies performed earlier were with ghosts prepared in phosphate buffer. However, when we considered evaluating the phospholipase activity by measuring phosphate release another buffer was needed. Since Tris-buffer was the basis for our incubation, we compared the cyclase activity of ghosts prepared in both buffers and subjected to preincubation and washing. In Fig. 6 it can be seen that the ghosts prepared with Tris were generally more responsive than those prepared with phosphate buffer. This was not true for NE stimulation of ghosts which were not preincubated and not washed or preincubated at 37° and washed. If the ghosts were *prepared* in Tris, it did not matter whether they were *incubated* in Tris or phosphate. Washing the ghosts one time markedly increased the stimulation by both F and NE of Tris prepared ghosts. Again, the NE stimulation of phosphate-prepared ghosts was not affected. Preincubation in an ice-bath for 30 min reduced the effect of washing in all cases. Since washing itself takes about 40 min to complete, it is possible that shorter periods of time would have yielded higher activities. The effect of washing was greater if glucose was present in the Tris-buffer.

Washing the ghosts removes about 2/3 of the associated protein and this may include inhibitory factors. The presence of phosphodiesterase was probably not the problem since the use of a potent inhibitor did not alter the results. It would be of interest to direct further studies to the mechanism of activation by washing.

The decreased response of the erythrocyte adenylate cyclase following preincubation at 37° for 30 min was the subject of further investigation. Was it possible that the presence of the substrate (ATP) or a stimulating agent (F or ISO) during the preincubation period would stabilize the system and protect it from deterioration? From the results in Table VII, it is apparent that some success was achieved. Both ISO and F in the preincubation medium resulted in elevated basal production of cyclic AMP which may have reflected some carry-over from the preincubation medium. In the presence of these elevated basal values, the stimulation by ISO was no longer significant. Fluoride stimulation of F-preincubated ghosts, however, was significantly greater than that seen with the Tris preincubation. It should be noted that the ISO concentration used here was supramaximal. When in a subsequent experiment it was reduced to a maximally stimulating concentration and appropriately diluted, the basal level fell and ISO stimulation was comparable to that of Tris-preincubated ghosts.

Both the ISO and F stimulation were protected in those situations where ATP was present. Cyclic AMP seemed to protect NE stimulation to a very slight extent but had little effect on F stimulation. The Mg^{++} on the other hand had little effect on the adenylate cyclase but as expected enhanced the adenosine production both in the presence and absence of F. The lack of specificity of the ATP effect can be seen in Fig. 8 where the triphosphates of uridine (UTP) and guanosine (GTP) were quite active. In fact, GTP maintained the ISO stimulation at the levels observed with the cold incubated samples.

The protection of the cyclase system by the nucleoside triphosphates as well as F suggests the possibility that a certain amount of phosphorylated protein may be essential.

It might be relevant that the preincubation of intact cells had no effect on the adenylate cyclase activity of subsequently prepared ghosts and this could be related to their ability to maintain an adequate intracellular concentration of ATP and thus a phosphorylated state of the membrane. The validity of this concept must await the results of studies now underway.

Oxidative Atmosphere

It was recognized that the presence of an oxidative atmosphere could result in undesirable oxidative reactions which could alter the state of lipids and/or proteins in the membrane. However, preparing and incubating the ghosts in N_2 had little or no effect on the activity. In addition, ghosts obtained from a vitamin E deficient rat had cyclase activity which differed little from those of a vitamin E supplemented animal. Thus, conditions which should alter the peroxidation of lipids in the membrane had little effect on the activity of the adenylate cyclase.

Effect of Age

In view of the reports in the literature concerning age-dependent changes in hormone-responsiveness of the adenylate cyclase of neurons (16,17,18) hepatic tissue (19,20) and thymocytes (21), we considered the possibility that age-dependent alterations in erythrocyte enzyme systems might exist. In Fig. 8, we see that at the ages of 25 and 11 days, the basal, as well as F and ISO stimulation, was much higher than that obtained with the mature animals. With the 25 day old animals, the ISO stimulation was the greatest. It is important to note that the 11 day old animals was still suckling and that the 74 day old animal was young but mature. It would seem therefore that the prepubertal period was one of enhanced β-receptor activity for the rat erythrocyte ghost. Although the actual time of peaking of adenylate cyclase activity for liver (19,20), brain (16,17,18) and lymphocytes (21) varied somewhat, these systems also appeared to be more active in the prepubertal animal. The inference, here, is that the development of this system may be under hormonal control.

Summary

It is apparent that the erythrocyte ghost offers a system for studying the properties of adenylate cyclase and the effects of a variety of forces operative in the intact animal. The relatively mild treatment used for obtaining the cell membrane preparations provides increased sensitivity to stimulating agents but also exposes the marked sensitivity of these responses to environmental factors. By working with such a system it may provide us with some hints for obtaining more active cyclases from tissues requiring more rigorous methods of preparation.

The erythrocyte adenylate cyclase contains a catecholamine sensitive receptor of a β-type which also responds to DA. It is more active in immature animals and is very sensitive to pH, preparation time and temperature. Purine and pyrimidine nucleoside triphosphates and possibly F offer some protection from the deteriorating effects of preincubation.

Presented by Herbert Sheppard

References

1. Klainer, L. M., Y. -M. Chi, S. L. Freidberg, T. W. Rall and E. W. Sutherland. Adenyl cyclase IV. The effects of neurohormones on the formation of adenosine 3',5'-phosphate

by preparations from brain and other tissues. J. Biol. Chem. 237:1239-1243 (1962).

2. Sheppard, H. and C. R. Burghardt. Adenyl cyclase in non-nucleated erythrocytes of several mammalian species. Biochem. Pharmacol. 18:2576-2578 (1969).

3. Sheppard, H. and C. R. Burghardt. The stimulation of adenyl cyclase of rat erythrocyte ghosts. Mol. Pharmacol. 6:425-429 (1970).

4. Sheppard, H. and C. R. Burghardt. The effect of alpha, beta, and dopamine receptor-blocking agents on the stimulation of rat erythrocyte adenyl cyclase by dihydroxyphenethylamines and their β-hydroxylated derivatives. Mol. Pharmacol. 7:1-7 (1971).

5. Goldberg, L. I., P. F. Sonneville and J. L. McNay. An investigation of the structural requirements for dopamine-like renal vasodilation: Phenylethylamines and apomorphine. J. Pharmacol. Exp. Ther. 163:188-197 (1968).

6. Ernst, A. M. The role of biogenic amines in the extrapyramidal system. Acta Physiol. Pharmacol. Neerl. 15:141-154 (1969).

7. Kebabian, J. W. and P. Greengard. Dopamine-sensitive adenyl cyclase: Possible role in synaptic transmission. Science 174:1346-1349 (1971).

8. Brown, J. H. and M. H. Makman. Stimulation by dopamine of adenylate cyclase in retinal homogenates and of adenosine-3,5'-cyclic monophosphate formation in intact retina. Proc. Nat. Acad. Sci. 69:539-543 (1972).

9. Weiss, B. and E. Costa. Selective stimulation of adenyl cyclase of rat pineal gland by pharmacologically active catecholamines. J. Pharmacol. Exp. Ther. 161:310-319 (1968).

10. Jester, J. and W. D. Horst. Influence of serotonin on adrenergic mechanisms. Biochem. Pharmacol. 21:333-338 (1972).

11. Weiss, B. Similarities and differences in the norepinephrine-and sodium fluoride-sensitive adenyl cyclase system. J. Pharmacol. Exp. Ther. 166:330-338 (1969).

12. Giles, R. E. and J. W. Miller. A comparison of certain properties of catechol-O-methyl transferase to those of adrenergic beta receptors. J. Pharmacol. Exp. Ther. 156:201-206 (1967).

13. Assicot, M. and C. Bohuon. Presence of two distinct catechol-O-methyltransferase activities in red blood cells. Biochimie 53:871-874 (1971).

14. Axelrod, J. and R. Tomchick. Enzymatic O-methylation of epinephrine and other catechols. J. Biol. Chem. 233:702-705 (1958).

15. Roelofsen, B., R. F. A. Zwaal, P. Comfurius, C. B. Woodward and L. L. M. Van Deenen. Action of pure phospholipase A_2 and phospholipase C on human erythrocytes and ghosts. Biochim. Biophys. Acta 241:925-929 (1971).

16. Schmidt, M. J., E. C. Palmer, W-D. Dettbarn and G. A. Robison. Cyclic AMP and adenyl cyclase in the developing rat brain. Develop. Psychobiol. 3:53-67 (1970).

17. Schmidt, M. J. and G. A. Robison. The effect of norepinephrine on cyclic AMP levels in discrete regions of the developing rabbit brain. Life Sci. 10:459-464 (1971).

18. Weiss, B. Ontogenetic development of adenyl cyclase and phosphodiesterase in rat brain. J. Neurochem. 18:469-477 (1971).

19. Bär, H-P. and P. Hahn. Development of rat liver adenylcyclase. Canadian J. Biochem. 49:85-89 (1971).

20. Bitensky, M. W., V. Russell and M. Blanco. Independent variation of glucagon and epinephrine responsive components of hepatic adenyl cyclase as a function of age, sex and steroid hormones. Endocrinology 86:154-159 (1970).

21. Makman, M. H. Properties of adenylate cyclase of lymphoid cells. Proc. Nat. Acad. Sci. USA 68:885-889 (1971).

TABLE I

METABOLISM OF ATP BY MAMMALIAN ERYTHROCYTE GHOSTS

Species	Stimulant	$\%^{14}C$ Found in:			
		ATP	ADP	AMP	Adeno- sine
Human	none	31.5	48.6	19.9	0.035
	F	67.2	24.2	8.6	0.023
	NE	40.6	39.3	20.1	0.043
Dog	none	48.4	33.7	17.6	0.048
	F	57.2	30.2	12.2	0.039
	NE	51.4	32.1	16.4	0.053
Cat	none	57.0	30.2	12.3	0.077
	F	70.6	19.5	5.7	0.021
	NE	60.2	28.6	11.2	0.066
Mouse	none	28.5	43.8	27.7	0.096
	F	34.3	46.0	18.9	0.058
	NE	24.8	44.8	30.0	0.093
Rat	none	38.2	35.4	25.7	0.112
	F	53.0	30.8	15.8	0.048
	NE	46.0	32.2	21.2	0.089

TABLE II

EFFECT OF VARIOUS INHIBITORS ON THE STIMULATION OF RAT
ERYTHROCYTE ADENYL CYCLASE BY D(-) NOREPINEPHRINE (NE),
D(-) EPINEPHRINE (E) AND N-METHYL DOPAMINE (NMD)

*Net production of C-Amp refers to the increase over basal
values obtained by the addition of the catecholamine.*

Addition	NMD (10^{-5}M)	NE (10^{-5}M)	E (10^{-6}M)
	pmoles C-AMP/30 min		
None[a]	306	315	304
Serotonin (2.5 x 10^{-4}M)	66	98	91
Chlorpromazine (5 x 10^{-5}M)	- 35	- 15*	- 16*
Haloperidol (5 x 10^{-5}M)	85	97	98
Phentolamine (5 x 10^{-4}M)	62	54	68
Propranolol (10^{-7}M)	7*	3*	8*

[a]*P values relative to basal C-AMP production: * > 0.05. All
other values were significantly different from basal production with p values < 0.05. P values for all results
relative to the stimulations obtained with no additions were
all highly significant (< 0.001).*

TABLE III

EFFECT OF NEURAMINIDASE (NAm) PHOSPHOLIPASE C (PL-C)
AND TRYPSIN (T) ON THE PRODUCTION OF C-AMP AND
ADENOSINE BY RAT ERYTHROCYTE GHOSTS

Addition ^{a,b}	C-AMP			Adenosine	
	Basal	F	NE	Basal	F
	nmoles/incubation				
None	0.08	1.67	0.44	1.42	0.49
NAm	0.09	1.64	0.37*	3.61*	1.10*
PL-C	0.20$^+$	1.99$^+$	0.57	18.84$^+$	0.85*
T	0.09	0.14	0.08	0.85*	0.44

^{a}The additions per incubation were NAm, 0.6 mg; PL-C, 0.02 mg; and T, 0.004 mg (0.72 units).

^{b}Compared to incubations with no enzymes the p values are:
* < 0.05; + < 0.01.

TABLE IV

EFFECT OF PHOSPHOLIPASE C ON THE PRODUCTION OF C-AMP
AND ADENOSINE BY RAT ERYTHROCYTE GHOSTS

*The ghosts were washed 1 X with Tris-glucose buffer but were
not preincubated with PL-C. The figures in parenthesis represent ± standard error of the mean.*

PL-C Ghosts		C-AMP			Adenosine		
		Basal	NE	F	Basal	NE	F
				nmoles product/incubation			
20 µg	+	0.71	1.92	7.07	50.70	51.02	1.68
		(0.01)	(0.01)	(0.29)	(1.9)	(1.0)	(0.04)
20 µg- *boiled*	+	0.28	1.64	4.87	2.07	2.03	0.76
		(0.05)	(0.08)	(0.07)	(0.10)	(0.16)	(0.03)
20 µg	-	0.16	0.18	0.19	0.88	0.85	0.63
		(0.02)	(0.03)	(0.02)	(0.01)	(0.00)	(0.10)

TABLE V

EFFECT OF INCREASING AMOUNTS OF PHOSPHOLIPASE C
ON THE PRODUCTION OF C-AMP AND ADENOSINE BY RAT
ERYTHROCYTE GHOSTS

Preincubation	PL-C µg	Basal	F	NE
		nmoles C-AMP/mg prot./incubation		
-	0	0.21 $\pm$ 0.04	4.67 $\pm$ 0.53	2.27 $\pm$ 0.11
+	0	0.18 $\pm$ 0.03	1.10 $\pm$ 0.02	0.46 $\pm$ 0.01
+	20	0.23 $\pm$ 0.03	1.61 $\pm$ 0.13	0.65 $\pm$ 0.02
+	40	0.34 $\pm$ 0.02	1.50 $\pm$ 0.06	0.69 $\pm$ 0.05
+	80	0.60 $\pm$ 0.04	1.53 $\pm$ 0.08	0.79*$\pm$ 0.06
+	160	0.70 $\pm$ 0.04	1.27 $\pm$ 0.06	0.80*$\pm$ 0.03
+	200	1.05 $\pm$ 0.10	1.26*$\pm$ 0.01	1.08*$\pm$ 0.02

Not significantly different from its basal production
(p > 0.05).

TABLE VI

COMPARISON OF THE PHOSPHOHYDROLASE ACTIVITY OF GHOSTS
EXPOSED TO PL-C DURING THEIR PREPARATION WITH THAT OF
NAIVE GHOSTS INCUBATED WITH ESTIMATED CARRY-OVER
QUANTITIES OF THE ENZYME

Sample	ATP	ADP	AMP	Ar
	cpm			
Naive ghosts	128,000	91,100	38,100	739
Naive ghosts + PL-C	134,000	89,300	39,300	1,090
PL-C exposed ghosts	18,000	58,600	93,500	89,500

TABLE VII

EFFECTS OF COMPONENTS OF INCUBATION MEDIUM ON
PREINCUBATION-LOSS OF STIMULATION OF CYCLASE ACTIVITY

Addition	Cyclic AMP			Adenosine	
	Basal (B)	F-B	ISO-B	B	F
	nmoles/incubation				
Tris[a]	0.21	0.49*	0.01	1.0	0.62
Cyclic AMP	0.33^{+}	0.62*	0.16*	0.73^{+++}	0.53
Cyclic AMP+Mg	0.38^{+}	0.59*	0.09	1.34^{++}	0.92^{++}
Cyclic AMP+ATP	0.26	1.18^{+++}*	0.22*	0.83^{+}	0.57
Cyclic AMP+ATP+Mg	0.39^{++}	1.29^{+++}*	0.31*	1.06	0.80^{+}
ATP+Mg	0.41^{++}	1.37^{+++}*	0.21*	1.27^{++}	0.92^{++}
F	0.64^{++}	1.44^{++}*	0.20	0.96	0.65
ISO	0.55^{++}	0.44*	0.16	1.01	0.65

[a]*Statistical significance is expressed by p values of ++<0.01; +++<0.001 when compared to Tris incubation or * <0.05, when compared to basal.*

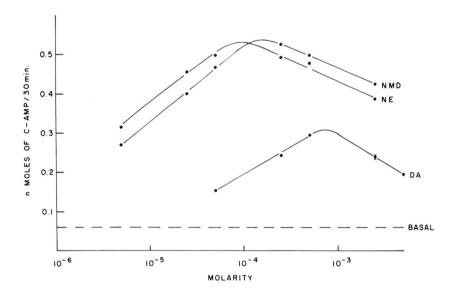

Fig. 1. Activation of rat erythrocyte adenylate cyclase by D (-)-norepinephrine (NE), dopamine (DA), and N-methyldopamine (NMD). The dashed line represents the basal production of C-AMP (cyclic AMP). Each incubation contained the equivalent of 0.2 ml of packed cells and was run in quadruplicate. All points represent the mean production of cyclic AMP minus the basal values. At any given concentration, the values in the presence of N-methyldopamine and norepinephrine were not significantly different.

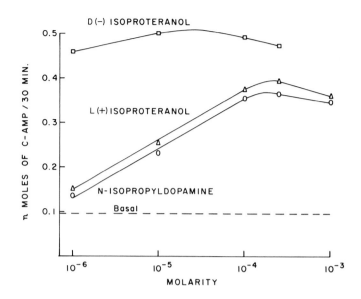

Fig. 2. *Activation of rat erythrocyte adenylate cyclase by N-isopropyldopamine and D(-)- and L(+)-isomers of isoproterenol.* Each incubation contained the equivalent of 0.2 ml of packed cells and was run in quadruplicate. All points represent the mean production of cyclic AMP minus the basal values. At any given concentration, the values in the presence of L(+)-isoproterenol and N-isopropyldopamine were not significantly different.

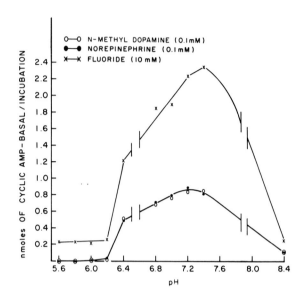

Fig. 3. *The effect of pH on the activation of rat erythro-cyte adenylate cyclase by fluoride, norepinephrine and N-methyldopamine.* The results are expressed in terms of the nmoles of cyclic AMP produced over the basal values. The break in the curves separates individual experiments. The buffer used was 0.04 M Tris adjusted to the appropriate pH with HCl.

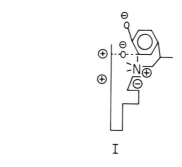

I

II   III

*Fig. 4. A pictorial representation of a possible mode of in-
teraction of catecholamines with a β-receptor component of
the adenylate cyclase system.*

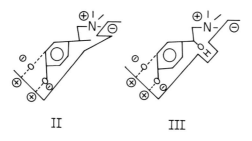

*Fig. 5. The levels of ATP, ADP, AMP and adenosine produced
by rat erythrocyte ghosts preincubated with 0-200 μg of PL-C
and incubated under basal conditions with ATP-8-^{14}C.*

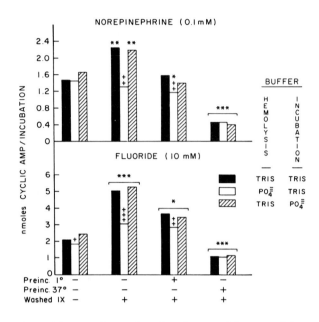

Fig. 6. The effect of preincubation and/or washing on the adenylate cyclase activity of rat erythrocyte ghosts prepared and incubated in either Tris or phosphate buffer (pH 7.4). The statistical significance of the results are designated by p values of < 0.05 (*,+); < 0.01 (**,++) or < 0.001 (***,+++). The "*" compares the cyclic AMP production with that of non-preincubated, unwashed conditions. The "+", however, compares the effects of buffers with those obtained by hemolysing and incubating in Tris.

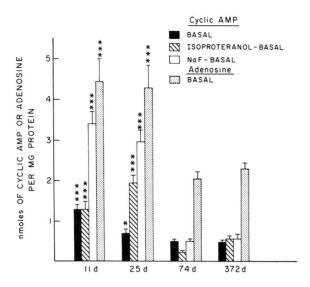

Fig. 7. *The influence of the age of female rats on the ability of fluoride and isoproterenol to stimulate the adenylate cyclase of erythrocyte ghosts.* The statistical significance of the results compared with those of the 74 day old rat are designated by p values of < 0.05 (*); < 0.001 (***).

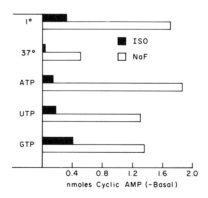

Fig. 8. *The effect of the triphosphates of adenosine, uridine and guanosine on the preincubation decrease of sensitivity of the adenylate cyclase to stimulation by 5 uM isoproterenol (ISO) and 5 mM NaF.* The concentration of each nucleotide was 0.49 mM.

IONIC EFFECTS IN THE REGULATION OF SUGAR TRANSPORT IN MUSCLE

Ivan Bihler

The mechanisms whereby insulin, muscular contraction, anoxia and other factors stimulate the specific membrane transport process for glucose and similar sugars in muscle are at present unknown. In the preceeding contribution Dr. Morgan has very ably discussed some aspects of this process, and I would like to continue by describing the effects of several factors modulating sugar transport in muscle and to propose a working hypothesis which attempts to provide a unified basis for the action of these agents.

The first thing to point out is that the membrane transport of glucose is rate-limiting for its utilization in those animal tissues in which the rate of glucose utilization is subject to large changes. In these tissues, which include various types of muscle and adipose tissue, the metabolic requirements vary greatly with contractile, synthetic or other activity, and it is significant that the stimuli for these functions are also activators of sugar transport. It would be consistent with the principle of economy of means we so often encounter in Nature that the various regulatory factors share in at least some aspects of a common mechanism. Starting from this premise, we have used a variety of pharmacological and metabolic interventions as tools in the study of regulation of the transport mechanism.

Since insulin and some of the other factors influence cellular metabolism, as well as membrane transport, we have chosen to follow the distribution in the tissue of non-metabolized glucose analogs, thus limiting ourselves to effects at the transport step exclusively. Most of the work was done with intact rat hemidiaphragms (1) incubated *in vitro* with ^{14}C-labelled 3-0-methyl-D-glucose. Langendorff-perfused rabbit hearts and preparations of the rabbit and the rat detrusor, a smooth muscle, were also used for comparative purposes. The data are given as percent sugar penetration, expressing sugar concentration in the intracellular water space

411

as percentage of its concentration in the incubation medium. This is not an accurate reflection of initial transport rates but provides a good semiquantitative measure of transport under a given set of conditions.

Following reports that ouabain and other digitaloids affect carbohydrate metabolism in the heart (2), skeletal muscle (3), and adipose tissue (4) in an insulin-like manner, we have investigated the effect of these drugs on the transport of non-metabolized sugars. These studies have led to the discovery (5) in the rat diaphragm, of a negative feedback from the aerobic Na^+-pump to sugar transport. Inhibition of the Na^+-pump either directly by digitaloids or a low-K^+ medium or indirectly by restricting oxidative energy supplies, $e.g.$ through anoxia or uncoupling of oxidative phosphorylation, activates the sugar carrier. Since the Na^+-pump in skeletal muscle depends largely on energy derived from oxidative metabolism, this relationship would also explain the increase in sugar transport caused by anoxia. It is consistent with this explanation that while ouabain did not affect sugar transport under anoxic conditions in the diaphragm, it did so in the detrusor (Bihler and Sawh, unpublished results), a smooth muscle which is able also to utilize anaerobic energy for Na^+-pumping (6). A physiological role for this negative feedback from the Na^+-pump to sugar transport could be the provision, during anoxia, of increased amounts of glucose for anaerobic glycolysis. It should be emphasized that it is essential for the operation of the Pasteur effect that the rate-limiting step, the membrane transport of glucose, be enhanced along with the activity of glycolytic enzymes.

The converse regulatory relationship was also demonstrated. Sugar transport in the diaphragm was inhibited when the Na^+-pump was stimulated by a high-K^+ medium (7), by very low concentrations of digitaloids (8) or by some anticonvulsant drugs such as diphenylhydantoin (9). Simultaneous measurements of Na^+ and K^+ concentrations in the tissue confirmed that stimulation of the Na^+-pump occurs under the conditions of our experiments. This relationship is illustrated in Fig. 1 showing the increments or decrements in sugar transport and the simultaneous changes in internal Na^+ measured in paired experiments with rat hemidiaphragms. These are pooled data from experiments with high-K^+ media and with various levels of diphenylhydantoin; che latter drug has a biphasic effect on the Na^+-pump and may be used to produce either a decrease or an increase in internal Na^+ and the associated changes in sugar transport. The correlation between these two changes is very strong and statistically highly significant, both with and without insulin. An identical but negative correlation is also seen with changes in K^+. At the present we have no way to vary one ion independently of the other.

These stimulatory and inhibitory effects do not depend on the activity of the Na^+-pump as such, nor on a direct association of Na^+ or K^+ with the sugar carrier. Rather, the effect is indirect, with the intracellular levels of Na^+ or K^+ affecting influx and efflux of sugar equally (10).

The earlier work of Holloszy and Narahara (11) indicated that, in frog skeletal muscle, the increase in sugar transport during muscular contraction depends on the frequency of stimulation but not on the work load. In contrast, as shown by Dr. Morgan, sugar transport in the perfused rat heart does depend on the work load. However, our studies with perfused non-working rabbit hearts (12) revealed that sugar transport in the heart and in skeletal muscle are very similar in other regards. Figure 2 shows L-arabinose transport in hearts stimulated at different frequencies or virtually arrested by cauterization of the AV-node (13,14). As in skeletal muscle, sugar transport increased progressively with the frequency of contraction, and a high, "toxic", dose of ouabain also stimulated transport, regardless of the frequency of stimulation. A "therapeutic" dose of ouabain stimulated transport only in the beating hearts, presumably because it increased the strength of contraction; an effect limited, of course, to cardiac muscle.

It is obvious that the relationship between internal levels of Na^+ and K^+ and sugar transport outlined above is unable to explain the stimulation of sugar transport by muscular exercise or insulin, neither of which cause large scale alterations in the intracellular levels of Na^+ and K^+. A more likely candidate for the role of mediator in the regulation of sugar transport would be calcium. On the one hand, it was shown by Holloszy and Narahara (11) that the stimulation of sugar transport by muscular contraction is linked to excitation-contraction coupling, a process known to depend on Ca^{++} and to involve its redistribution between cellular compartments. On the other hand, owing to the existence of a $Na^+ - Ca^{++}$ exchange system in the cell membrane (15,16), alterations in internal or external Na^+ will also affect Ca^{++} distribution. An increase in internal Na^+

will increase Ca^{++} influx, and so will a decrease in external Na^+ (unless counteracted by a decrease in internal Na^+). The observed flux of ^{45}Ca into rat hemidiaphragms (17) agrees with these predictions, first increasing and then decreasing as Na^+ in the incubation medium is progressively lowered. As shown by these authors and by our data in Table I, sugar transport shows a similar course, first increasing when about 1/3 of the Na^+ is omitted and then decreasing to below the control rate when Na^+ is reduced to a low level.

While the above data seem compatible with a role of Ca^{++} in the regulation of sugar transport, the role of Ca^{++} in the effect of insulin is less clear. Our data (18) indicate that the stimulation of sugar transport by insulin is strongly inhibited in a Ca^{++}-free medium (Table II). This effect is enhanced by Ca^{++}-chelators such as EGTA (ethyleneglycol-bis(β-amino-ethyl ether) N'N-tetraacetic acid). Furthermore, ions antagonistic to Ca^{++}, such as La^{+++} and Ni^{++} as well as Zn^{++}, Mn^{++} and Co^{++} (not shown), have a similar inhibitory effect which may be partially overcome by increasing the Ca^{++} concentration. These ions act like partial agonists and stimulate sugar transport in the absence of Ca^{++}. These experiments, and some of the data of Gould and Chaudry (19), support a role of Ca^{++} in mediating the effect of insulin. However, Mg^{++} also appears to play an important, if obscure role (19).

The evidence briefly outlined above has led us to formulate a working hypothesis according to which the various regulatory influences on sugar transport in muscle and perhaps other insulin-sensitive tissues are mediated by a particular membrane pool of Ca^{++}. As shown in Fig. 3, it is thought that inhibition of the Na^+-pump stimulates Na^+ - Ca^{++} exchange, and this increases the binding of Ca^{++} to some specific membrane sites. The same Ca^{++}-pool is affected by ions antagonistic to Ca^{++} and may be also linked to the "trigger Ca" of excitation-contraction coupling. Attachment of insulin to its membrane receptors may also be followed by interaction with the Ca^{++}-dependent regulatory sites. It is hard to be more specific at present but it is not difficult to imagine that increased Ca^{++}-binding at certain sites could alter membrane structure of conformation and thus exert an allosteric effect on the sugar carrier which we perceive as an increase in its "mobility".

Another physiologically important regulatory mechanism is the inhibition of sugar transport by the oxidation of fatty acids. It may serve to limit glucose utilization when

an alternate source of energy is available. The glucose-
fatty acid competition is most prominent in the heart and
was shown by Neely *et al.* (20) to involve interaction at the
glucose transport step. Regarding skeletal muscle, the
evidence is contradictory and it has even been suggested (21)
that any inhibition seen is due to insulin antagonists in
the added serum albumin. In our experiments on the effect
of palmitic acid on the transport of 3-0-methyl-D-glucose
in rat hemidiaphragms (22), we have, therefore, added the
same concentration of bovine serum albumin to control and
experimental tissues and we have kept a constant molar ratio
of FFA/albumin when varying the FFA concentration. We have
found that the stimulation of sugar transport by insulin,
muscular contraction, ouabain and several other stimulatory
factors is inhibited by palmitate in a dose-dependent manner.
This inhibitory effect was absent in anoxia and, as shown
in Fig. 4, was antagonized by 2-bromostearate, an inhibitor
of fatty acid oxidation (23). It thus depends on the oxidation of fatty acids, and may be considered as another negative feedback from cellular metabolism to the membrane transport of glucose. While the availability of oxidative substrates, including fatty acids, is a prerequisite for the
operation of the feedback from Na^+-pump, the effect of fatty
acids is not fully explained on this basis. Firstly, the
addition of fatty acids affects sugar transport even when
endogenous metabolism adequately supports ion transport;
secondly, fatty acid oxidation antagonizes the effects of
all stimulatory factors tested; and thirdly, it is not accompanied by any significant changes in internal Na^+ and K^+
levels. We have therefore tentatively concluded that fatty
acid oxidation acts at a distal step in the chain of regulatory events, perhaps as the Ca^{++}-dependent regulatory site.
This is shown schematically in Fig. 5 which also indicates
some of the other stimulatory and inhibitory influences and
their proposed relationship in sugar transport regulation.

The usefulness of any such model depends mainly on
whether it suggest new experiments which add to our factual
knowledge and bring us a step closer to the full understanding of the problem at hand. Referring to fatty acid
oxidation, for example, the question arises if the effect
on sugar transport could be explained on the basis of a
shift of Ca^{++} from membrane sites to the mitochondria.
This and other aspects of the interaction between Ca^{++}
and various regulatory factors are presently being studied.

Presented by Ivan Bihler. The work reported was supported by grants from the Medical Research Council (Canada), the Manitoba Heart Foundation and the Canadian Diabetes Association. The author is an Associate of the Medical Research Council.

References

1. Kono, T. and S.P. Colowick. Stereospecific sugar transport caused by uncouplers and SH-inhibitors in rat diaphragm. Arch. Biochem. Biophys. 93:514-519 (1961).
2. Kreisberg, R.A. and J.R. Williamson. Metabolic effects of ouabain in the perfused rat heart. Am. J. Physiol. 207:347-351 (1964).
3. Clausen, T. The relationship between the transport of glucose and cations across cell membranes in isolated tissue. I. Stimulation of glycogen deposition and inhibition of lactic acid production in diaphragm induced by ouabain. Biochim. Biophys. Acta 109:164-171 (1965).
4. Ho, R.J. and B. Jeanrenaud. Insulin-like action of ouabain. I. Effect of carbohydrate metabolism. Biochim. Biophys. Acta 144:61-73 (1967).
5. Bihler, I. The action of cardiotonic steroids of sugar transport in muscle *in vitro*. Biochim. Biophys. Acta 163:401-410 (1968).
6. Munson, J. L. and D. M. Paton. Metabolic requirements for sodium pumping in rabbit detrusor muscle. Proc. Can. Fed. Biol. Soc. 14: 47 (1971).
7. Bihler, I. and P. C. Sawh. Regulation of sugar transport in muscle: Effect of increased external potassium *in vitro*. Biochim. Biophys. Acta 241: 302-309 (1971).
8. Bihler, I. The sodium pump and regulation of sugar transport in skeletal muscle. Pharmacologist 10: 198 (1968).
9. Bihler, I. and P. C. Sawh. Effects of diphenylhydantoin on the transport of Na^+ and K^+ and the regulation of sugar transport in muscle *in vitro*. Biochim. Biophys. Acta 249: 240-251 (1971).
10. Bihler, I. and P. C. Sawh. The effect of alkali metal ions on sugar transport in muscle: Interaction with the sugar carrier or indirect effect. Biochim. Biophys. Acta 225: 56-63 (1971).

11. Holloszy, J. O. and H. T. Narahara. Studies of tissue permeability X. Changes in permeability to 3-methyl-glucose associated with contraction of isolated frog muscle. J. Biol. Chem. 240: 3493-3500 (1965).

12. Elbrink, J. and Bihler, I. The effects of ouabain and of frequency of contraction on sugar penetration in cardiac muscle. Proc. Can. Fed. Biol. Soc 12: 57 (1969).

13. Pruett, J. K. and E. F. Woods. Technique for experimental complete heart block. J. Appl. Physiol. 22: 830-831 (1967).

14. Macdonald, I. B. A simple method of producing experimental heart block in dogs. J. Thorac. Cardiovasc. Surg. 53: 695 (1967).

15. Baker, P. F. and M. P. Blaustein. Sodium-dependenct uptake of calcium by crab nerve. Biochim. Biophys. Acta 150: 167-170 (1968).

16. Reuter, H. In: L. Bolis, A. Katchalsky, R. D. Keynes, W. R. Loewstein and B. A. Pethica (Editors), Permeability and Function of Biological Membranes, North-Holland Publ. Co., Amsterdam (1970), p. 342-347.

17. Ilse, D. and S. Ong. Studies on the sugar carrier in skeletal muscle. Biochim. Biophys. Acta 211: 602-604 (1970).

18. Bihler, I. and P. C. Sawh. Nature of the ionic effect regulating sugar transport in muscle. Proc. Can. Fed. Biol. Sox. 13: 75 (1970).

19. Gould, M. K. and Chaudry, I. H. The action of insulin on glucose uptake by isolated rat soleus muscle. I. Effects of cations. Biochim. Biophys. Acta 215: 249-257 (1970).

20. Neely, J. R., R. H. Bowman and H. E. Morgan. Effects of ventricular pressure development and palmitate on glucose transport. Am. J. Physiol. 216: 804-811 (1969).

21. Schonfeld G. and D. M. Kipnis. Effect of fatty acids on carbohydrate and fatty acid metabolism of rat diaphragm. Am. J. Physiol. 215: 513 (1968).

22. Bihler, I. and P. C. Sawh. Effect of fatty acid oxidation on sugar transport in muscle. Fed. Proc. 31: 287 abs. (1972).

23. Randle, P. J. Apparent reversal of insulin resistance in cardiac muscle in alloxan -diabetes by 2-bromostearate. Nature 221: 777 (1969).

24. Byrne, J. E. and P. E. Dresel. The effect of temperature and calcium concentration on the action of ouabain in quiescent rabbit atria. J. Pharm. Exp. Ther. 166:

354-363 (1969).

Table I

EFFECT OF EXTERNAL Na$^+$ ON THE TRANSPORT
OF 3-O-METHYL-D-GLUCOSE (5mM).

The figures are means (N = 6 or more) of differences in paired experiments. Na$^+$ was isosmotically replaced by mannitol. Insulin (0.25 m unit/ml) was added to all flasks. Preincubation was for 20 min and incubation for 30 min.

Na$^+$	Δ Penetration
mM	*%*
145 (Krebs control)	--
110	+14.7
90	+21.8
75	+13.1
45	+ 6.2
0	-15.9

Table II

EFFECT OF Ca^{++} ON THE STIMULATION OF 3-0-METHYL-D-GLUCOSE
(5 mM) TRANSPORT BY INSULIN

Insulin, as indicated; La^{+++}, 0.5 mM; Ni^{++}, 2 mM; Ca^{++}, 5.0 mM is double the standard concentration. Preincubation was for 20 min and incubation for 30 min except where indicated. N = 6 or more. Other details as in Table I.

Additions		Δ% penetration	% change
to both hemidiaphragms	to one only		
Insulin, 0.5 m unit/ml (no preincubation)	Ca^{++}-free	-10.4	-27.2
Insulin, 0.5 m unit/ml	Ca^{++}-free	-39.5	-61.0
Insulin, 1.0 m unit/ml	La^{+++}	-30.8	-62.0
Insulin + La^{+++}	Ca^{++}, 5 mM	+ 5.1	+37.6
La^{+++}	Ca^{++}-free	+ 4.2	+22.6
Insulin, 1.0 m unit/ml	Ni^{++}	-44.6	-68.1
Insulin + Ni^{++}	Ca^{++}, 5 mM	+ 2.7	+19.2
Insulin + Ni^{++}	Ca^{++}-free	+ 6.7·	+25.9

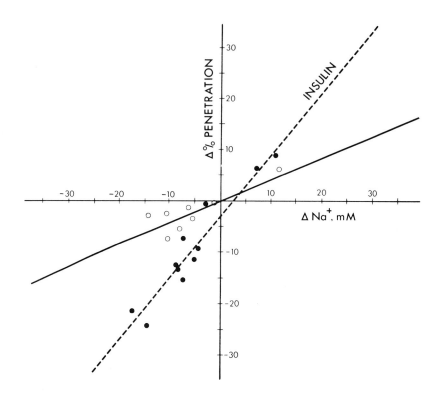

Fig. 1. *Correlation between 3-0-methyl-D-glucose (5 mM) transport and internal Na⁺ levels.* Means of differences from control values (paired experiments, N = 6 to 31) are shown. The lines were calculated by the method of least squares and the coefficient of correlation, r is 0.952 (P < 0.001) and 0.844 (P < 0.01), with and without 0.5 m unit/ml insulin, respectively. For other details see Bihler and Sawh (9).

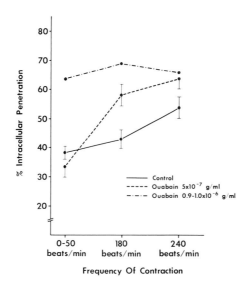

Fig. 2. *The dependence of L-arabinose transport in perfused rabbit hearts on the frequency of contraction and on ouabain.* The low and high concentrations of ouabain were shown to be "inotropic" and "toxic" in rabbit heart (24). N = 5 or more.

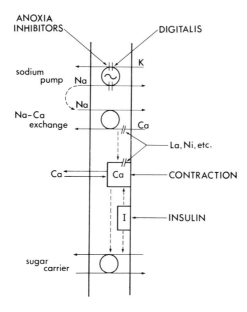

Fig. 3. *Relationship of ion fluxes in the membrane to sugar transport in muscle.*

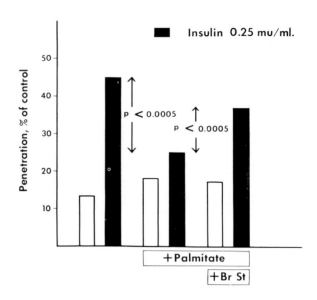

Fig. 4. *Effect of palmitate oxidation on the transport of 3-0-methyl-D-glucose (5 mM).* Palmitate, 8 mM; 2-bromo-stearate, 4 mM; molar ratio FFA/albumin = 7.5. The p values refer to means of differences in paired experiments, N = 6 to 10.

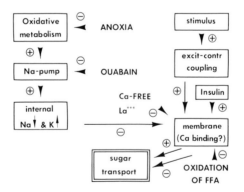

Fig. 5. *Scheme of some regulatory factors on sugar transport in muscle.* ⊕ and ⊖ indicate stimulatory and inhibitory influences, respectively.

SUBJECT INDEX

A

A23187, 111, 153
  uncoupling by, 113
Acetoacetate, 183
Acetylcholine, 65
  receptor, 77
Acrylamide gels, 25
ACTH((*see* Adrenocorticotropic
  hormone)
Activated diffusion, 1
Active transport, 287
Acyl CoA esters, long chain, 165, 168
  accumulation in liver of diabetic and
    fasting
    animals, 165
Adenine nucleotide(s), 140
  translocation of, 165, 169
Adenosine, 390
Adenosine-3,5'-monophosphate, 80, 242,
  249, 349
  hepatic, 333
Adenosine triphosphate, 295, 394
  metabolism of, 386
Adenosine triphosphatase, 24, 25
  mitochondrial, inhibition of, 116
  sodium and potassium activated, 295
Adenyl cyclase, 84, 261
Adenylate cyclase, 249, 349, 385
  in erythrocytes, 393
Adenylate kinase, 367, 370
Adipose tissue, 167, 238
Adrenalectomy, 330
α-Adrenergic receptor, 65
β-Adrenergic receptor, 65, 261, 386
Adrenocorticotropic hormone, 84, 239,
  313, 321

Agarose-ACTH, 318
Agarose-glucagon, 367, 370
Age, effect of, 393
Agonist(s), activity of, 71
  cholinergic, 66
  full, 68
  induction of receptor desensitization,
    82
  partial, 68
Amino acids, 287
α-Aminoisobutyric acid, 249
Amphipathic molecules, 2
Anoxia, 135, 411
Apomorphine, 388
ATP (*see* Adenosine triphosphate)
Azalomycin F, 113

B

2-Bromostearate, 415
Buoyant density, 168

C

Calcium, 111
  alteration of potential dependent ion
    channels, 62
  binding, effect of hormones, 84
  dependent voltage shift, 62
  depleted membrane areas, 81
  in excitation-contraction coupling, 59
  external, 60, 61, 65, 67
  flux, 116
  induced neurotransmitter release at
    skeletal neuromuscular junction, 65